Task Analysis

An Individual, Group, and Population Approach

3rd Edition
Sylvia A. Wilson, MSc, OT(C),
and Gregg Landry, MHA, OT

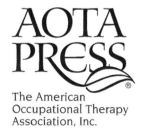

AOTA PRESS

The American
Occupational Therapy
Association, Inc.

AOTA Centennial Vision
We envision that occupational therapy is a powerful, widely recognized, science-driven, and evidence-based profession with a globally connected and diverse workforce meeting society's occupational needs.

Mission Statement
The American Occupational Therapy Association advances the quality, availability, use, and support of occupational therapy through standard-setting, advocacy, education, and research on behalf of its members and the public.

AOTA Staff
Frederick P. Somers, *Executive Director*
Christopher M. Bluhm, *Chief Operating Officer*

Chris Davis, *Director, AOTA Press*
Ashley Hofmann, *Development/Acquisitions Editor*

Rebecca Rutberg, *Director, Marketing*
Amanda Goldman, *Marketing Manager*
Jennifer Folden, *Marketing Specialist*

American Occupational Therapy Association, Inc.
4720 Montgomery Lane
Bethesda, MD 20814
Phone: 301-652-AOTA (2682)
TDD: 800-377-8555
Fax: 301-652-7711
www.aota.org
To order: 1-877-404-AOTA or store.aota.org

Disclaimers
This publication is designed to provide accurate and authoritative information in regard to the subject matter covered. It is sold or distributed with the understanding that the publisher is not engaged in rendering legal, accounting, or other professional service. If legal advice or other expert assistance is required, the services of a competent professional person should be sought.
—*From the Declaration of Principles jointly adopted by the American Bar Association and a Committee of Publishers and Associations*

It is the objective of the American Occupational Therapy Association to be a forum for free expression and interchange of ideas. The opinions expressed by the contributors to this work are their own and not necessarily those of the American Occupational Therapy Association.

ISBN: 978-1-56900-534-7

Library of Congress Control Number: 2014933153

Cover Design by Debra Naylor, Naylor Design, Inc., Washington, DC
Composition by Manila Typesetting Company, Manila, Philippines
Printed by Automated Graphic Systems, Inc., White Plains, MD

Dedication

I quote George Santayna as saying, "The family is one of nature's masterpieces." Throughout the years of my career and the orchestration around family life I have had support and insights from Ron, Kelsey, Nicole, Karlee, Gregory, Jason, Dan, Suzy, Claudia, Cleo and Oliver, every one of them brilliant in their own way and dropping seeds of wisdom along life's path that are woven into my work. Diane Watson and Gregg Landry have always been there in support of many life activities, including writing to teaching—to me they are family. There are those that stimulated me to reach for higher goals and achieve them—Dr. Helen Madill, Sharon Brintnell, Dorethea Bott Banner, Dr. Charlene Robertson, and Dr. John White—they taught me that focus on process leads to the best outcome. And all the clients that entered into my life as teachers—I honour them.

—*Sylvia A. Wilson*

Diane, You are my inspiration. You continue to raise the bar for me and then help me over it. Austin, once upon a time . . . your patient and thoughtful discussions always begin when I need them most. Moraya, your creativity and humour are an absolute joy and welcome relief in the busyness of life. Dad, thank you for your tireless support. You have shown me what can be accomplished with hard work and determination. Steven, your selfless encouragement has meant more to me than you could ever know. Patty, you are and always will be wonderful. Sylvia, thank you for talking me into this. I could never have done it without you.

—*Gregg Landry*

Contents

Items on the Flash Drive
- Client Profile and Task Analysis Form
- AOTA Position Paper: Purposeful Activity
- Occupational Therapy's Role in Sleep
- Occupational Therapy's Role in Health Promotion
- Case Examples
- Assignments

Acknowledgments

A few key people have heavily influenced the occupation of writing this book, and the contexts in which we have lived our lives laid the foundation on which this book was written. We address the former and the latter together, as people and contexts are inseparable in their influence on our lives.

Diane Watson wrote the first edition of this text, bringing to the profession an instrument and strategies to conduct task analysis. This formative concept was further developed in the second edition through her leadership with the co-author (Wilson) in expanding the text to consider emerging areas of practice.

We also credit the many people involved in the creation of the Person–Environment–Occupation model of occupational performance, integration of the concept of enabling occupation in client-centered practice, and the Cardinal Hill Occupational Participation Process in client-centered care. They must be congratulated for "simplifying the recipe." Many other scholars have influenced this work, and they are cited in the reference lists.

The first edition of *Task Analysis* acknowledged 30 different people for their valued contribution to that text. As this work builds on theirs, we continue to owe credit. The first edition was created out of a collaborative effort between one author, Diane Watson, and the occupational therapy graduating class of 1998 from the University of Scranton in Pennsylvania. These practitioners, and Dr. Jack Kasar, who was the department chairperson at that time, contributed to the success of the first edition and have laid the foundation used to create the second edition.

Occupations as intense and all-consuming as writing a book also require supportive performance contexts at work and home. The second edition of *Task Analysis* was led by Diane Watson and coauthored by Sylvia Wilson. Anonymous reviewers provided extensive feedback that enhanced the text. Gregg Landry, the coauthor of the third edition, assisted with the second edition by framing its breadth and scope. The editors and staff at the American Occupational Therapy Association contributed substantially to the quality and completion of all three editions.

We owe tremendous gratitude to Kelsey Wilson, who provided numerous hours reviewing the readability of the text and providing editorial comments. She applied her skills as a graduate of political science, university book buyer, and writer, always thinking about how the student would use the textbook optimally for developing knowledge, skills, and self-directed learning. Gregory Wilson applied his design capacity to an updated figure for the text that provides an integrated illustration of the task analysis process. Sharon Kirkham, an occupational therapist with extensive experience in life care planning and knowledge of medical legal consultation, provided input for Chapter 6, "Care Planning: Needs Analysis and Use in Consultation," a new addition to *Task Analysis*.

The authors have over 60 years of experience as occupational therapy practitioners in diverse practice environments across Canada, the United States, and Australia. It would be impossible to count the clients we have collectively served, but it is they who have taught us the art of applying task analysis to occupational therapy practice.

We would also like to thank AOTA Press for encouraging us to take the challenge of writing another *Task Analysis* book. They provided us access to their literary resources, including the *Occupational Therapy Practice Framework, 3rd Edition*. They also provided us access to peer reviewers. These resources, along with the editorial input of Ashley Hofmann, helped us create a textbook that builds on but is truly unique from the prior editions of the *Task Analysis* books. Ashley, we particularly want to thank you for sometimes pushing us during this project in directions we didn't always want to go. You helped us create a better product.

About the Authors

Sylvia A. Wilson, MSc, OT(C), earned her bachelor of science in occupational therapy, followed by a master's degree of science in occupational therapy (thesis based), from the University of Alberta, Edmonton. Her initial professional focus was in the area of pediatrics at the Glenrose Rehabilitation Hospital (GRH), Edmonton. During her tenure at the GRH she had the opportunity to contribute to specialized programs for children with cerebral palsy, developmental delay, brain injury, muscular dystrophy, learning disabilities, autism, fetal alcohol spectrum disorder, and neonatal and infant assessment.

While working at the GRH, she also held an adjunct professor position at the University of Alberta teaching two pediatric courses. She was the first occupational therapist to work in a neonatal follow-up program headed by Dr. Charlene Robertson. Subsequently, her graduate thesis was a study of more than 3,000 children she followed from birth to 8 years of age, with the research focus on early predictors of learning disability in high-risk infants.

At the GRH she progressed from clinician to clinical supervisor, with a term as acting coordinator of a department of 28 therapists. Her experience at the GRH was the springboard for her recruitment by the Arbutus Society for Children and Perkes Centre in Victoria, British Columbia. Her role as clinical supervisor was to establish and coordinate a school-based rehabilitation program serviced by occupational, physical, and speech therapists. A key challenge was to design and implement a school-based program that would cost less than a facility-based program—it was successful in accomplishing this fiscal goal.

She returned to the University of Alberta to assume the role of clinical practice coordinator, organizing local, national and international placements for occupational therapy students. Concurrent with this position, her proposal to Health Canada to design and implement a community-based rehabilitation service for 16 First Nation communities was accepted and implemented within the capped budget. The community-based model was implemented, outcome measures reported, and community stewardship achieved within 5 years of introduction of the community-based rehabilitation model.

Wilson next worked in Oregon as Assistant Professor in the School of Occupational Therapy at Pacific University in Forest Grove. It was here that her interest was piqued in the value of inquiry-based teaching. The experience fostered much of the approach taken in the second and third editions of *Task Analysis*.

Returning to Canada, Wilson took the position of Centre Coordinator at the Centre for Health Promotion Studies at the University of Alberta for the graduate program and research projects, leading to work with Alberta Health and Wellness as research manager. The nexus of these experiences was that of university research and harnessing university intellectual assets for government research.

In 2008, after a number of years "dabbling" in medical–legal consultation, she went into private practice and is now the director of Sylvia A Wilson & Associates Ltd. Her role is disability analysis, life care planning, and cost-of-future-care determination. She has been qualified in the Court of Queen Bench to testify as an expert witness in the field.

Gregg Landry, MHA, OT, graduated with a bachelor of science from the University of Puget Sound, Tacoma, Washington, and a master's degree in Health Administration at the University of British Columbia, Vancouver. He has earned a Diploma of Quality Auditing; a Certificate IV in Occupational Health and Safety; and a Certificate IV in Training, Assessment, and Evaluation in the states of New South Wales and Queensland, Australia. He is currently completing an advanced diploma in Work Health and Safety.

Landry was an adjunct clinical professor at the University of Scranton and helped design its inaugural industrial rehabilitation and hand therapy curriculum. Prior to co-authoring this book, he contributed to four occupational therapy textbooks, including *Clinical Cases for Learning Pediatric Occupational Therapy: A Problem-Based Approach; Task Analysis: An Occupational Performance Approach; Evaluating Outcomes: Demonstrating the Value of Rehabilitation Services; and Task Analysis: An Individual and Population Approach* (2nd ed.).

Occupational therapy has given Landry a world of opportunities. He has worked throughout both the United States and Canada and now works in Sydney, Australia. His occupational therapy clinical experiences include acute care from the emergency room through the hospital wards and intensive care units. He has worked in neurologic and orthopaedic inpatient rehabilitation and long-term care. As an outpatient therapist, he specialized in hand therapy and return-to-work rehabilitation. For nearly a decade he worked in the insurance sector as a rehabilitation consultant and a worker's compensation case manager.

In Australia, Landry's passion turned to injury prevention. Initially, he was a people manual handling specialist in the home care sector and is now a project manager in work health and safety for a community care organization of 23,000 workers located across New South Wales. His safety work focuses on strategic planning, designing and implementing corporate health and safety training, writing policies and procedures, overseeing corporate projects, and making strides to change best practices for services delivery in state and national community care sectors in order to keep tens of thousands of workers and their clients safe.

List of Figures, Tables, Exhibits, Case Examples, and Assignments

Figures

Tables

Exhibits

Case Examples

Assignments

Introduction

Sylvia A. Wilson, MSc, OT(C), and
Gregg Landry, MHA, OT

Occupational therapy practitioners seek to use meaningful and purposeful activities to create experiences that clients value. Aligned with this tradition, we wrote this new edition of *Task Analysis: An Individual, Group, and Population Approach* to create a meaningful and purposeful context for learning.

Task analysis is the process of analyzing the dynamic relation among a client, a selected task, and specific contexts—in other words, persons, occupations, and environments. Task analysis involves breaking down an occupation or activity into the smallest, identifiable, essential, and complete piece. This text focuses on the use of task analysis as a clinical reasoning tool that provides a stepping stone to developing and refining the art and science of occupational performance analysis.

Occupational performance analysis requires a broad understanding of the full range of a client's current and desired occupations; client factors, performance skills, and performance contexts; and an appreciation for the complexity of how these determinants of health interact. This understanding and appreciation are the primary clinical reasoning talents of occupational therapy practitioners.

TERMINOLOGY

We derived the task analysis framework from the *Occupational Therapy Practice Framework: Domain and Process* (3rd ed.; hereinafter, the *Framework*; American Occupational Therapy Association [AOTA], 2014), which outlines the terminology we use in this volume. Occupational therapy practitioners have historically used the term *activity analysis* to describe the analysis of the demands inherent in engagement in purposeful activities, but this is only one step in the process of conducting task analysis—the part that focuses on an activity or occupation. The purpose of activity analysis is to determine whether an activity has restorative potential or value and how to grade therapeutic activities (Moyers & Dale, 2007; Watson, 1997). This text uses the term *activity analysis* to refer to the skill of analyzing an occupation, activity, or process to determine whether it motivates and fulfills a client's needs and enhances occupational performance analysis.

In occupational therapy, the term *client* has evolved to include any entity that receives services. The *Framework* defines *client* as a "person or persons (including those involved in the care of a client), group (collective of individuals, e.g., families, workers, students, or community members), or population (collective of groups or individuals living in a similar locale—e.g., city, state, or country—or sharing the same or like concerns)" (AOTA, 2014, p. S41).

Although the most common form of service delivery is directed toward individual clients, practitioners increasingly serve clients at the group and population levels and are involved in community development initiatives. Many practitioners do not have experience applying task analysis to organizations and populations, but increasingly, occupational therapy practitioners serve these groups. We designed this text in part as an introductory guide for those practice areas and the broadened understanding of what our clients are.

DEVELOPMENT OF THE
THIRD EDITION

We elected to use problem- and inquiry-based approaches to learning, because we believe it creates a realistic and rewarding context for developing clinical reasoning. The people, organizations, and circumstances in this text's case examples are hypothetical and are intended to provide meaningful contexts for learning; any similarity to real persons, organizations, community groups or events is purely coincidental. Although the cases in this book are hypothetical, they reflect what occupational therapy students may experience in their professional roles.

Problem-based learning should refine readers' skills in narrative, interactive, procedural, and conditional clinical reasoning (Van Leit, 1995). The case examples are intended to enable readers to practice the cognitive steps and professional behaviors that are required of knowledgeable and skilled practitioners. The learning experiences are developmental and integrative, and assignment questions throughout each chapter provide opportunities for readers to determine the focus of their learning experience.

The problem- and inquiry-based approaches to learning complements the occupational therapy profession's belief that meaningful engagement sanctions diversity and flexibility in learning

and adaptation (Watson, 1997). It parallels the profession's tradition of using purposeful activity to promote learning, insight, skills, and independent and self-directed performance.

The first edition of this book, *Task Analysis: An Occupational Performance Approach* (Watson, 1997), included a section on how to use task analysis to guide services to individuals and communities. The second edition (Watson & Wilson, 2003) added the concept of applying task analysis to working with populations. Since then, our understanding of this area of practice has been enriched by the work of several scholars and practitioners who work in the areas of community development, public health, population health, and insurance and legal industries. This new edition is also aligned the latest edition of the *Framework's* (AOTA, 2014) use of the term *population*.

HOW THIS BOOK IS ORGANIZED

Aligned with the latest *Framework* (AOTA, 2014), this *Task Analysis* has two parts. Part I, "Domain and Process of Occupational Therapy," discusses occupational therapy's distinct approach; outlines its domains and dimensions; describes its process; explains service delivery to individuals, groups, and populations; and examines care planning in terms of needs analysis and consultation.

Part II, "Occupation and Intervention Strategies," considers occupation across the lifespan, play, education, activities of daily living, adolescence and emerging adulthood, adulthood and maintaining meaningful lifestyles, older adults and transitions for successful aging, and healthy communities. These chapters explore how task analysis applies to occupational therapy intervention in these areas.

Also included is a Client Profile and Task Analysis Form (Appendix A), which is used throughout this text. The flash drive included with this publication contains an electronic, fillable version of this form. Other appendixes include three AOTA documents referred to in chapter assignment questions: *Position Paper: Purposeful Activity* (Appendix B), *Occupational Therapy's Role in Sleep* (Appendix C), and *Occupational*

Therapy in the Promotion of Health and Well-Being (Appendix D). Assignments challenge readers' reasoning skills, and case examples encourage real-world application.

SUMMARY

This text reflects the authors' experiences in the areas of community health promotion, as well as the insurance and legal industries. Over the past 20 years, one author (Wilson) has worked closely with communities to promote health in their customary contexts and in medical–legal consultation that involves life care planning and cost of care. The second author (Landry) has extensive experience in the areas of return-to-work rehabilitation and workers compensation insurance. Drawing on that experience, *Task Analysis: An Individual, Group, and Population Approach, 3rd Edition,* aims to provide students and practitioners with a clear understanding of how task analysis applies to everyday practice, whether they work with individuals, groups, or populations.

REFERENCES

American Occupational Therapy Association. (2014). Occupational therapy practice framework: Domain and process (3rd ed.). *American Journal of Occupational Therapy, 68*(Suppl. 1), S1–S48. http://dx.doi.org/10.5014/ajot.2014.682006

Moyers, P. A., & Dale, L. M. (2007). *The guide to occupational therapy practice* (2nd ed.). Bethesda, MD: AOTA Press.

Van Leit, B. (1995). Using the case method to develop clinical reasoning skills in problem-based learning. *American Journal of Occupational Therapy, 49,* 349–353. http://dx.doi.org/10.5014/ajot.49.4.349

Watson, D. E. (1997). *Task analysis: An occupational performance approach.* Bethesda, MD: American Occupational Therapy Association.

Watson, D. E., & Wilson, S. A. (2003). *Task analysis: An individual and population approach* (2nd ed.). Bethesda, MD: AOTA Press.

Part I. Domain and Process of Occupational Therapy

Historical Perspective: Intervention Through Activity

1

By virtue of our biological endowment, people of all ages and abilities require occupation to grow and thrive; in pursuing occupation, humans express the totality of their being, a mind–body–spirit union. Because human existence could not otherwise be, humankind is, in essence, occupational by nature.

—Hooper & Wood (2014, p. 38, as cited in American Occupational Therapy Association, 2014, p. S3)

LEARNING OBJECTIVES

At the completion of this chapter, readers will be able to

- Understand a historical perspective on the framing of occupational therapy and how its core concepts have evolved and continue to evolve and
- Describe occupational therapy's contribution to health and wellness.

KEY TERMS

Activity
Activity analysis
Activity limitations
Co-occupations
Dimensions
Disability
Domain
Fit
Frames of reference
Health
Impairments
International Classification of Functioning, Disability and Health

Involvement
Occupation
Occupational performance
Occupational therapy
Occupational Therapy Practice Framework
Occupations
Participation
Participation restrictions
Person–Environment–Occupation model
Task
Task analysis
Wellness
World Health Organization

Occupational therapy has a long tradition of helping clients improve their health and wellness. This tradition has been shaped over generations by its practitioners' enduring commitment to promoting their clients' engagement in occupations and participation in context. This chapter frames occupational therapy's contribution to health and wellness by describing key concepts that start with services and end with health and wellness. Occupational therapy offers a distinct approach to the promotion of health and wellness, providing services that enable clients to engage in occupations to support participation in contexts.

EVOLUTION OF A PROFESSIONAL FOCUS

Activities are "designed and selected to support the development of performance skills and performance patterns that will enhance occupational engagement" (American Occupational Therapy Association [AOTA], 2014, p. S41). The belief that engagement in activity has healing power has its roots in the Arts and Crafts movement of the late 19th century and in the philosophies of the founders of occupational therapy. Early occupational therapy theorists acknowledged the unity among mind, body, and spirit and the connection among engagement, self-fulfillment, and health (Atwood, 1907; Meyer, 1922; Moher, 1907). Goal-directed activities to instill craftsmanship and workplace skills were used as diversions as well as for therapeutic, vocational, and motivational benefit.

Terms used to describe early occupational therapy included *work treatment, work therapy, occupational reeducation,* and *work cure* (Hall, 1910; Hopkins, 1988). The term *occupational therapy* was coined by George Barton, who saw therapists as curing people through the use of work (Dunlop, 1933). Barton was an architect who experienced disabling conditions that led him to pursue studies in the field of rehabilitation. Through these pursuits he made contact with the contemporary leaders of the field—Dr. William R. Dutton, Eleanor Clarke Slagle, Susan Tracey, and Susan Cox

Johnson (Sabonis-Chafee & Hussey, 1998). As Polatajko (2001) observed,

> Our evolution started with a concept of occupation that was akin to the present day concept of work, not necessarily paid work, but work none the less. . . . It was considered that the absence of work, in and of itself, resulted in the deterioration of the human condition and that the only remedy was work. (p. 204)

Other early theorists saw the potential domain of occupational therapy as much broader and more health related than vocational training (Friedland, 2001; Kidner, 1923). In 1921, the following definition of *occupational therapy* was proposed: "any activity, mental or physical, definitely prescribed and guided for the distinct purpose of contributing to and hastening recovery from disease or injury" (Hall, 1922, p. 61). This broader conceptualization of the domain of occupational therapy soon dominated the field.

Although early scholars wrote about the concept of occupation until the 1930s, the only consistent use of the term *occupation* between the 1940s and 1980s was in the title of the profession. The profession's literature during that period focused on the term *activity* and the therapeutic use of activity. Occupational therapy practitioners today continue to struggle with the terms *occupation* and *activity*. Practically speaking, these terms are synonymous, as discussed later in this chapter.

During the 1960s and 1970s, occupational therapy leaders advocated a focus not only on returning patients to previous activities but also on helping people engage in meaningful occupations and participate in life (Polatajko, 2001). By 2002, the focus on participation was ratified in the official definition of the *domain* of the profession: "engagement in occupation to support participation in context or contexts" (AOTA, 2002, p. 611). The core belief in the positive relation between occupation and health and the emphasis on people as occupational beings were articulated in the second and third editions of the *Occupational Therapy Practice Framework: Domain and Process* (hereinafter, the *Framework;* AOTA, 2008, 2014).

OCCUPATIONS, ACTIVITIES, AND TASKS

Activity analysis has been used as an approach to determining whether an occupation or activity is meaningful, motivates the client and fulfills his or her needs, and can be used to help the client attain the therapeutic aims of developing or restoring skills and abilities. Activity analysis "addresses the typical demands of an activity, the range of skills involved in its performance, and the various cultural meanings that might be ascribed to it" (Crepeau, 2003, p. 192, as cited in AOTA, 2014, p. S12). It enables occupational therapy practitioners to determine whether an activity has therapeutic potential or value and to select and design an activity to treat a disability or functional limitation (Trombly, 1995a). The purpose of activity analysis is to determine whether an activity has restorative potential or value and to grade therapeutic activities (Watson, 1997).

Occupational therapy practitioners and educators incorporated activity analysis into practice and educational programs during World War I (Creighton, 1992). Joint position, action, and muscle strength were of primary interest, as was analysis of the abilities required to engage in a specific activity. Haas (1922) suggested a system of activity analysis and rating. Activities were classified according to their therapeutic benefits between 1920 and the 1940s, and through the 1960s, analyses included physical requirements and emotional and social properties. During the 1970s, 1980s, and 1990s, several frames of reference influenced activity analysis methods, requiring practitioners to recognize sensorimotor, affective, cognitive, biomechanical, volitional, contextual, and spiritual parameters (Canadian Association of Occupational Therapists [CAOT], 1997; Creighton, 1992).

In the *Framework*, the term *occupation* is used to capture the breadth and meaning of "daily life activities in which people engage" (AOTA, 2014, p. S43). *Occupation* encompasses *activity*, and a *task* is a subset of an activity or occupation.

Throughout the 20th century, occupational therapy practitioners developed their skills in activity analysis to select and design therapeutic activities as modalities for use in enabling client goals. Early in the century, Gilbreth (1911) introduced the concept of *job analysis* through motion studies.

Motion studies involved analysis of characteristics of the worker, the worker's surroundings, and the motion requirements of the job. These studies enabled practitioners to recommend adaptations to improve efficiency. Friedman (1916) recommended that health professionals seeking to match clients with a vocation consider the physical, mental, and psychological requirements of the particular occupation. Thus, occupational therapy leaders have historically recognized the significance of a fit among persons, environments, and occupations, and this tenet continues to dominate the profession to this day (see Figure 1.1). Activities are deemed to be purposeful when they

- Are relevant, meaningful, and goal directed;
- Elicit coordination among sensorimotor, cognitive, psychological, and psychosocial systems; and
- Promote mastery and feelings of competence (AOTA, 1993; Fidler & Fidler, 1978; Trombly, 1995b).

Occupational therapy practitioners examine occupations and activities and are interested in the complexity of factors that make it possible for a client to participate in a meaningful occupation or activity. Thus, breaking down an occupation or activity into the smallest identifiable, essential, and complete piece of an activity seeded task analysis. *Task analysis* is an examination of differentiating details that are interdependent and contribute to performance. By analyzing the features, characteristics, and qualities of activities, occupational therapy practitioners realized that they could grade and modify activities through task analysis, taking into account the client's residual capabilities, and prescribe purposeful activities as therapeutic modalities (Hinojosa, Sabari, & Rosenfeld, 1983; Kidner, 1930).

OCCUPATIONS, PARTICIPATION, AND OCCUPATIONAL PERFORMANCE

Occupations occur in context and are influenced by client factors, performance skills, and performance patterns. Occupations "occur over time; have purpose, meaning, and perceived utility to the client; and can be observed by others (e.g., preparing a meal) or be known only to the person involved (e.g., learning through reading a textbook)" (AOTA, 2014, p. S6). Occupations can involve the execution of multiple activities for completion and can result in various outcomes. The *Framework* recognizes and categorizes occupations as activities of daily living, instrumental activities of daily living (IADLs), rest and sleep, education, work, play, leisure, and social participation (AOTA, 2014).

Occupations are often shared and may be termed *co-occupations* (e.g., feeding an infant). The experience of engaging in an occupation generally has a distinct, subjective meaning for each person. For example, one person may view doing laundry as work, and another may consider it an IADL (AOTA, 2014). By engaging clients' minds, spirits, and bodies in occupations, occupational therapy practitioners facilitate optimal engagement and participation. This approach distinguishes occupational therapy from verbal therapy (CAOT, 1993).

Participation, which is "involvement in a life situation" (World Health Organization [WHO], 2001, p. 193), was incorporated as a tenet of occupational therapy by the early 1990s and through to the present (AOTA, 2014; CAOT, 1997; Polatajko, 1992). Definitions of the profession place a strong value on the occupational therapy practitioner's role in supporting participation in context through engagement in occupations or activities:

> *Occupational therapy* is the art and science of directing an individual's participation in selected tasks to restore, reinforce, and enhance performance; facilitate learning of those skills and functions essential for adaptation and productivity; diminish or correct pathology; and promote and maintain health. (AOTA, 1995, p. 89)

Occupational therapy strives to enable clients to participate in occupations that provide meaningful engagement in their lives. Participation can be a disabling tool rather than an enabling tool if the practitioner loses focus on occupation or on client participation (Townsend & Polatajko, 2007). Occupational therapy practitioners should

take a client-centered approach and encourage and invite clients to take an active part in implementing required occupational changes.

In the early 1970s, AOTA proposed that the role, function, and domain of concern of occupational therapy practitioners be termed *occupational performance* (AOTA, 1973, 1974). *Occupational performance* is the level of accomplishment of a selected occupation, task, or activity resulting from

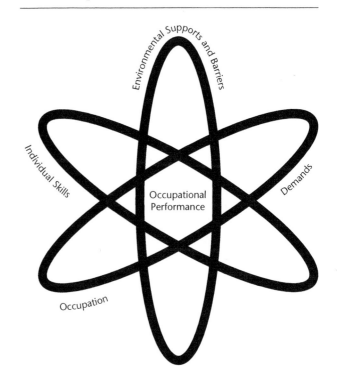

FIGURE 1.1

Person–Environment–Occupation model of occupational performance.
Note. From "The Person–Environment–Occupation Model: A Transactive Approach to Occupational Performance," by M. Law, B. Cooper, S. Strong, D. Steward, P. Rigby, & L. Letts, 1996, *Canadian Journal of Occupational Therapy, 63,* p. 15. Copyright © 1996 by the Canadian Association of Occupational Therapists. Used with permission.

the dynamic interaction among persons, their environments, and their occupations (AOTA, 1994). In response to regulatory requirements for uniform reporting systems, a national uniform terminology system was first developed and approved in 1979. This document started to frame the profession's view of the determinants of occupational performance and the domain of concern to the profession (AOTA, 1979).

The third edition of this document, *Uniform Terminology for Occupational Therapy* (hereinafter, *Uniform Terminology;* AOTA, 1994), described practice as focusing on three domains: (1) performance areas, (2) performance components, and (3) performance contexts. At that time, optimal occupational performance was deemed to occur when there was a fit, or match, among persons, activities, and environments that resulted in enhanced participation. The purpose of intervention was seen as the creation of a *fit* among the person, the activity, and the environment by aligning "the skills and abilities of the individual; the demands of activity; and the characteristics of the physical, social, and cultural environments" (AOTA, 1994, p. 277).

As part of the review process to update and revise the *Uniform Terminology,* the AOTA Commission on Practice again updated the profession's domain of concern. In 2002, AOTA developed a new *Framework,* which superseded the *Uniform Terminology* and adhered to the concept of interaction and fit among person, environment, and occupation:

> Execution of a performance skill occurs when the performer, the context, and the demands of the activity come together in the performance of the activity. Each of these factors influences the execution of a skill and may support or hinder actual skill execution. (AOTA, 2002, p. 612)

An occupational performance approach to evaluation and intervention focuses on the dynamic, interdependent, and transactional relations among persons (i.e., clients), environments (i.e., contexts), and occupations. The *Person–Environment–Occupation (PEO) model* holds that occupational performance is shaped by the continuous and simultaneous interaction among these aspects (CAOT, 1993; Law, 2002; Law et al., 1996; Law, Polatajko, Baptiste, & Townsend, 1997). The person and environment are connected through occupational performance and participation (Christiansen, Baum, & Bass-Haugen, 2005).

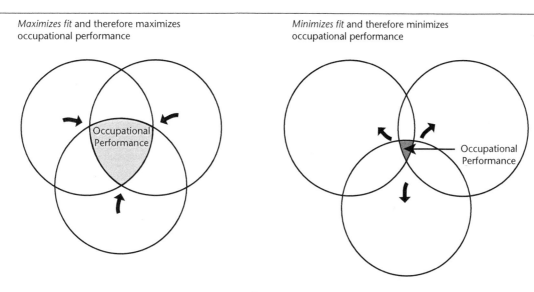

FIGURE 1.2

Changes to occupational performance as a consequence of variations in fit among person, environment, and occupation.
Note. From "The Person–Environment–Occupation Model: A Transactive Approach to Occupational Performance," by M. Law, B. Cooper, S. Strong, D. Steward, P. Rigby, & L. Letts, 1996, *Canadian Journal of Occupational Therapy, 63,* p. 18. Copyright © 1996 by the Canadian Association of Occupational Therapists. Used with permission.

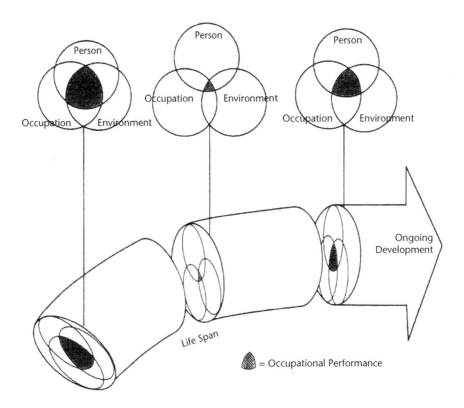

FIGURE 1.3

The Person–Environment–Occupation model of occupational performance across the lifespan.
Note. From "The Person–Environment–Occupation Model: A Transactive Approach to Occupational Performance," by M. Law, B. Cooper, S. Strong, D. Steward, P. Rigby, & L. Letts, 1996, *Canadian Journal of Occupational Therapy, 63,* p. 15. Copyright © 1996 by the Canadian Association of Occupational Therapists. Used with permission.

Figure 1.1 shows the three aspects of the PEO model, with occupational performance represented in the overlap among the aspects. This model provides a holistic perspective on the domain of occupational therapy and increases the scope of assessment options and intervention strategies available to practitioners beyond activity analysis (Dunn, Brown, & McGuigan, 1994; Law et al., 1996; Letts et al., 1994).

The PEO model of occupational performance clarifies the conceptualization of fit by focusing attention on the interaction among aspects of the model. As depicted in Figure 1.2, separate but interconnected spheres represent the person, the environment, and the occupation. Overlap among the spheres represents occupational performance. Optimal occupational performance occurs when the overlap among the spheres is maximized and the person, environment, and occupation appear inseparable.

When the interaction of the three aspects of the model is harmonious or compatible and the client engages in occupations within his or her context and capacity, occupational performance can be deemed the best possible. As depicted in Figure 1.3, the interactions among the dimensions vary across time and are reflected in clients' changing performance patterns (i.e., habits, roles, and routines; Law et al., 1996). The factors that contribute to temporal changes in the interactions are those conditions or situations that contribute to or influence health.

OCCUPATIONAL THERAPY'S CONTRIBUTION TO HEALTH AND WELLNESS

Occupational therapy has a long tradition of helping clients improve their health and wellness. How does one define what it is like to experience

---

Assignment 1.2. Health and Wellness

Reflect on your personal experience, values, and beliefs about health and wellness to better understand WHO and AOTA definitions of these important concepts. (A) What is it like to feel healthy and to experience well-being? (B) Describe what "state of health and well-being" means to you. (C) Identify and list things that contribute to a state of health. Cluster these items into one or more of the following three categories: (1) person, (2) environment, and (3) occupation. For example, if you describe health and well-being as including a sense of personal security and identify public safety as a determinant of this state of health, then write *sense of security* in the person category and *safe public places* in the environment category.

---

health and wellness? AOTA (2014) uses WHO's (1986) definition of *health*, which is a state of physical, mental, and social well-being, as well as a positive concept emphasizing social and personal resources and physical capacities. AOTA (2014) uses Hettler's (1984) definition of *wellness* as "an active process through which individuals [groups or populations] become aware of and make choices toward a more successful existence" (p. 1170).

International Classification of Functioning, Disability and Health

WHO is the United Nations' specialized agency for health, and as such it has produced guidelines that provide a unifying and standard language and framework to understand, describe, and study health and health-related states, outcomes, and determinants. These guidelines are known as the *International Classification of Functioning, Disability and Health* (ICF; WHO, 2001). Broad constructs of health and well-being include the following conditions and resources as fundamental determinants: peace, shelter, education, food, income, a stable ecosystem, sustainable resources, social justice, and equity (WHO, 1986). The components of health and health-related states include body functions and structures, engagement in activities and participation in life situations, and environmental factors (WHO, 2001). In the *ICF*, emphasis is on health and functioning rather than disability; previously, disability began where health ended (WHO, 2002). A major innovation in the *ICF* is classification of environmental factors that enable identification of barriers and enablers for both capacity and performance (p. 8).

WHO (2013) uses the term *disability* as an "umbrella term for impairments, activity limitations, and participation restrictions" that are a part of the human condition. Almost everyone will have a disability at some point in life, and as people age they face greater functional challenges (WHO, 2011). *Impairments* are problems in body function (i.e., physiology) and structure (i.e., anatomy) that result in significant deviation or loss in what are considered normal functions or structures. *Activity limitations* "are difficulties in executing a task," and *participation restrictions* "are problems experienced in involvement in life situations" (WHO, 2011, p. 5). The term *involvement* means the state of "taking part, being included or engaged in an area of life, being accepted, or having access to needed resources," and it can be gauged through performance (WHO, 2001, p. 15).

The *ICF* is based on the conceptual framework of functioning and disability as a dynamic interaction between health conditions and contextual factors, both personal and environmental. Disability results from the interaction between people with impairments and societal barriers that hinder their participation on an equal basis with others (WHO, 2011). WHO's focus on engagement and participation is echoed in the definition of the targeted outcome of occupational therapy provided in the *Framework* (AOTA, 2014).

Occupational Therapy Practice Framework: Domain and Process

Frames of reference provide structure to help people organize and apply knowledge. In 2002, AOTA published the first edition of the *Framework,* which established "engagement in occupation to support participation" as one of the profession's necessary objectives. The *Framework*

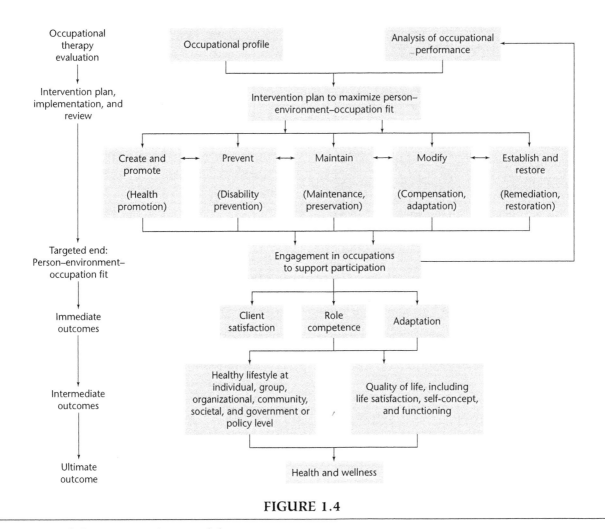

FIGURE 1.4

Occupational therapy services model.

Note. From *Task Analysis: An Individual and Population Approach* (2nd ed.), by D. E. Watson and S. A. Wilson, 2003, p. 5. Copyright © 2003 by the American Occupational Therapy Association. Used with permission.

articulated the profession's current thinking on the domain and process of the profession. Youngstrom (2002), a member of the AOTA Commission on Practice, explained the commission's choices of terms used in the *Framework:*

> The phrase "engagement in occupation to support participation" was purposefully chosen to point out several key ideas that describe the profession's understanding of occupation and its contribution to health. . . . Positioning occupational therapy in this domain makes a clear statement about occupational therapy's contribution to health—a focus on helping clients (individuals, groups, or organizations) to engage in occupations (i.e., daily life activities that are purposeful,

meaningful, and important to the client) that enable their participation in life situations. (p. 608)

This publication uses the approach to occupational therapy described in the *Framework* and examines domain as the foundation of task analysis. *Domain* refers to the occupational therapy profession's purview, areas in which its members have an established body of knowledge and expertise to support health and participation in life through engagement in occupation (AOTA, 2014). *Dimensions* referred to in this text are the components of task analysis and include occupations, client factors, activity demands, performance skills, performance patterns, and contexts and environments. Intertwined with the discussion in this book are

---

Assignment 1.3. Meaningful Activity

Interview a person to determine what he or she does that is meaningful. (A) How does he or she set priorities on what is most important? (B) What are the environments or contexts in which he or she engages or participates? (C) How would the sudden inability to bend the right knee affect his or her ability to engage or participate?

---

case studies that guide student learning of the task analysis process used in the delivery of occupational therapy. Figure 1.4 depicts the occupational therapy services model through a logic chain that starts with services and ends with health and wellness.

SUMMARY

Throughout its history, the occupational therapy profession has helped clients improve their health and wellness through engagement in occupation and participation in context. Activity analysis and task analysis are used by occupational therapy practitioners in determining whether an occupation or activity is meaningful, motivating, and useful for helping clients achieve the therapeutic goals.

REFERENCES

American Occupational Therapy Association. (1973). *The roles and functions of occupational therapy personnel.* Bethesda, MD: Author.

American Occupational Therapy Association. (1974). *A curriculum guide for occupational therapy educators.* Bethesda, MD: Author.

American Occupational Therapy Association. (1979). *Occupational therapy product output reporting system and uniform terminology for reporting occupational therapy services.* Bethesda, MD: Author.

American Occupational Therapy Association. (1993). Position paper: Purposeful activity. *American Journal of Occupational Therapy, 47,* 1081–1082. http://dx.doi.org/10.5014/ajot.47.12.1081

American Occupational Therapy Association. (1994). *Uniform terminology: Application to practice.* Bethesda, MD: Author.

American Occupational Therapy Association. (1995). *Essentials and guidelines for an accredited educational program for the occupational therapist.* Bethesda, MD: Author.

American Occupational Therapy Association. (2002). Occupational therapy practice framework: Domain and process. *American Journal of Occupational Therapy, 56,* 609–639. http://dx.doi.org/10.5014/ajot.56.6.609

American Occupational Therapy Association. (2008). Occupational therapy practice framework: Domain and process (2nd ed.). *American Journal of Occupational Therapy, 62,* 625–683. http://dx.doi.org/10.5014/ajot.62.6.625

American Occupational Therapy Association. (2014). Occupational therapy practice framework: Domain and process (3rd ed.). *American Journal of Occupational Therapy, 68*(Suppl.), S1–4. http://dx.doi.org/10.5014/ajot.2014.682006

Atwood, C. E. (1907). The favorable influence of occupation in certain nervous disorders. *New York Medical Journal, 86,* 1101–1103.

Canadian Association of Occupational Therapists. (1993). *Occupational therapy guidelines for client centred mental health practice.* Toronto, ON: Author.

Canadian Association of Occupational Therapists. (1997). *Enabling occupation: An occupational therapy perspective.* Ottawa, ON: Author.

Christiansen, C., Baum, C., & Bass-Haugen, J. (Eds.). (2005). *Occupational therapy: Enabling function and well-being* (3rd ed.). Thorofare, NJ: Slack.

Creighton, C. (1992). The origin and evolution of activity analysis. *American Journal of Occupational Therapy, 46,* 45–48. http://dx.doi.org/10.5014/ajot.46.1.45

Crepeau, E. (2003). Analyzing occupation and activity: A way of thinking about occupational performance. In E. Crepeau, E. Cohn, & B. A. B. Schell (Eds.), *Willard and Spackman's occupational therapy* (10th ed., pp. 189–198). Philadelphia: Lippincott Williams & Wilkins.

Dunlop, W. J. (1933). A brief history of occupational therapy. *Canadian Journal of Occupational Therapy, 1,* 6–11.

Dunn, W., Brown, C., & McGuigan, A. (1994). The ecology of human performance: A framework for considering the effect of context. *American Journal of Occupational Therapy, 48,* 595–607. http://dx.doi.org/10.5014/ajot.48.7.595

Fidler, G. S., & Fidler, J. (1978). Doing and becoming: Purposeful action and self-actualization. *American Journal of Occupational Therapy, 32,* 305–310.

Friedland, J. (2001). Knowing from where we came: Reflecting on return-to-work and interpersonal relationships. *Canadian Journal of Occupational Therapy, 68,* 266–271.

Friedman, H. M. (1916, September 23). Occupational specialization in the defective. *New York Medical Journal*, pp. 587–592.

Gilbreth, F. B. (1911). *Motion study*. New York: Nostrand.

Haas, L. J. (1922). Crafts adaptable to occupational need: Their relative importance. *Archives of Occupational Therapy, 1*, 443–445.

Hall, H. J. (1910). The work cure. *JAMA, 54*, 12.

Hall, H. J. (1922). Occupational therapy in 1921. *Modern Hospital, 18*, 61–63.

Hettler, W. (1984). Wellness—The lifetime goal of a university experience. In J. D. Matarazzo, S. M. Weiss, J. A. Herd, N. E. Miller, & S. M. Weiss (Eds.), *Behavioral health: A handbook of health enhancement and disease prevention* (pp. 1117–1124). New York: Wiley.

Hinojosa, J., Sabari, J., & Rosenfeld, M. S. (1983). Purposeful activities. *American Journal of Occupational Therapy, 37*, 805–806.

Hooper, B., & Wood, W. (2014). The philosophy of occupational therapy: A framework for practice. In B. A. Boyt Schell, G. Gillen, & M. Scaffa (Eds.), *Willard and Spackman's occupational therapy* (12th ed., pp. 35–46). Philadelphia: Lippincott Williams & Wilkins.

Hopkins, H. L. (1988). A historical perspective on occupational therapy. In H. L. Hopkins & H. D. Smith (Eds.), *Willard and Spackman's occupational therapy* (7th ed., pp. 16–37). Philadelphia: Lippincott.

Kidner, T. B. (1923). President's address. *Archives of Occupational Therapy, 2*, 415–424.

Kidner, T. B. (1930). *Occupational therapy: The science of prescribed work for invalids*. Stuttgart, Germany: W. Kohlhammer.

Law, M. (2002). Participation in the occupations of everyday life. *American Journal of Occupational Therapy, 56*, 640–649. http://dx.doi.org/10.5014/ajot.56.6.640

Law, M., Cooper, B., Strong, S., Stewart, D., Rigby, P., & Letts, L. (1996). The Person–Environment–Occupation model: A transactive approach to occupational performance. *Canadian Journal of Occupational Therapy, 63*, 9–23.

Law, M., Polatajko, H., Baptiste, W., & Townsend, E. (1997). Core concepts of occupational therapy. In Canadian Association of Occupational Therapists (Ed.), *Enabling occupation: An occupational therapy perspective* (pp. 29–56). Ottawa, ON: Canadian Association of Occupational Therapists.

Letts, L., Law, M., Rigby, P., Cooper, B., Stewart, D., & Strong, S. (1994). Person–environment assessments in occupational therapy. *American Journal of Occupational Therapy, 48*, 608–618. http://dx.doi.org/10.5014/ajot.48.7.608

Meyer, A. (1922). The philosophy of occupational therapy. *Archives of Occupational Therapy, 1*, 1–10.

Moher, T. J. (1907). Occupation in the treatment of the insane. *JAMA, 158*, 1664–1666.

Polatajko, H. J. (1992). Naming and framing occupational therapy: A lecture dedicated to the life of Nancy B. *Canadian Journal of Occupational Therapy, 59*, 184–200.

Polatajko, H. J. (2001). The evolution of our occupational perspective: The journey from diversion through therapeutic use to enablement. *Canadian Journal of Occupational Therapy, 68*, 203–207.

Sabonis-Chafee, B., & Hussey, S. M. (1998). *Introduction to occupational therapy* (2nd ed.). St. Louis, MO: Mosby.

Townsend, E. A., & Polatajko, H. J. (2007). *Enabling occupation II: Advancing an occupational therapy vision of health, well-being, and justice through occupation*. Ottawa, ON: CAOT Publications.

Trombly, C. A. (1995a). Occupation: Purposefulness and meaningfulness as therapeutic mechanisms [Eleanor Clark Slagle Lecture]. *American Journal of Occupational Therapy, 49*, 960–972. http://dx.doi.org/10.5014/ajot.49.10.960

Trombly, C. A. (1995b). Purposeful activity. In C. A. Trombly (Ed.), *Occupational therapy for physical dysfunction* (pp. 237–253). Baltimore: Williams & Wilkins.

Watson, D. E. (1997). *Task analysis: An occupational performance approach*. Bethesda, MD: American Occupational Therapy Association.

Watson, D. E., & Wilson, S. A. (2003). *Task analysis: An individual and population approach* (2nd ed.). Bethesda, MD: AOTA Press.

World Health Organization. (1986). *The Ottawa Charter for Health Promotion*. Ottawa: Health and Welfare Canada and Author. Retrieved from www.who.int/healthpromotion/conferences/previous/ottawa/en/

World Health Organization. (2001). *International classification of functioning, disability and health*. Geneva: Author.

World Health Organization. (2002). *Towards a common language for functioning, disability and health (ICF)*. Geneva: Author.

World Health Organization. (2011). *World report on disability*. Geneva: Author.

World Health Organization. (2013). *Health topics: Disabilities*. Retrieved from www.who.int/topics/disabilities/en/

Youngstrom, M. J. (2002). The *Occupational Therapy Practice Framework*: The evolution of our professional language. *American Journal of Occupational Therapy, 56*, 607–608. http://dx.doi.org/10.5014/ajot.56.6.607

Occupational Therapy Services: A Distinct Approach

2

In its simplest terms, occupational therapists and occupational therapy assistants help people across the lifespan participate in the things they want and need to do through the therapeutic use of everyday activities (occupations).

—American Occupational Therapy Association (2012)

LEARNING OBJECTIVES

At the completion of this chapter, readers will be able to

- Describe the occupational therapy profession's focus on engagement in occupations and participation in contexts;
- Define the terms *client* and *client-centered service*;
- Explain and differentiate activity analysis and task analysis; and
- Understand the Client Profile and Task Analysis form as the task analysis template to be used throughout this publication's case examples and assignments.

KEY TERMS

Activity
Activity analysis
Canadian Occupational Performance
    Measure
Cardinal Hill Occupational Participation
    Process
Client
Client-centered service
Contexts
Co-occupations

Dimensions
Domain
FIM™
Goal attainment scaling
Models of practice
Occupations
Participation
Person–Environment–Occupation model
Task analysis

Occupational therapy practice is based on the premise that people with disabilities or activity limitations can achieve optimal engagement and participation leading to changes in health and well-being. Occupational therapy offers a distinct approach to the promotion of health and wellness.

OCCUPATIONAL THERAPY CONCEPTS

The occupational therapy profession provides services that enable people to engage in *occupations*—the normal activities of life—and that support participation in their *contexts*—their external and internal environments. The World Health Organization (WHO; 2001) defined *participation* as "involvement in a life situation" (p. 123), and Law (2002) defined it as "involvement in formal and informal everyday activities" (p. 641). Townsend and Polatajko (2007) quoted Thomas Jefferson's observation that "it is neither wealth nor splendor; but tranquility and occupation which give us happiness" (p. 15). Occupational therapy enables occupational engagement within the context of the spirit and needs of the person, organization, or population. Essentially, occupation brings meaning to life, and occupational therapy practitioners aim to enable activity through therapeutic strategies that are client centered and client directed. The key measurement is the degree of fit among persons, environments, and occupations.

Changes in the nature and distribution of health and illness risks, coupled with an enhanced understanding of the determinants of health and illness, have led occupational therapy practitioners to offer services not only to individuals but also to groups and populations of people to support everyday life and contribute to health and well-being. For any of these entities, occupational therapy practitioners target their evaluation and intervention to optimize the engagement of people, within their environments, as participants in personally meaningful occupations. It is this interaction that ultimately supports the health of clients, whether they are individuals, organizations, or populations.

Occupational therapy practice is a *client-centered service* in that practitioners collaborate with clients and their proxies and focus priorities on the issues clients identify. The term *client* refers to the entity that receives services, and a client may be

> persons (including those involved in care of the individual), groups (collective individuals, e.g., families, workers, students, or community), and populations (collective groups of individuals living in a similar locale, e.g., city, state, or country residents, people sharing same or like concerns). (AOTA, 2014, p. S3)

Often other professionals work with occupational therapy clients, and clients are best served when their occupational therapy practitioners establish partnerships and work in collaboration with interdisciplinary teams.

In the client-centered service model, occupational therapy practitioners work with clients to understand their occupational repertoires and patterns of living for the purpose of constructing solutions to enable engagement and participation at an optimum level. In work with organizations (e.g., community development initiatives), the occupational therapy consultant considers the engagement of the organization, the environment to be influenced, and the goals or outcomes targeted. In population health, the occupational therapy researcher examines the interaction of a specific population with the geographic and sociocultural environment and identifies the occupational needs of that population. In summary,

> Occupational therapy is the art and science of enabling engagement in everyday living, through occupation; of enabling people to perform the occupations that foster health and well-being; and of enabling a just and inclusive society so that all people may participate to their potential in the daily occupations of life. (Townsend & Polatajko, 2007, p. 89)

Developing an occupational profile, analyzing performance, and using this information to plan and review intervention require a broad understanding of the client. The practitioner must consider the client's current and desired occupations, tasks, activity demands, and contexts and

---

Assignment 2.1. Defining Terms

Define the terms *client* and *client-centered service,* and describe how occupational therapy is a client-centered service.

---

analyze the complex interactions among these dimensions (AOTA, 2014). In addition, the practitioner must take into account that occupations are idiosyncratic or personal and can be adaptive or maladaptive; "not all occupations lead to health, well-being and justice, or have therapeutic value" (Townsend & Polatajko, 2007, p. 22). Many occupations (e.g., home management, feeding a child) are shared, involving two or more people, and are termed *co-occupations* (AOTA, 2014).

Models of practice are individual occupational therapy practitioners' unique guides to day-to-day practice and illustrate how they think about what they do as practitioners. Models help practitioners sort and categorize complex relations among concepts and dimensions and articulate the basis of their clinical reasoning about clients and their needs (Canadian Association of Occupational Therapists, 2002). The *Person–Environment–Occupation (PEO) model* of occupational performance, introduced in Chapter 1, "Historical Perspective: Intervention Through Activity," describes what occupational therapy practitioners think about in their day-to-day practice when they seek to promote engagement and participation (Law et al., 1996).

Theories, approaches, and models of practice direct occupational therapy evaluation and intervention. This book does not focus on theories but provides ample opportunity for readers to apply their theoretical knowledge to the case studies in each chapter. As illustrated in Figure 1.4, occupational therapy practitioners choose from among several approaches to intervention, including health promotion, disability prevention, maintenance, compensation or adaptation, and remediation or restoration. They use different types of interventions within each of these approaches. Although engagement in occupations to support participation is the targeted end of service delivery, other intervention outcomes are expected that reflect client priorities and goals.

ACTIVITY ANALYSIS: DEFINITIONS AND USE

Activity is a state of being active or engaging in natural and normal functions. *Occupation* and *activity* are synonymous concepts within occupational therapy models; in the *Occupational Therapy Practice Framework: Domain and Process* (hereinafter referred to as the *Framework;* AOTA, 2014), the term *occupation* encompasses *activity. Activity analysis* is an approach used by an occupational therapy practitioner to determine whether restoring or developing an activity or occupation is meaningful to a client and is achievable. Activities and occupations that are within the domain of occupational therapy practice include activities of daily living (ADLs), instrumental activities of daily living, rest and sleep, education, work, play, leisure, and social participation.

TASK ANALYSIS: DEFINITIONS AND USE

Varying views exist on the coexistence of *activity analysis* and *task analysis.* Some practitioners and authors use the terms interchangeably, but this book does not. A *task* is a subset of the broader category of *activity* or *occupation* and is the smallest identifiable, essential, and complete piece of an activity. For example, the task of dressing is a subset of the activity of self-care, the task of vacuuming is a subset of the activity of housekeeping, the task of mowing the lawn is a subset of the activity of gardening, the task of golfing is a subset of the occupation of leisure and social participation, and so forth.

Task analysis is a clinical reasoning tool practitioners use to analyze occupational performance and related activities for the purpose of designing interventions targeted at people, environments, and activities or occupations. Task analysis focuses on the performance of a specific subset of an activity or occupation—for example, the subset of dressing for the activity of ADLs. The practitioner breaks the task down into its components to understand individual performance in the context of the client's environment and takes into consideration environmental

Assignment 2.2. Understanding Occupation and Activity vs. Tasks

1. Describe the cultural context in which fishing is seen as a work occupation, and describe the cultural context in which fishing is seen as a leisure activity. How are the meaning and purpose of a task or occupation influenced by context?

2. Using the "Tasks Analyzed" section of the CPTA form (Appendix A), list the array of tasks nested in fishing as a work occupation and as a leisure activity. How do the tasks differ between these two occupations? How are the basic needs of people met through fishing as work vs. fishing as leisure? In answering the latter question, consider the 4 functions of occupations identified by Wilcock (1998): (1) to provide for immediate bodily needs of sustenance, self-care, and shelter; (2) to develop skills, social structures, and technology aimed at safety and superiority over predators and the environment; (3) to maintain health by balanced exercise and personal capacities; and (4) to enable individual and social development so that each person and species will flourish.

3. Select 1 activity required in fishing as a work or leisure occupation. What are the demands of this activity (i.e., required actions, body functions, and body structures)?

4. Describe the differences between *activity analysis* and *task analysis*.

facilitators and barriers. This analysis in turn aids problem solving and suggests intervention strategies for areas of need.

For example, dressing consists of the tasks of upper- and lower-body dressing. Lower-body dressing is broken down into the smaller actions of donning and doffing underwear, pants, socks, and shoes. Task analysis focuses on the minute details of the interaction between the person and his or her environment during the performance of each action that is part of the overall task of dressing.

The Client Profile and Task Analysis (CPTA) form located in Appendix A and provided on the flash drive included with this publication is used throughout this text and for chapter assignment questions. The case examples provided in this chapter (and throughout this publication) are designed to build on students' understanding of the process of task analysis and eventually integrate it into their professional process.

Frame of Reference

The focus of this book is on teaching a model of practice and its application through task analysis when services are directed toward individuals, organizations, and populations. The frame of reference used in this book includes the following:

- *Domain* refers to engagement in occupation to support participation in context across areas of self-care, productivity, and leisure and is the foundation of task analysis.
- *Dimensions* are the components of analysis, including areas of occupation, performance skills, performance patterns, contexts, activity demands, and client factors, that provide detail for the analysis.
- The PEO model emphasizes the fit among the person, his or her environment, and the occupation or activity in support of optimal participation and engagement.

Occupational therapy practitioners apply their art and science in using this information to direct a client's involvement in selected tasks, and it is the sum of these engagements in tasks that constitutes engagement in occupations and participation in contexts. Occupational therapy services begin with evaluation, during which the occupational therapist focuses on establishing the client's occupational profile and analyzing his or her occupational performance.

Exhibit 2.1 shows an example of task analysis using the CPTA form for a client, Fred, a student with aquaphobia (i.e., fear of water).

(text continues on page 24)

EXHIBIT 2.1. CLIENT PROFILE AND TASK ANALYSIS FORM: FRED

CLIENT PROFILE

Name: Fred Fish **Advocates:** Fred Fish Sr. **Diagnoses:** Aquaphobia	**Birthdate:** **Age at assessment:** 21 **Education:** Third year at university **Work occupation:** Student **Current interventions:** Coaching engagement in new activities Setting goals for social participation

Referral Source: Student health

Fred is from a Midwest farm region and has moved to the Great Lakes area for school. Much of the socialization revolves around water-based activities. He has an extreme fear of water, which is restricting his participation with fellow students and developing friendships. He is feeling socially isolated from peer participation out of school.

PERSONAL INFORMATION

Family Unit	Parents and siblings living in the Midwest
Caregiver(s)	None
Roles and responsibilities (e.g., student, spouse, parent, friend, worker)	1. Student 2. Working part time at retail store selling fishing gear
Home environment (e.g., home design, number of people living in the home)	Sharing an apartment with one other student. The apartment is located one block from a lake.
Community context (e.g., rural, urban, metro; single-family home, residential care)	Small urban location that is a popular year-round resort area.
School or work context (e.g., public, special, or private school; stationary or travel location for work)	Social participation centers on using the lake for fishing, boating, and swimming.
Client priorities	1. Decrease fear of water. 2. Fish off the dock. 3. Work toward learning how to swim.
Values/beliefs/spirituality (e.g., principles, standards, beliefs, personal quest)	Values success but avoids novel challenges for fear of failing.

(Continued)

EXHIBIT 2.1. CLIENT PROFILE AND TASK ANALYSIS FORM: FRED (Cont.)

SUMMARY, PLAN, AND GOALS

Assessments completed (formal and observational):
Practitioner–client plan (e.g., further formal and observational assessments, inclusion of others): The practitioner will assist Fred with locating university and community resources and will periodically meet with him for progress updates.
Tasks requiring assessment or intervention

Short-term goals (Primarily client-driven, measurable, global task or activity achievements)	Long-term objectives (Primarily practitioner driven, measurable, incremental, stepwise or mini achievements)
1. Fred will spend time walking along the dock to build his tolerance for being near water. He will start by taking a short walk (5–10 minutes) and building his walk to up to 1 hour over 2–3 weeks.	1.a. The practitioner will accompany Fred on his first two attempts to walk along the dock and then will get a report from Fred on a weekly basis to check on his success.
2. Fred will enroll in a beginning swimming program for adults during the same period as in goal #1. He will keep a journal of his feelings during and after each swimming session to track his adaptive or maladaptive responses to the challenge.	2.a. The practitioner will assist with locating a program if Fred avoids the task. 2.b. During the weekly review with Fred, the practitioner will check on his progress in the swim program.
3. Fred will engage a peer to go fishing with him within 4–6 weeks.	3.a. During the weekly review with Fred, the practitioner will work with Fred on keeping momentum in his short-term goals so that he is ready to go fishing with a peer. 3.b. If Fred is not progressing past his fear of water by the 4th week of the program, the practitioner will refer him to additional psychological counseling.

TASKS ANALYZED

Occupation or Activity	Tasks (specific activity component)	Context or Environment (external and internal)
Leisure Fishing	1. Finding dock location or where to fish (e.g., water depth, safety railings) 2. Learning when to fish from local fisherman (e.g., water warming trends) 3. Securing loaner equipment 4. Learning to cast rod and reel in and dehook a fish	1. The lake is in close proximity to the university and has developed and natural areas around it (e.g., fishing can occur off a dock or off a bank). 2. Fishing is a common activity in the community and advice can be acquired from a local fisherman or from a retail store. 3. There are rental equipment businesses along the dock. 4. There are fishing lessons offered at the university and within the community.
Swimming	1. Learn to swim.	1. Beginning classes for adults at a local pool to decrease peer observance

ANALYSIS (OF PERFORMANCE SKILLS)

Performance Skills	Client Challenges (performance qualifier)
Rating: 0 = *no restriction*, 1 = *mild limitation*, 2 = *moderate restriction*, 3 = *severe restriction*, 4 = *complete impairment*	
Motor and praxis	**Rating**
Posture	0
Mobility	0
Coordination	1
Strength	0
Effort	2
Energy	0
Execution	2
Process skills	**Rating**
Mental energy	0
Knowledge	0
Organization	0
Adaptation	3
Social interaction skills	**Rating**
Communication posture	0
Gestures	0
Initiation	2
Information exchange	1
Acknowledging	0
Taking turns	0

ANALYSIS (OF PERFORMANCE PATTERNS)

Performance Patterns	Daily Life Activities	Client Challenges (skill deficits and context restrictions)
Habits (Automatic and integrated behaviors)	Within normal limits	None

(Continued)

EXHIBIT 2.1. CLIENT PROFILE AND TASK ANALYSIS FORM: FRED *(Cont.)*

Routines (Regular activities that provide daily structure)	Routines are based on his class and part-time work schedule.	He does not include leisure and social participation activities in his routines and has become isolated from his peers and community activities.
Roles (Expected behaviors and responsibilities)	Integration into the university and local community.	Extreme difficulty participating within the resort community related to his fear of water when most activities are centered around the local lake.
Rituals (Customary cultural/social activities)	None during the last three university years.	He has not integrated into his school and community but stays to himself other than engaging with his roommate.

Synopsis of performance skills and performance patterns (strengths, deficits and challenges):
Fred has the functional abilities to learn to swim and to engage in fishing. However, he has substantial fear of water and performance anxiety about trying new activities and meeting new people.

OCCUPATIONAL PROFILE AND ANALYSIS OF NEEDS

Functional ability (i.e., how strengths and deficits affect ability to perform activities and tasks)	Fred describes feelings of great anxiety when faced with trying new activities near the water and has used many avoidance strategies, including lonely isolation. He knows swimming, fishing, and boating bring great joy to others in his community. He no longer wants to be socially isolated and wants to overcome this fear. He wants to learn to swim and fish, despite a substantial fear of deep water.
Activity tolerance (e.g., physical and mental fatigue levels, energy to complete activities and tasks, temporal and environmental contexts)	There are no apparent problems with activity tolerance at this stage of analysis. Once Fred is engaged in the activities, it will be important to determine whether they cause any mental fatigue, because of his performance anxiety.
Impact on occupational performance: (i.e., reflecting on client roles, responsibilities, and priorities)	He is socially isolated from his peers in this lakeside resort community as a result of his phobia.
Intervention needs (e.g., physical, cognitive, emotional, social)	Although yet to be further determined through observation in context, there is a possibility that he will need occupational coaching and psychological counseling to meet his goals.
Resource needs (e.g., assistive devices, equipment, technology)	None
Program needs (e.g., day programs, return-to-work, socialization)	Classes that provide a learning environment and supportive socialization are indicated (e.g., community recreational classes).

Outlook (i.e., practitioner projection of long-term needs and life care planning)	It is too early to provide an opinion on long-term needs regarding Fred's capacity to overcome his phobia to develop and integrate healthy leisure and social participation routines into his lifestyle.

GUIDELINES AND CHECKLIST FOR TASK ANALYSIS

Areas of Occupation

Activities of Daily Living
- ☐ Bathing or showering
- ☐ Bowel or bladder management
- ☐ Dressing
- ☐ Swallowing and eating

- ☐ Feeding
- ☐ Functional mobility
- ☐ Personal device care
- ☐ Personal hygiene and grooming
- ☐ Sexual activity
- ☐ Toileting and toilet hygiene

Instrumental Activities of Daily Living
- ☐ Care of others
- ☐ Care of pets
- ☐ Child rearing
- ☐ Communication management

- ☐ Driving and community mobility
- ☐ Financial management
- ☐ Home establishment
- ☐ Home management and maintenance
- ☐ Meal preparation and cleanup
- ☐ Religious and spiritual observance
- ☐ Safety and emergency maintenance
- ☐ Shopping

Rest and Sleep
- ☐ Rest and relaxation
- ☐ Sleep participation
- ☐ Sleep preparation

Play
- ☐ Peer interaction
- ☐ Play exploration
- ☐ Play participation

Leisure
- ☐ Customary activities or hobbies
- ☑ Leisure exploration
- ☑ Leisure participation

Social Participation
- ☑ Community
- ☐ Family
- ☑ Peer or friend

Education
- ☐ Formal education participation
- ☐ Informal personal education or exploration
- ☐ Informal personal education participation

Work
- ☐ Employment interests or pursuits
- ☐ Employment seeking or acquisition
- ☐ Job performance
- ☐ Retirement preparation and adjustment
- ☐ Volunteer exploration
- ☐ Volunteer participation

Client Factors

Body Functions and Structures
Physical
- ☐ Cardiovascular or hematological systems
- ☐ Digestive, metabolic, or endocrine systems
- ☐ Genitourinary or reproductive functions
- ☐ Movement-related functions
- ☐ Respiratory or immunological systems
- ☐ Skin and related structure functions
- ☐ Voice and speech functions

Body Functions and Structures
Sensory and pain
- ☐ Hearing functions
- ☐ Pain grading and description
- ☐ Seeing and related functions
- ☐ Tactile functions
- ☐ Taste and smell functions
- ☐ Temperature and pressure reception
- ☐ Vestibular and proprioceptive functions

(Continued)

EXHIBIT 2.1. CLIENT PROFILE AND TASK ANALYSIS FORM: FRED *(Cont.)*

Body Functions: Mental
Specific mental functions
☐ Attention
☑ Emotional
☐ Experience of self and time
☐ Higher level cognitive
☐ Motor sequencing
☐ Memory
☐ Perception
☐ Thought

Body Functions: Mental
Global mental functions
☐ Consciousness
☐ Energy and drive
☐ Orientation
☐ Sleep
☐ Temperament and personality

Values, Beliefs, and Spirituality

Values
☐ Meaningful qualities
☐ Principles
☐ Standards

Beliefs and Spirituality
☐ Cognitive content health as true
☐ Guiding actions
☐ Life meaning and purpose

Activity and Occupational Demands

Objects and Their Properties
☐ Inherent properties (e.g., heavy, light)
☐ Required tools, materials, equipment

Space Demands
☐ Size, arrangement, surface, lighting

Social Demands
☑ Cultural context
☑ Social environment

Sequence and Timing
☐ Sequence and timing of steps
☐ Specific steps

Required Actions and Performance Skills
☐ Cognitive
☐ Communication and interaction
☑ Emotional and social
☐ Motor and praxis
☐ Sensory–perceptual

Required Body Functions and Structures
☐ Anatomical parts
☐ Level of consciousness
☐ Mobility of joints

Performance Skills

Motor and Praxis Skills
☐ Movement actions and behaviors
☐ Skilled purposeful movements
☐ Ability to carry out learned movement

Process Skills
☐ Judgment
☐ Select and sequence objects or tools
☐ Organize and prioritize
☐ Create and problem solve
☐ Multitask

Performance Patterns

Habits
☐ Automatic behavior
☐ Repeated activities
☐ Good, bad, or impoverished

Routines
☐ Observable patterns of behavior
☐ Time commitment
☐ Satisfying, promoting, or damaging

Roles	Rituals
☐ Set of expected behaviors	☐ Symbolic actions
☐ Socially or culturally	☐ Spiritual, cultural, or social
☐ Within context	☐ Link to values and beliefs

Contexts and Environments

Cultural	Personal
☐ Customs and beliefs	☐ Age and gender
☐ Activity patterns	☐ Socioeconomic status
☐ Expectations	☐ Educational status

Temporal	Virtual
☐ Location of performance in time	☐ Communication environment
☑ Experience shaped by engagement	

Physical	Social and Political
☑ Natural environment (e.g., geography)	☐ Relationship to individuals
☐ Built environment (e.g., building, furniture)	☐ Relationship to organizations and systems

TASK ANALYSIS TEMPLATE
(An individual form required for each task that is examined.)
Task:

Task Demands	Action Demands (What is required of the person to do the task)	Client Challenges (Availability of required body functions and structures)
Objects used (e.g., equipment, technology)	Use of fishing rod and equipment	No learning restrictions
Space demands (e.g., physical context)	Fishing requires proximity to water from a dock or bank.	Fred has substantial fear of getting near water and this is one of his greatest challenges.
Social demands (e.g., social environment and context)	Accessing information and learning options within the university and/or community	Fred has substantial fear of water and water activities. He is challenged to address these fears and to work to resolution.
Sequence and timing (e.g., process to carry out the task)		
Required actions and performance skills (e.g., basic requirements)		

Fred has identified his fear of water, including decreased tolerance of being near an open water environment. Much of the socialization in his new community revolves around water-based activities, and his fear of water is restricting his participation with fellow students. He is feeling socially isolated and is looking for a resolution of his fear of water.

Assessments for Client-Centered Task Analysis

Task analysis is an important evaluation and intervention tool. Evaluation enables the occupational therapist to understand the client and his or her environments and occupations and to design an intervention to optimize the fit among these areas. Clients describe or demonstrate the meaningful occupations that they have difficulty with but would like to perform. The therapist uses task analysis, clinical observations, and formal and standardized assessments to evaluate the dimensions of occupational performance. Strengths and limitations across dimensions underpin intervention strategies. Ongoing assessment of progress toward the client's goals and shifts in intervention enable the practitioner to accommodate changes in a step-by-step, incremental progression. Three assessments can facilitate client-centered task analysis:

1. Canadian Occupational Performance Measure (COPM; Law et al., 2005),
2. Goal attainment scaling (GAS; Kiresuk, Smith, & Cardello, 1994), and
3. Cardinal Hill Occupational Participation Process (CHOPP; Skubik-Peplaski, Paris, Boyle, & Culpert, 2009).

Canadian Occupational Performance Measure

The early editions of the COPM were specifically designed to facilitate goal setting and can be used with children and families. Using a semistructured interview and a structured scoring method, the occupational therapist guides the client or caregiver in selecting areas in which he or she is dissatisfied with performance and rating the perceived current level of performance on a 10-point scale. The COPM has been referred to as the *Canadian Model of Occupational Performance and Engagement (CMOP–E)* and may be adopted in subsequent publications and is interchangeable with the use of COPM (Townsend & Polatajko, 2007). The COPM has been used in more than 35 countries and has been translated into more than 20 languages.

Goal Attainment Scaling

Like the COPM, GAS is a client-centered measurement tool that focuses on the client's view of his or her own needs (Ertzgaard, Ward, Wissel, & Borg, 2011; Mailloux et al., 2007; Turner-Stokes, 2009). GAS is often used with people who have chronic conditions because it allows the measurement of incremental change. In GAS, goals are broken down into a series of small, achievable steps that show that the client is making progress (Occupational Therapy Australia, 2012).

For example, a client who needs assistance with self-feeding could create goals that demonstrate small performance improvements toward independence, such as to eat mashed vegetables independently using a spoon after setup. Small goals also help ensure success by providing quick feedback on whether an intervention is effective or whether interventions or goals require altering (Occupational Therapy Australia, 2012).

Cardinal Hill Occupational Participation Process

Following development of the *Framework*, occupational therapists at the Cardinal Hill Healthcare System developed an application of the *Framework* to guide occupational analysis and intervention planning that exemplifies a shift from a component-based to an occupation-based focus (Skubik-Peplaski et al., 2009). The CHOPP consists of an occupational analysis, an occupational profile, and intervention planning with protocols; case studies are provided to illustrate consistent use of the documentation process.

CHOPP draws conceptually from the COPM and the FIM™ (Wright, 2000). The FIM is the most widely accepted functional assessment measure used by the rehabilitation community. It is based on the uniform measurement of disability described in the *International Classification of Impairment, Disabilities and Handicaps* (WHO, 1980).

SUMMARY

Task analysis is a clinical reasoning tool that, when integrated in the professional process of the occupational therapy practitioner, ensures thorough examination of the basic features of an occupation or activity required to achieve the highest level of independence possible. Developing an occupational profile, analyzing performance, and using task analysis to establish an intervention plan are key functions of occupational therapy.

REFERENCES

American Occupational Therapy Association. (2012). *About occupational therapy.* Retrieved from www.aota.org/Consumers.aspx

American Occupational Therapy Association. (2014). Occupational therapy practice framework: Domain and process (3rd ed.). *American Journal of Occupational Therapy, 68*(Suppl.), S1–48. http://dx.doi.org/10.5014/ajot.2014.682006

Canadian Association of Occupational Therapists. (2002). Models and evidence in occupational therapy. *Canadian Journal of Occupational Therapy, 64,* 186.

Ertzgaard, P., Ward, A. B., Wissel, J., & Borg, J. (2011). Practical considerations for Goal Attainment Scaling during rehabilitation following acquired brain injury. *Journal of Rehabilitation Medicine, 43,* 8–14.

Kiresuk, T. J., Smith, A., & Cardello, J. E. (Eds.). (1994). *Goal Attainment Scaling: Applications, theory, and measurement.* Hillsdale, NJ: Erlbaum.

Law, M. (2002). Participation in the occupations of everyday life. *American Journal of Occupational Therapy, 56,* 640–649. http://dx.doi.org/10.5014/ajot.56.6.640

Law, M., Baptiste, S., Carswell, A., McColl, M. A., Polatajko, H., & Pollock, N. (2005). *Canadian Occupational Performance Measure.* Ottowa, ON: CAOT Publications.

Law, M., Cooper, B., Strong, S., Stewart, D., Rigby, P., & Letts, L. (1996). The Person–Environment–Occupation model: A transactive approach to occupational performance. *Canadian Journal of Occupational Therapy, 63,* 9–23.

Mailloux, Z., May-Benson, T. A., Summers, C. A., Miller, L. J., Brett-Green, B., Burke, J. P., . . . Schoen, S. A. (2007). The Issue Is—Goal Attainment Scaling as a means of meaningful outcomes for children with sensory integration disorders. *American Journal of Occupational Therapy, 61,* 254–259. http://dx.doi.org/ 10.5014/ajot.61.2.254

Occupational Therapy Australia. (2012). *Goal Attainment Scaling—GAS.* Available at http://otalautismcpd.com.au/modulethree/31occupationaltherapyprocess/gas

Skubik-Peplaski, C., Paris, C., Boyle, D. C., & Culpert, A. (Eds.). (2009). *Applying the Occupational Therapy Practice Framework: The Cardinal Hill Occupational Participation Process in client-centered care.* Bethesda, MD: AOTA Press.

Townsend, E. A., & Polatajko, H. J. (2007). *Enabling occupation II: Advancing an occupational therapy vision of health, well-being, and justice through occupation.* Ottawa, ON: CAOT Publications.

Turner-Stokes, L. (2009). Goal Attainment Scaling (GAS) in rehabilitation: A practical guide. *Clinical Rehabilitation, 23,* 362–370.

Wilcock, A. A. (1998). *An occupational perspective of health.* Thorofare, NJ: Slack.

World Health Organization. (1980). *International classification of impairments, disabilities, and handicaps: A manual of classification relating to the consequences of disease.* Geneva: Author.

World Health Organization. (2001). *International classification of functioning, disability and health.* Geneva: Author.

Wright, J. (2000). *The FIM.* San Jose, CA: Center for Outcome Measurement in Brain Injury.

Domain and Dimensions of Occupational Therapy

3

Occupations are the "activities . . . of everyday life, named, organized, and given value and meaning by individuals and a culture."

—Law, Polatajko, Baptiste, & Townsend (1997, p. 32, italics added)

LEARNING OBJECTIVES

At the completion of this chapter, readers will be able to

- Define the domain and dimensions of concern to occupational therapy practitioners;
- Define *occupations;* and
- Identify and define the types of performance skills and patterns, contexts, activity demands, and client factors that influence engagement and participation.

KEY TERMS

Activities of daily living
Activity demands
Beliefs
Body functions
Body structures
Client factors
Clinical reasoning
Context and environment
Co-occupations
Dimension
Domain
Education
Habits
Instrumental activities of daily living
Leisure
Leisure participation
Motor skills

Occupation
Performance patterns
Performance skills
Play
Process skills
Rest and sleep
Rituals
Roles
Routines
Service delivery process
Social interaction skills
Social participation
Spirituality
Task analysis
Tasks
Values
Work

DOMAIN OF OCCUPATIONAL THERAPY

In the late 1990s, the Commission on Practice of the American Occupational Therapy Association (AOTA) undertook a review and consultation process to develop a framework for practice that defines and communicates the domain of the profession and the process of service delivery. The first edition of the *Occupational Therapy Practice Framework: Domain and Process* (AOTA, 2002; hereinafter referred to as the *Framework*) described the domain of concern to the profession and built on a historic AOTA document that established a uniform terminology for occupational therapy (AOTA, 1994). The *Framework* incorporated terminology from the *International Classification of Functioning, Disability and Health (ICF)* developed by the World Health Organization (WHO; 2001). As noted in Chapter 1, "Historical Perspective: Intervention Through Activity," this international classification system provided a unified and standard framework for describing health and health-related status, fostering better communication among health practitioners nationally and internationally.

A *domain* refers to the profession's established body of knowledge or expertise or area of professional influence. The domain of the occupational therapy profession is "achieving health, well-being, and participation in life through engagement in occupation" (AOTA, 2014, p. S4). This domain of practice provides the foundation on which practitioners construct their activities (Law, 2002). In addition, "all aspects of the domain, including occupations, client factors, performance skills, performance patterns, and the context and environment, are of equal value, and together they interact to affect the client's occupational identity, health, well-being, and participation in life" (AOTA, 2014, p. S4).

In the *Framework,* the term *occupation* encompasses "daily life activities in which people engage" (AOTA, 2014, p. S6).

> *Occupation* refers to groups of activities and tasks of everyday life, named, organized, and given value and meaning by individuals and a culture. Occupation is everything people do to occupy themselves, including looking after themselves (self-care), enjoying life (leisure), and contributing to the social and economic fabric of their communities (productivity). (Law et al., 1997, p. 32, italics added)

Occupations structure everyday life and are intrinsically necessary for health and well-being, and engagement in occupations and participation in contexts are driven by the need for mastery, competence, self-identity, sense of competence, and group acceptance (AOTA, 2014; Law et al., 1997; Polatajko, 1994). Occupations that are shared—for example, between a caregiver and the recipient of care—are called *co-occupations.* The complexities lie in the fact that people and their environments and occupations are indivisible. Although occupation is a complex construct, it is a concept people readily understand because everyone engages in it in their daily lives.

The occupational therapy profession views the client's engagement in occupation both as a means to an end (i.e., a process of intervention) and as an end in itself (i.e., an outcome of service). Engagement in occupation may be done individually or with others and involves both subjective (i.e., emotional and psychological) and objective (i.e., physically observable) aspects of performance (AOTA, 2008a, 2014). The targeted outcome of the occupational therapy intervention process occurs when the client attains maximum engagement in occupations and participation in contexts.

By comparison, the *service delivery process* involves the therapeutic use of purposeful activity and involvement in daily life activities as a means or method of changing levels of engagement and participation. Occupational therapy practitioners use their expertise to contribute to clients' health by enabling them to choose and engage in occupations that give their lives meaning and purpose (AOTA, 2014; Canadian Association of Occupational Therapists [CAOT], 1993, 1997). Important to the process is *clinical reasoning,* which occupational therapy practitioners use to analyze the transactional connection of the information a client brings to the therapeutic relationship (e.g., knowledge about

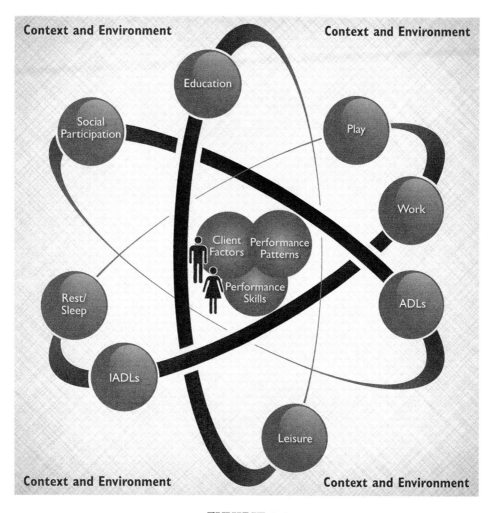

EXHIBIT 3.1

Aspects of Occupational Therapy's Domain

Note. From *Occupational Therapy Practice Framework: Domain and Process, 3rd Edition,* by the American Occupational Therapy Association, 2014, *American Journal of Occupational Therapy, 68*(Suppl. 1), p. S4. Copyright © 2014 by the American Occupational Therapy Association. Used with permission.

his or her life experiences, hopes and dreams for the future, and needs and priorities) and apply their own knowledge and skills to interventions (e.g., observe, analyze, describe, and interpret human performance; AOTA, 2014).

The domain and its dimensions frame the focus of practitioners' attention during the evaluation and intervention process—namely, the interaction of persons, environments, and occupations. The extent and quality of this interaction determine the client's levels of engagement and participation. Occupational therapy practitioners are trained to evaluate the interaction of persons, environments, and occupations using task analysis and to apply the knowledge they gain through this analysis to planning and reviewing interventions to facilitate their clients' engagement in occupations. Occupational therapy assistants participate in this process under the supervision of an occupational therapist.

Assignment 3.1. *Framework* **Definitions**

Define the domain of occupational therapy and its aspects and process. Refer to the *Framework* (AOTA, 2014) for guidance with completing this assignment.

OCCUPATIONS

When occupational therapy practitioners work with an individual, organization, or population to promote engagement in occupations, they take into account all of the occupations identified in Exhibit 3.1: *activities of daily living (ADLs*, sometimes called *basic activities of daily living), instrumental activities of daily living (IADLs), rest and sleep, education, work, play, leisure,* and *social participation.* Each of these areas includes several tasks, and a single task may apply to more than one area of occupation. As discussed in Chapter 2, "Occupational Therapy Services: A Distinct Approach," *tasks* are a subset of occupation or activity and make up the smallest identifiable, essential, and complete piece of an activity. Practitioners bear in mind that "the ways in which clients prioritize engagement in selected occupations may vary at different times" (AOTA, 2014, p. S6).

Reflect on Question 3 in Assignment 2.1, "Understanding Occupation and Activity vs. Tasks" (located in Chapter 2, "Occupational Therapy Services: A Distinct Approach"), in which the occupation of fishing is considered from the perspectives of the leisure fisherman and the professional fisherman. The importance of this occupation is different to each of them, and so are their needs and interests in carrying out the tasks that comprise the occupation of fishing. Each fisherman prioritizes participation and engagement in that occupation differently.

ADLs and IADLs

ADL occupations include the basic and personal activities a person engages in for the purpose of taking care of his or her own body, such as bathing and showering, bowel and bladder management, dressing, eating and feeding, functional mobility, personal device care, personal hygiene and grooming, sexual activity, and toilet hygiene (AOTA, 2014). The *IADL* area of occupation includes tasks required for effective interaction with the environment, such as care of others, care of pets, child rearing, communication management, community mobility, financial management, health management and maintenance, home establishment and management, meal preparation and cleanup, religious observance, safety and emergency maintenance, and shopping (AOTA, 2014).

Rest and Sleep

Rest and *sleep* includes tasks related to these activities (AOTA, 2014). Rest and sleep are achieved through engagement in the quiet time for rest, sleep preparation (routines), going to sleep, and staying asleep (cessation of activity). Sleep is a resource related to stress management and self-regulation. The relevance to the occupational therapy practitioner is that sleep is an active process of the brain, and it plays an important part in memory, concentration, and emotional processing. Normal sleep patterns can be impaired, for example, by injury-related pain, psychosocial issues, mental illnesses, or side effects of medications. Disrupted sleep patterns can lead to impaired cognitive processes, irritability, reduced coping skills, and an increase in anxiety about returning to bed to repeat the disrupted sleeping pattern (Centers for Disease Control and Prevention, 2012).

Education

Education includes engagement in student roles, participation in learning environments, formal educational participation, and informal personal education participation (AOTA, 2014). The key role of occupational therapy practitioners in the school system is reframing the expectations placed on a child with learning challenges through identification of a match between the student's skills and abilities and learning expectations (Whalen, 2002). Interventions include task adaptation, task modification, and assistive devices.

Work

Work occupations include both remunerative employment and volunteer activities (AOTA, 2014). This area entails identification and selection of work opportunities (interests and pursuits), employment seeking and acquisition, and job performance (initiation, productivity, compliance and sustaining of work, retirement preparation and adjustment, volunteer exploration and participation). Occupational therapy services are designed to enable clients' integration or reintegration into the work force or a specific workplace (CAOT, 2009). Occupational therapy practitioners provide task analysis of workplace demands, vocational evaluation, evaluation of work or functional capacity, work-hardening or occupational rehabilitation interventions, workplace stress management, ergonomics, and more. Practitioners may work with employers to provide disability information, strategies for reduction of absenteeism, time loss prevention, return-to-work strategies, and related services.

WHO's (2011) *World Report on Disability* reported that employment rates for persons with disabilities are below those of the overall population, and great variability exists among persons with different disabilities. Employment rates for persons with disabilities among several Western countries include

- United States: 38.1%
- Canada: 56.3%
- Australia: 41.9%
- United Kingdom: 38.9%
- Germany: 46.1%
- Switzerland: 62.2%.

These statistics highlight the work to be done by occupational therapy practitioners and other disciplines, along with industry, to support increasing employment for persons with disabilities.

Play

Play refers to spontaneous or organized activities that are purely for enjoyment, entertainment, amusement, or diversion and includes the exploration and social participation in these components of play (CAOT, 1997; Parham & Fazio, 1997). According to AOTA (2008b), to impede children from playing deprives them of optimal development and learning, and for that reason occupational therapy practitioners support and enhance children's participation in play. The rationale for using play as a therapeutic intervention is that play and playful learning enhance children's academic, social, and emotional outcomes (Rushton, Juoloa-Rushton, & Larkin, 2010; Whitebread, Coltman, Jameson, & Lander, 2009).

Leisure

Leisure includes "nonobligatory activity that is intrinsically motivated and engaged in during discretionary time, that is, time not committed to obligatory occupations such as work, self-care, or sleep" (Parham & Fazio, 1997, p. 250). Leisure is generally associated with freedom from work, and leisure activities are unique to each individual. *Leisure exploration* refers to "identifying interests, skills, opportunities, and appropriate leisure activities" (AOTA, 2014, p. S21). *Leisure participation* includes planning and participating, maintaining balance between leisure and other occupations, and obtaining and using equipment and supplies (AOTA, 2014).

The importance of leisure to well-being is often undervalued. According to a study by Hyyppä, Mäki, Impivaara, and Aromaa (2005) of participants from the general population in Finland, people with abundant leisure survived longer than those with intermediate and low quality of leisure.

Social Participation

Social participation includes the patterns of behaviors that are characteristic and expected of people sharing or taking part in a social group or system. According to Kang et al. (2010), participation creates avenues to form friendships, develop self-concept, and determine a sense of the meaning of life. This area includes activities that result in successful interaction within communities and with society, as well as with family, peers, and friends (Mosey, 1996). Social participation includes engagement in community activities, in expected family roles, and in peer and friend activities (AOTA, 2014).

A strong link has been found between cultural and social participation and survival (Hyyppä et al., 2005). Social isolation occurs when people become withdrawn and disconnected from social groups and activities. The reasons for social isolation are multifactorial and can result from causes such as physical or psychological conditions that hinder access to social events, divorce, death of a spouse, loss of employment, increased use of the Internet and media devices, and longer work hours and commutes.

According to Liptak (2008), disability is a form of social restriction, and removing social barriers can improve health and well-being. The effects of social isolation can have a negative impact on the affective state of a person, which in turn can lead to social withdrawal and further social isolation (Kawachi & Berkman, 2001).

DIMENSIONS OF OCCUPATIONAL PERFORMANCE

Dimension refers to a characteristic, property, or quality used in analysis and includes client factors, activity demands, performance skills, performance patterns, and context and environment. To develop a holistic client profile, task analysis requires considering all of these dimensions. Readers should refer to the Client Profile and Task Analysis (CPTA) form (Appendix A) as they read the next sections.

Assignment 3.2. How Does a Cast Affect Performance?

You have just returned from the doctor with a cast that covers your dominant hand and extends to your upper forearm but leaves your thumb and fingers free to move. Review the content found in Exhibit 3.1. Provide an example of how the cast would affect your ability to perform in ADLs, education, routines, and sequencing.

Client Factors

Client factors are specific abilities, characteristics, and beliefs that reside within the client. Client factors influence clients' ability to engage in occupations, and conversely engagement in occupations can also influence client factors (AOTA, 2014). For example, arthritis might limit participation in walking, but walking can help a client maintain joint mobility.

Client factors include values, beliefs, and spirituality and body functions and structures. These factors may be substantially different at the person, group, and population levels (AOTA, 2014).

Values, beliefs, and spirituality

Values, beliefs, and spirituality influence the participation in occupations of individuals, organizations, and populations. *Values* are beliefs tied intrinsically to emotion, rather than objective ideas, that hold importance in people's lives and are motivational. *Beliefs* are strongly held ideas about the way things are and are often impervious to logic. *Spirituality* is "the personal quest for understanding answers to ultimate questions about life, about meaning, and about relationship with the sacred or transcendent" (Moreira-Almeida & Koenig, 2006, p. 844). It is both a trait embedded in personality and a state; exists across cultures, time, and geography; and is influenced by the environment and by events (McColl, 2011).

Values, beliefs, and spirituality are related to *occupational justice*, or the power of individuals, groups, or populations to be acknowledged and respected relative to social structures that affect occupation and enable occupational empowerment (Townsend & Polatajko, 2007).

Values and beliefs underpin individual perceptions of life, including roles, responsibilities, and rituals; indeed, values and beliefs are woven into the fabric of who the person is within his or her environment. In addition, people faced with the challenges of disadvantage, disability, and chronic health conditions may seek answers in religious or spiritual terms, especially when they are unable to find a rational explanation for their circumstances. As McColl (2011) noted, "The nature and degree of the relationship among occupation, spirituality and health is at the root of occupational therapists' interest in spirituality as part of our professional domain of concern" (p. 100). At the core of occupational therapy practice is viewing people as humans, safeguarding their dignity, and appreciating their uniqueness (McColl, 2011).

Body functions and structures

Body functions and structures are attributes that provide foundation abilities that may enhance or limit participation and performance in occupations. WHO (2001) considers *body functions* to be the cognitive, sensory, physical, psychosocial, and affective attributes that promote or restrict engagement in occupations. *Body functions* involve "physiological function of body systems (including psychological functions)," such as mental functions (e.g., attention, memory, emotion), sensory functions (e.g., seeing, hearing, vestibular), movement-related functions (e.g., muscles, movement), and cardiovascular systems, among others. *Body structures* are "anatomical parts of the body such as organs, limbs, and their components" and include the nervous system and sensory and motor organs (WHO, 2001, p. 10).

Client factors for organizations

Organizations are macro social environments guided by a vision statement, code of ethics, or other formal and informal values and beliefs and influence the individuals in them through institutional policies, funding, or legislation (Townsend & Polatajko, 2007). Within the organization, functions include planning, organizing, coordinating, and operationalizing its mission, products, and productivity. Structures include departments, leadership and management, human resources, and business processes. For example, workers' compensation boards have business processes that guide claims adjudicators on whether to accept a claim for compensation. These adjudicators have team leaders and managers who act as resources and supports to help them complete their job tasks in a productive manner that is in keeping with the mission of the organization. Behind the scenes of customer interaction is a body of people who are involved in a vast array of activities such as planning future policies and economic scenarios, organizing training for employee health, providing safety and continuing education, and coordinating payments and services.

Understanding the foundational components of an organizational client enables occupational therapy practitioners to successfully engage in client-centered practice within an organizational context. For example, practitioners may provide health promotion strategies or ergonomic assessment in the workplace. They may be involved in the development of policies and programs to address issues related to the physical environment, the psychosocial environment, and the culture of the organization (Bachmann, 2000, p. i). They may also be involved in mobilizing community action and working with community and government bodies to develop an integrated approach to community-driven and community-directed services.

Activity Demands

Activity demands are the

> aspects of an activity or occupation [that] include the relevance to the client, objects used and their properties, space demands, social demands, sequencing and timing, required actions and performance skills, and required underlying body functions and body structures. (AOTA, 2014, p. S32)

To better understand a client's engagement in areas of occupation, practitioners apply their analysis skills to determine the demands placed on a client and the influence of those demands on engagement and participation. Any activity involves required actions that are dependent on performance skills and performance patterns. Furthermore, these actions place demands on body functions and structures. Activity demands are also a function of the objects used and their properties, as well as sequencing and timing processes. In addition, social demands, external to clients, place performance expectations on them, and space demands are an important environmental parameter of engagement and participation.

Performance Skills

Performance skills are "goal-directed actions that are observable as small units of engagement in daily life occupations. They are learned and developed over time and are situated in specific contexts and environments" (Fisher & Griswold, 2014, as cited in AOTA, 2014, p. S44). Occupational therapy practitioners observe and analyze performance skills to understand the factors that support or hinder engagement in occupations and occupational performance (pp. 639–640). Addressing performance in the areas of occupation requires knowledge of the skills needed and patterns used to accomplish task components. Performance skills are actions or features of what one does (e.g., walk, choose, reach, handle), not underlying abilities, capabilities, or body functions (e.g., joint mobility, visual acuity): "Skills are observable elements of action that have implicit functional purposes" (Fisher & Kielhofner, 1995, p. 113).

There are multiple ways of approaching, categorizing, and analyzing performance skills. *Task analysis* comes into play as a fundamental approach to observing and understanding action demands, performance skills, and the fit of individual capacity to required performance. Performance skills are learned and developed over time, starting in infant routines and continuing through play, education and vocational training, home management, and so forth. Performance skills are small, measurable units in a chain of activities (and embedded tasks) that occur when a person performs activities and tasks (Fisher, 2006).

The *Framework* (2014) describes three categories of performance skills:

1. Motor skills
2. Process skills
3. Social interaction skills.

Motor skills enable people to move and interact with objects and environments and include posture, mobility, coordination, strength, and effort. *Process skills* are observed as a person selects, interacts with, and uses task tools and materials; carries out individual actions and steps; and modifies performance when problems are encountered

(AOTA, 2014). *Social interaction skills* are those skills "observed during the ongoing stream of a social exchange" (AOTA, 2014, p. S26).

Because body functions and structures underlie and enable performance, practitioners must analyze the impact of the client's mental, sensory, neuromuscular, and movement functions as described in the *ICF* (WHO, 2001; see also Rogers & Holm, 2008). Other factors, such as context, values, and beliefs, must also factor into the analysis of performance skills and meaning to the client (AOTA, 2014).

Performance Patterns

Performance patterns refer to the habits, routines, roles, and rituals people adopt as they engage in occupations; patterns change over time and are influenced by contexts (AOTA, 2014). *Habits* are specific, automatic behaviors that are integrated into complex patterns of conduct that support or

---

Assignment 3.3. Meaningful Occupations

1. Prepare a short list of the occupations or activities and related tasks that you find most meaningful. Occupations and activities consist of self-directed, functional tasks in which a person engages over his or her life span. How does engagement in the occupations or activities and tasks you have listed lead to your personal sense of health and well-being? How does engagement in occupations enable you to participate in life situations?
2. What are some tasks specifically required for engagement in the occupation of being a student?
3. Examine the task of using a printed textbook. Describe the activity demands required for engagement (i.e., required actions, body structures, body functions).
4. Using the CPTA form, identify and define the different client factors, performance skills and patterns, contexts, and activity demands that influence engagement in using a textbook while studying.

interfere with a person's ability to function on a day-to-day basis (Neistadt & Crepeau, 1998). Habits can be useful, impoverished, or dominating (Dunn, 2000). *Routines* are "established sequences of occupations or activities that provide a structure for daily life" (AOTA, 2014, p. S8). *Roles* organize behavior, communicate expectations, and evolve across the life span; they represent unique configurations of tasks, and some tasks fall into more than one role. "*Rituals* are symbolic actions with spiritual, cultural, or social meaning" (AOTA, 2014, p. S8) that are part of the internal context of the client. These rituals are manifested in the home and community through engagement and participation in socially and culturally defined activities and tasks (e.g., holiday celebrations).

Context and Environment

Context and environment influence engagement in occupations. Occupations happen everywhere, and contexts and environments shape choice, influence health and well-being, and affect occupational performance (Townsend & Polatajko, 2007, p. 48). When occupational therapy practitioners attempt to understand performance skills and patterns, they need to consider the context and environment in which the actions are being undertaken. Environments are external to the client (e.g., physical, social, institutional, or virtual) and "are so embedded in the day-to-day experience as to become almost imperceptible" (Townsend & Polatajko, 2007, p. 52). Other contexts are internal (e.g., personal and spiritual) and are major contributing factors to engagement in occupations. Some contexts (e.g., culture) have external features that are influenced by society and that shape internal features through indoctrination and internalization. Temporal contexts have time dimensions, such as time of day, age, and history (AOTA, 2014).

SUMMARY

Engagement in occupations and participation in contexts promote health and well-being. Engagement and participation influence and are influenced by characteristics of persons, environments, and occupations. This notion is at the heart of the profession's primary philosophical beliefs and aligns with concepts proposed by WHO (2001). According to the *ICF*, health domains include human function and participation:

> A person's functioning . . . is conceived as a dynamic interaction between health conditions (i.e., diseases, disorders, injuries, traumas, etc.) and contextual factors. . . . [Participation] is an individual's involvement in life situations in relation to their health condition, body function and structures, activities, and contextual factors. (WHO, 2001, pp. 8, 14)

As Law (2002) observed, participation in the everyday occupations of life is a vital part of human development and lived experience, including acquisition of skills and competencies, social connection, and integration into the community (p. 640). Therefore, the paradigms of the profession and WHO are connected philosophically and in practice and are used to navigate the task analysis process of evaluating persons, environments, and occupations and identifying interventions to maximize fit among them.

REFERENCES

American Occupational Therapy Association. (1994). *Uniform terminology: Application to practice.* Bethesda, MD: Author.

American Occupational Therapy Association. (2002). Occupational therapy practice framework: Domain and process. *American Journal of Occupational therapy, 56,* 609–639. http://dx.doi.org/10.5014/ajot.56.6.609

American Occupational Therapy Association. (2008a). Occupational therapy practice framework: Domain and process (2nd ed.). *American Journal of Occupational Therapy, 62,* 625–683. http://dx.doi.org/10.5014/ajot.62.6.625

American Occupational Therapy Association. (2008b). Societal statement on play. *American Journal of Occupational Therapy, 62,* 707–708. http://dx.doi.org/10.5014/ajot.62.6.707

American Occupational Therapy Association. (2014). Occupational therapy practice framework: Domain and process (3rd ed.). *American Journal of Occupational therapy, 68*(Suppl.), S1–48. http://dx.doi.org/10.5014/ajot.2014.682006

Bachmann, K. (2000). *More than just hard hats and safety boots: Creating healthier work environments.* Ottawa, ON: Conference Board of Canada.

Canadian Association of Occupational Therapists. (1993). *Occupational therapy guidelines for client centred mental health practice.* Toronto, ON: Author.

Canadian Association of Occupational Therapists. (1997). *Enabling occupation: An occupational therapy perspective.* Ottawa, ON: Author.

Canadian Association of Occupational Therapists. (2009). *Position statement on occupational therapy in return-to-work.* Ottawa, ON: Author.

Centers for Disease Control and Prevention. (2012). *About sleep.* Retrieved from www.cdc.gov/sleep/about_sleep/index.htm

Dunn, W. (2000). *Best practice occupational therapy in community service with children and families* (2nd ed.). Thorofare, NJ: Slack.

Fisher, A. (2006). Overview of performance skills and client factors. In H. Pendleton & W. Schultz-Krohn (Eds.), *Pedretti's occupational therapy: Practice skills for physical dysfunction* (pp. 372–402). St. Louis, MO: Mosby/Elsevier.

Fisher, A. G., & Griswold, L. A. (2014). Performance skills: Implementing performance analyses to evaluate quality of occupational performance. In B. A. Boyt Schell, G. Gillen, & M. Scaffa (Eds.), *Willard and Spackman's occupational therapy* (12th ed., pp. 249–264). Philadelphia: Lippincott Williams & Wilkins.

Fisher, A., & Kielhofner, G. (1995). Skill in occupational performance. In G. Kielhofner (Ed.), *A model of human occupation: Theory and application* (2nd ed., pp. 113–128). Philadelphia: Lippincott Williams & Wilkins.

Hyyppä, M. I., Mäki, J., Impivaara, O., & Aromaa, A. (2005). Leisure participation predicts survival: A population-based study in Finland. *Health Promotion International, 21,* 5–12.

Kang, L. J., Palisano, R. J., Orlin, M. N., Chiarello, L. A., King, G. A., & Polansky, M. (2010). Determinants of social participation—with friends and others who are not family members—for youths with cerebral palsy. *Physical Therapy, 90,* 1743–1757.

Kawachi, I., & Berkman, L. F. (2001). Social ties and mental health. *Journal of Urban Health: Bulletin of the New York Academy of Medicine, 78*(3), 458–467.

Law, M. (2002). Participation in the occupations of everyday life. *American Journal of Occupational Therapy, 56,* 640–649. http://dx.doi.org/10.5014/ajot.56.6.640

Law, M., Polatajko, H., Baptiste, W., & Townsend, E. (1997). Core concepts of occupational therapy. In Canadian Association of Occupational Therapists (Ed.), *Enabling occupation: An occupational therapy perspective* (pp. 29–56). Ottawa, ON: Canadian Association of Occupational Therapists.

Liptak, G. S. (2008). Health and well being of adults with cerebral palsy. *Current Opinion in Neurology, 21,* 136–142.

McColl, M. A. (2011). *Spirituality and occupational therapy.* Ottawa, ON: CAOT Publications.

Moreira-Almeida, A., & Koenig, H. G. (2006). Retaining the meaning of the words religiousness and spirituality: A commentary on the WHOQOL SRPB group's "A cross-cultural study of spirituality, religion, and personal beliefs as components of quality of life" (62:6, 2005, 1486–1497). *Social Science and Medicine, 63,* 843–845.

Mosey, A. C. (1996). *Applied scientific inquiry in health professions: An epidemiological orientation* (2nd ed.). Bethesda, MD: American Occupational Therapy Association.

Neistadt, M. E., & Crepeau, E. B. (Eds.). (1998). *Willard and Spackman's occupational therapy* (9th ed.). Philadelphia: Lippincott.

Parham, L. D., & Fazio, L. S. (1997). *Play in occupational therapy for children.* St. Louis, MO: Mosby.

Polatajko, H. J. (1994). Dreams, dilemmas, and decisions or occupational therapy practice in the new millennium: A Canadian perspective. *American Journal of Occupational Therapy, 48,* 590–594. http://dx.doi.org/10.5014/ajot.48.7.590

Rogers, J. C., & Holm, M. B. (2008). The occupational therapy process: Evaluation and intervention. In E. B. Crepeau, E. S. Cohn, & B. A. Boyt Schell (Eds.), *Willard and Spackman's occupational therapy* (11th ed., pp. 478–518). Baltimore: Lippincott Williams & Wilkins.

Rushton, S., Juoloa-Rushton, A., & Larkin, E. (2010). Neuroscience, play and early childhood education: Connections, implications and assessment. *Early Childhood Education Journal, 37,* 351–361.

Townsend, E. A., & Polatajko, H. J. (2007). *Enabling occupation II: Advancing an occupational therapy vision of health, well-being, and justice through occupation.* Ottawa, ON: CAOT Publications.

Whalen, S. S. (2002). How occupational therapy makes a difference in the school system: A summary of the literature. *OT Now, 4*(3), 15–18.

Whitebread, D., Coltman, P., Jameson, H., & Lander, R. (2009). Play, cognition and self-regulation: What exactly are children learning when they learn to play? *Educational and Child Psychology, 26,* 40–52.

World Health Organization. (2001). *International classification of functioning, disability and health.* Geneva: Author.

World Health Organization. (2011). *World report on disability.* Geneva: Author.

Occupational Therapy Process

4

Occupational therapy practitioners engage in a collaborative process with clients to identify clients' strengths and barriers to health and participation in society.

—American Occupational Therapy Association (2010, p. S57)

LEARNING OBJECTIVES

At the completion of this chapter, readers will be able to

- Understand the relationship between engagement in occupation and participation in contexts and the concept of fit among persons, environments, and occupations and
- Describe the collaborative service delivery process of occupational therapy.

KEY TERMS

Action demands
Analysis
Capacity building
Client-centered practice
Collaboration
Collaborative consultation
Enablement
Evaluation
Intervention implementation
Intervention plan
Intervention process
Intervention review

Occupational performance approach
Occupational profile
Occupation-based activity
Person–Environment–Occupation model
Preparatory methods
Purposeful activity
Targeted outcomes
Task analysis
Therapeutic use of occupations and activities
Therapeutic use of self

Occupational therapy practitioners see health as being shaped and influenced by the fit or transaction among the person, environment, and occupation. The *Person–Environment–Occupation (PEO) model* of occupational performance clarifies this conceptualization of fit by focusing attention and analysis on the interaction and overlap among these three aspects (Law et al., 1996). The PEO model identifies six constructs:

1. Person
2. Environment
3. Activity
4. Task
5. Occupation
6. Occupational performance.

The model highlights that the intersections among people, their environments, and their occupations occur at the points of engagement and participation.

This chapter describes the relationship between engagement in occupation and participation in contexts and the concept of fit among persons, environments, and occupations and discusses the collaborative service delivery process of occupational therapy.

ENABLEMENT

Enablement, or the provision of interventions that improve the ability of individuals or groups to participate in activities, is another core construct of occupational therapy (Townsend & Polatajko, 2007, p. 89). The primary competency of an occupational therapy practitioner is to facilitate clients' engagement in everyday living through occupation. Engagement in occupations and participation in contexts is maximized when there is a close fit among these aspects. How the areas in the PEO model relate to each other varies across time and is reflected in people's changing performance patterns (e.g., habits, roles, routines). Figure 4.1 depicts the transactional connection required in task analysis and critical thinking, which requires practitioner attention to the necessary *action demands,* or the "doing" required by the practitioner, to achieve a therapeutic aim that meets the client's goal. Action

is also required on the part of the client to achieve a therapeutic goal.

COLLABORATIVE PROCESS

Collaboration involves working with others for a common purpose. *Others* can include the client, other clinicians, employers, insurers, lawyers, unions, community groups, and government organizations. Collaboration provides opportunities for better outcomes by increasing the number of participants and hence broadening the collective knowledge pertaining to issues, assessment tools, analyses and ideas, planning, and intervention options.

For the occupational therapy practitioner, the collaborative process may include working with several stakeholders with varying views and needs that are sometimes at odds with one another. The practitioner must bear in mind who the client is (e.g., individual, group, organization); who the paying customer is (e.g., funder, agency); and what the therapy's purpose is, as defined by the individual, group, or organization. The practitioner must strike the right balance between these sometimes competing forces while maintaining a client-centered and preferably client-directed approach to intervention.

Client intervention begins with developing the client's understanding of the therapeutic aims so that the approach can in fact be client directed relative to the client's goals. Placing priority on client-directed goals over practitioner-determined goals helps ensure that clients are engaged in the process and readily participate in activities that have direct meaning to them, thus helping them achieve their objectives.

Client-centered collaboration can be viewed as "power sharing" (Townsend & Polatajko, 2007, p. 107). In a paternalistic paradigm, the practitioner holds the power and determines the goals and interventions. With a client-centered, collaborative approach, power is shared, and the client and practitioner agree to goals and interventions that are consistent with the expert advice and guidance from the practitioner. Together, the client and practitioner problem solve the methods they will use to address the areas of concern.

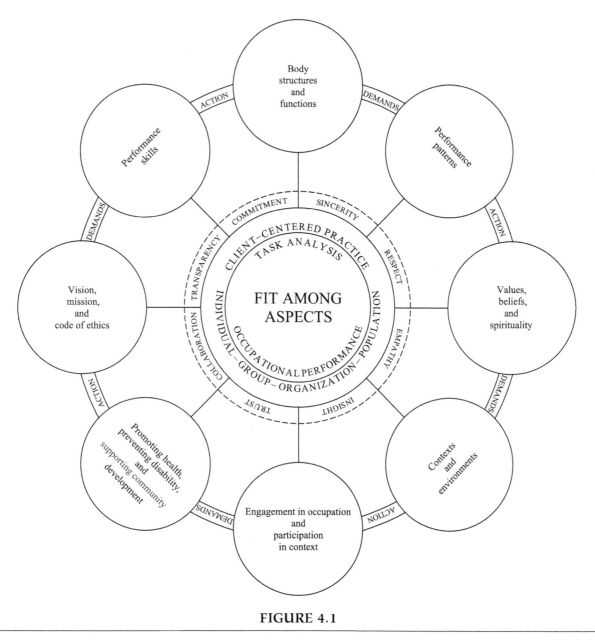

FIGURE 4.1

The transactional connection required in task analysis and critical reasoning.

According to the Canadian Model of Client-Centered Enablement (Townsend & Polatajko, 2007), the practitioner's key occupational therapy enablement competencies include

- Facilitation of adaptation,
- Advocacy for the client,
- Client coaching,
- Collaboration,
- Consultation,
- Coordination,
- Design or building and development of intervention plans,
- Education,
- Engagement in context, and
- Specialization in areas of practice.

Throughout this text, these skills are described in the context of task analysis in client-centered practice.

EVALUATION AND ANALYSIS

Evaluation is the process of obtaining information and deciphering its meaning, and *analysis* refers to the methods the occupational therapy practitioner uses to interpret the information gathered from the evaluation (American Occupational Therapy Association [AOTA], 2014). Evaluation and analysis are the initial steps an occupational therapist takes for purposes of service intervention. Evaluation is the responsibility of an occupational therapist, and occupational therapy assistants contribute to the process on the basis of established competencies and under an occupational therapist's supervision (AOTA, 2014).

Occupational Profile

Occupational therapy practitioners start the service delivery process by developing an *occupational profile*, which describes the client's patterns of daily living, interests, values, and needs, and conducting an analysis of occupational performance (Figure 4.2). The occupational profile enables the practitioner to develop "a working hypothesis regarding possible reasons for identified problems

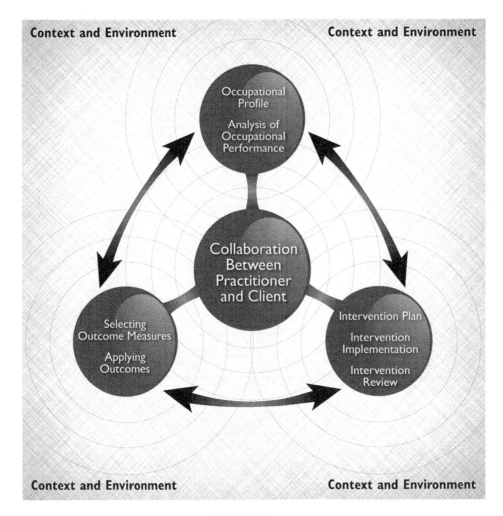

FIGURE 4.2

Occupational therapy's process. Collaboration between the practitioner and the client is central to the interactive nature of service delivery.

Note. From *Occupational Therapy Practice Framework: Domain and Process, 3rd Edition,* by the American Occupational Therapy Association, 2014, *American Journal of Occupational Therapy,* 68(Suppl. 1), p. S10. Copyright © 2014 by the American Occupational Therapy Association. Used with permission.

and concerns" and identifies the client's strengths and weaknesses (AOTA, 2014, p. S13). The *Occupational Therapy Practice Framework: Domain and Process* (AOTA, 2014) aptly describes some of the intake information that is learned from the referral source, the file review, and the initial interview with the client or carer:

- "Why is the client seeking service, and what are the client's current concerns relative to engaging in occupations and in daily life activities?
- In what occupations does the client feel successful, and what barriers are affecting his or her success?
- What aspects of the environments or contexts does the client see as supporting engagement in desired occupations, and what aspects are inhibiting engagement?
- What is the client's occupational history (i.e., life experiences)?
- What are the client's values and interests?
- What are the client's daily life roles?
- What are the client's patterns of engagement in occupations, and how have they changed over time?" (AOTA, 2014, p. S13)

Upon gathering this information, the practitioner considers the evaluation tools and methods that will best enable him or her to assess the client's occupational performance in the targeted areas of concern. During the evaluation, the practitioner uses observational skills, physical facilitation techniques, and ongoing discussions with the client as part of the information-gathering process.

Analysis of Occupational Performance

Occupational therapy practitioners conduct an analysis of occupational performance to more clearly specify the client's assets, problems, and potential problems. The analysis of occupational performance focuses on clients' characteristics, engagement in occupations, and participation in contexts. The client's assets, problems, or potential problems are identified, levels of participation and engagement may be observed or recorded through interview, and dimensions of performance are evaluated.

An *occupational performance approach* to service delivery requires the use of task analysis to evaluate and maximize the dynamic, (text continues on page 49)

CASE EXAMPLE 4.1. JOSH: STROKE

Josh, age 52 years, had a stroke 2 weeks ago and has just been admitted to the stroke unit. Upon review of his chart, the occupational therapy practitioner notes that Josh is right-hand dominant. He is a big man with partial paralysis of his left side and requires moderate assistance for all aspects of mobility. He can feed himself after set up and is on a soft-food diet with thickened liquids. He has known visual deficits, but there are no definitive notes on his chart to pinpoint his visual–perceptual or visual–spatial abilities. He was seen by physical therapy and speech therapy in the acute care hospital but apparently not by occupational therapy, because there is no occupational therapy transfer summary and no mention of occupational therapy in the file. The practitioner completes the initial assessment.

During the assessment process, the practitioner learns more about Josh's professional and social contexts. Josh has been a farmhand as long as he can remember. He grew up on a farm. As a little boy, Josh's job was to mind the chickens and gather their eggs for his family to sell to the local grocer and at the Saturday Farmer's Market. As he got older, his responsibilities increased to managing the pigs, cattle, and horses. When the family sold the farm, he continued working in agriculture and has worked for just about every farmer in the county. He has operated heavy equipment in canola fields and worked in granaries, feed lots, dairy farms, slaughterhouses, and pig farms. He has helped raise beef cattle and bison and, as he says, "Done just about any job you can do in this business with your hands, your back, and a good old pickup truck."

Josh has been married to Margi for 25 years. Margi says that Josh has never been one for reading if he didn't have to, and she has always managed the family finances. She tends their tiny farm, which keeps them fed year round with duck, chicken, and quail meat; eggs; fruits; and vegetables. They trade their poultry meat and eggs with local farmers for beef and pork meat and fresh milk. Margi says, "The farm isn't much, but it provides for all of our basic needs, and it's been bought and paid for, for over 15 years."

EXHIBIT 4.1. CLIENT PROFILE AND TASK ANALYSIS FORM: JOSH

CLIENT PROFILE

Name: Josh	Birthdate:	Age at assessment: 52
Advocates: Himself, his wife	**Education:** High school but trained in numerous job-specific tasks, equipment and vehicle uses **Work occupation:** Farmhand	
Diagnoses: Stroke	**Current interventions:** 1. Occupational therapy 2. Physical therapy 3. Speech therapy	
Referral source: Josh received initial treatment in acute care and was referred to the home care occupational therapist for a home assessment and to begin a treatment program that will link to intensive treatment in a rehabilitation hospital (he's waiting for placement).		

PERSONAL INFORMATION

Family Unit	Self and spouse
Caregiver(s)	Wife, Margi
Roles and responsibilities (e.g., student, spouse, parent, friend, worker)	1. Husband 2. Farmhand 3. Friend 4. Community member
Home environment (e.g., home design, number of people living in the home)	Lives with wife in a one-story detached home on a small rural farm. Four steps with right-hand rail into the home from front and walkout rear entrance. All entrances accessible via paved walkway. Main bathroom with stall shower and spare bathroom with tub and shower.
Community context (e.g., rural, urban, metro; single-family home, residential care)	Lived in same rural farming community his entire life. Supportive friends and work associates.
School or work context (e.g., public, special, or private school; stationary or travel location for work)	Capable of all manner of manual farm work. Must be capable of standing, walking, lifting, carrying, and operating manually controlled vehicles and heavy equipment. Assists wife with household & farm maintenance and repairs.
Client Priorities	1. Regain full ability to use left arm and leg. 2. Return to work in full capacity.
Values/Beliefs/Spirituality (e.g., principles, standards, beliefs, personal quest)	Love of his wife. Worked hard his entire life to achieve results. Believes in the power of positive thinking, prayer, and his own responsibilities to bring about change in his life.

SUMMARY, PLAN, AND GOALS

Assessments completed (formal and observational): Acute care facility provided formal assessments of cognitive capacity prepared by the neurologist, physical therapist, and psychologist.

Practitioner–client plan (e.g., further formal and observational assessments, inclusion of others): Interview with the couple, plus home and community accessibility assessment

Tasks Requiring Assessment or Intervention

Short-term goals (Primarily client driven, measurable, global task, or activity achievements)	Long-term objectives (Primarily practitioner driven, measurable, incremental, stepwise, or mini achievements)
1. Josh will engage in planning a step-by-step plan to maximize the function of his left arm and left leg in everyday functions around his home.	1.a. Josh does not have insight into the extent of his poststroke outcome and will need ongoing assistance with adaptation to his residual performance restrictions and limitations, as it is unlikely that he will regain full physical capacity. 1.b. Josh will achieve maximum independence in all areas of ADLs within 3 months of hospital discharge. 1.c. Reassessment of progress is to be conducted monthly for 3 months to identify additional needs and strategies.
2. Josh will practice transfers to and from the toilet using the provided support bars.	
3. Josh will manage his eating, grooming, and hygiene with minimal cuing while maintaining a consistent routine within 3 months of hospital discharge.	
4. Josh will dress himself with moderate assistance within 2 weeks with the longer term goal to achieve maximum independence within 3 months of discharge.	
5. Josh will shower with standby assistance using the provided equipment. His wife will learn how to provide standby assistance in a consistent and safe manner.	

TASKS ANALYZED

Occupation or Activity	Tasks (specific activity component)	Context or Environment (external and internal)
Dressing	Don and doff undershorts, socks, jogging pants, shoes, T-shirt	Sitting in chair in bedroom

(Continued)

EXHIBIT 4.1. CLIENT PROFILE AND TASK ANALYSIS FORM: JOSH *(Cont.)*

Showering	Wash and dry hair, upper body, back, genital and buttocks regions, legs, and feet.	On shower chair with armrests in wheelchair-accessible shower
Grooming and hygiene	Shave face, comb hair, brush teeth, and wash face.	Sitting in chair with armrests, bedside table, supplies, and mirror
Toileting	Transfer on and off over-toilet frame, have movement, clean front and rear, and flush toilet.	Over-toilet frame in bathroom
Bed mobility	Rolling left and right, lying to and from sitting, and edge-of-bed sitting.	On adjustable-head, -feet, and -height bed with bilateral upper side rails
Functional mobility in bedroom and bathroom	Bed, chair, toilet, and shower chair transfers.	On adjustable-height bed, on chair with armrests, over-toilet aid, and on shower chair with armrests
Feeding	Pierce and cut food, bring food to mouth, and bring cup and glass to mouth.	Chair, table, utensils, and compartmentalized meal tray

ANALYSIS (OF PERFORMANCE SKILLS)

Performance Skills	Client Challenges (Performance qualifier)
Rating: 0 = *no restriction*, 1 = *mild limitation*, 2 = *moderate restriction*, 3 = *severe restriction*, 4 = *complete impairment*	
Motor and praxis	**Rating**
Posture	2
Mobility	2
Coordination	2
Strength	2
Effort	1
Energy	2
Execution	2
Process skills	**Rating**
Mental energy	0
Knowledge	0
Organization	0
Adaptation	0

Social interaction skills	Rating
Communication posture	0
Gestures	I
Initiation	0
Information exchange	0
Acknowledging	0
Taking turns	0

Assessments completed (formal and observational): Basic ADLs, functional mobility in bedroom and bathroom	
Assessments required (formal and observational): Visual–perceptual testing, kitchen assessment, car transfers, and predischarge home assessment.	

ANALYSIS (OF PERFORMANCE PATTERNS)

Performance Patterns	Daily Life Activities	Client Challenges (skill deficits and context restrictions)
Habits (Automatic and integrated behaviors)	Personal care and care of animals	Impaired functional mobility, coordination, and strength cause him to require assistance for personal care and unable to care for animals.
Routines (Regular activities that provide daily structure)	Up at 4:00 a.m. with wife, showers, drinks coffee, and eats breakfast. Arrives at work by 5:30 a.m., calls wife at lunch, and is home by 7:00 p.m. Eats dinner, prepares for next day, chats with wife, goes to bed.	In hospital and unable to carry out home and work routines.
Roles (Expected behaviors and responsibilities)	Husband, worker, farm-equipment operator, driver, provider, friend	Currently able to carry out role of husband and friend in modified capacity
Rituals (Customary cultural and social activities)	Saturday breakfast at the café; church on Sunday	In hospital and unable to participate in customary rituals

Synopsis of performance skills and performance patterns (strengths, deficits and challenges): Within the first week at home, Josh showed insight into the difficulties he will have in returning to his customary lifestyle, but he continued to be optimistic about redeveloping skills. He has a moderate motor limitation related to ADLs, and he must relearn to manage many tasks unilaterally and to adapt to ways of accomplishing tasks. Of concern is how the cognitive limitations affect his capacity to self-regulate and to follow an ADL routine without cuing.

(Continued)

EXHIBIT 4.1. CLIENT PROFILE AND TASK ANALYSIS FORM: JOSH *(Cont.)*

GUIDELINES AND CHECKLIST FOR TASK ANALYSIS

Occupations	
Activities of daily living ☑ Bathing and showering ☐ Bowel and bladder management ☑ Dressing ☑ Eating and swallowing ☐ Feeding ☑ Functional mobility ☐ Personal device care ☑ Personal hygiene and grooming ☐ Sexual activity ☑ Toileting and toilet hygiene	**Instrumental activities of daily living** ☐ Care of others ☐ Care of pets ☐ Child rearing ☐ Communication management ☐ Driving and community mobility ☐ Financial management ☐ Home establishment ☐ Home management and maintenance ☐ Meal preparation and cleanup ☐ Religious and spiritual observance ☐ Safety and emergency maintenance ☐ Shopping
Rest and sleep ☐ Rest and relaxation ☐ Sleep participation ☐ Sleep preparation	**Play** ☐ Peer interaction ☐ Play exploration ☐ Play participation
Leisure ☐ Customary activities or hobbies ☐ Leisure exploration ☐ Leisure participation	**Social participation** ☑ Community ☑ Family ☐ Peer or friend
Education ☐ Access issues ☐ Formal education participation ☐ Informal personal education or exploration ☐ Informal personal education participation ☐ Level of education	**Work** ☐ Employment interests and pursuits ☐ Employment seeking and acquisition ☐ Job performance ☐ Retirement preparation and adjustment ☐ Volunteer exploration ☐ Volunteer participation
Client Factors	
Body functions and structures *Physical* ☐ Cardiovascular and hematological systems ☐ Digestive, metabolic, and endocrine systems ☐ Genitourinary and reproductive functions ☑ Movement-related functions ☐ Respiratory and immunological systems ☐ Skin and related structure functions ☐ Voice and speech functions	**Body functions and structures** *Sensory and pain* ☐ Hearing functions ☐ Pain grading and description ☐ Seeing & related functions ☑ Tactile functions ☐ Taste & smell functions ☑ Temperature & pressure reception ☑ Vestibular & proprioceptive functions

Body functions: Mental
Specific mental functions
- ☑ Attention
- ☑ Emotional
- ☑ Experience of self and time
- ☐ Higher level cognitive
- ☑ Motor sequencing
- ☑ Memory
- ☑ Perception
- ☑ Thought

Body functions: Mental
Global mental functions
- ☐ Consciousness
- ☑ Energy and drive
- ☑ Orientation
- ☐ Sleep
- ☑ Temperament and personality

Values, Beliefs, and Spirituality

Values
- ☑ Meaningful qualities
- ☑ Principles
- ☑ Standards

Beliefs and spirituality
- ☐ Cognitive content health as true
- ☑ Guiding actions
- ☐ Life meaning and purpose

Activity and Occupational Demands

Objects and their properties
- ☑ Inherent properties (e.g., heavy, light)
- ☑ Required tools, materials, equipment

Space demands
- ☑ Size, arrangement, surface, and lighting

Social demands
- ☑ Cultural context
- ☑ Social environment

Sequence and timing
- ☑ Sequence and timing
- ☑ Specific steps

Required actions and performance skills
- ☑ Cognitive
- ☑ Communication and interaction
- ☑ Emotional and social
- ☑ Motor and praxis
- ☑ Sensory–perceptual

Required body functions and structures
- ☑ Anatomical parts
- ☑ Level of consciousness
- ☑ Mobility of joints

Performance Skills

Motor skills
- ☑ Movement actions or behaviors
- ☑ Skilled purposeful movements
- ☑ Ability to carry out learned movement

Process skills
- ☑ Judgment
- ☑ Select and sequence objects or tools
- ☑ Organize and prioritize
- ☐ Create and problem solve
- ☐ Multitask

Social and interaction skills
- ☑ Identify, manage, and express feelings
- ☑ On a one-to-one basis
- ☐ In groups
- ☑ Communication and interaction skills

(Continued)

EXHIBIT 4.1. CLIENT PROFILE AND TASK ANALYSIS FORM: JOSH *(Cont.)*

Performance Patterns

Habits	Routines
☑ Automatic behavior	☑ Observable patterns of behavior
☑ Repeated activities	☑ Time commitment
☑ Good, bad, or impoverished	☑ Satisfying, promoting, or damaging

Roles	Rituals
☑ Set of expected behaviors	☐ Symbolic actions
☐ Social or cultural	☐ Spiritual, cultural, or social
☑ Within context	☐ Link to values and beliefs

Contexts and Environments

Cultural	Personal
☐ Customs and beliefs	☑ Age and gender
☐ Activity patterns	☐ Socioeconomic status
☑ Expectations	☐ Educational status

Temporal	Virtual
☑ Location of performance in time	☐ Communication environment
☑ Experience shaped by engagement	

Physical	Social and political
☐ Natural environment (e.g., geography)	☑ Relationship to individuals
☑ Built environment (e.g., building, furniture)	☐ Relationship to organizations or systems

TASK ANALYSIS TEMPLATE

An individual form is required for each task that is examined.
Task: Bath and toilet transfers

Task Demands	Action Demands (What is required of the person to do the task)	Client Challenges (Availability of required body functions and structures)
Objects used (e.g., equipment, technology)	Josh requires assistive devices to support transfers on to the toilet and a wheeled shower chair to access the stall shower.	Josh must learn to use his unaffected side with some assistance from his affected side.
Space demands (e.g., physical context)	The bathroom with the stall shower is small.	Moving a shower chair in and out of a small space will be challenging.
Social demands (e.g., social environment and context)	Josh's wife needs him to gain as much independence as possible.	The couple cannot finance a personal care assistant.
Sequence and timing (e.g., process to carry out the task)	Developing new motor plans for transfers is required by Josh to effectively and efficiently manage toileting and bathing.	Josh's spatial perception has been affected by the stroke and may affect motor planning, sequencing, and timing of movements needed in toilet and shower transfers.

Required actions and performance skills (e.g., basic requirements)	Ability to make a standing transfer from his wheelchair to the toilet using toilet support bars. Ability to move his one-hand drive wheeled shower chair into the shower stall and out.	Transition will be required from standby assistance to independent transfers. Standby assistance may be needed in the long term if bathroom renovations cannot be made.
Note. ADLs = activities of daily living; TBD = to be determined.		

interdependent, and transactional interaction of persons, environments, and occupations and to enable occupational performance through prompting engagement and participation using therapeutic strategies, modalities, and assistive devices. *Task analysis* is the process of analyzing the dynamic interaction among a client, his or her environments, and selected tasks (a subset of occupation) and designing intervention to optimize the fit among these three dimensions. Task analysis is used as part of the occupational performance analysis to assess the contribution of

- Performance skills,
- Performance patterns,
- Context or contexts,
- Activity demands, and
- Client factors.

Additionally, task analysis helps the occupational therapy practitioner determine which activities and tasks a particular client must perform to assume a lifestyle or level of participation that he or she values. The therapist may specifically assess only selected aspects deemed relevant because they contribute to or limit occupational performance (AOTA, 2014). The therapist does not formulate a medical diagnosis but rather develops a disability profile through a functional analysis that describes the client's circumstances and contexts in relation to engagement and participation. Although not intended to be diagnostic, the information adds to the practitioner's understanding of the impairment.

The information collected from the assessments is then considered together with information from other sources, such as the client's goals, the environment or context in which the occupations occur, normative data (e.g., range of movement of joints, scores on standardized cognitive assessments), and the client's

self-reported historical performance of occupations vs. current performance. The practitioner considers his or her own prior experiences with other clients who faced similar issues. Information gathered during progress measurement is analyzed and then incorporated into future interventions.

A useful resource for analysis is the Cardinal Hill Occupational Participation Process in Client-Centered Care (CHOPP; Skubik-Peplaski, Paris, Boyle, & Culpert, 2009). The CHOPP provides examples that reflect disability analysis for a cross-section of impairments, disabilities, and conditions that may be encountered in a hospital setting by an occupational therapy practitioner. The purpose is to measure goal achievement from initial assessment to discharge outcome and whether interventions have led to functional improvement for the client. Consistency in applying the CHOPP process can enable the organization to measure the effectiveness of service procedures or protocols, ensure client safety by avoiding injuries or harm while the client is in care, provide efficient and equitable service, and reduce wait time for service implementation across disciplines (Skubik-Pelaski et al., 2009).

Targeted outcomes, which are the achievements expected to result from intervention, are then identified. When the client is an individual, the practitioner maps the client's participation in areas of occupation and the relevance and meaningfulness of different activities and tasks relative to performance.

When the client is an organization, the practitioner seeks to identify variations in levels of participation consistency across the organization and combined efforts of its members to learn the best methods for obtaining stakeholder buy-in, engagement, and participation.

Assignment 4.1. Developing an Occupational Profile

1. One of the first stages in developing an occupational profile is to develop an understanding of the client's occupational history, patterns of daily living, interests, values, and needs. Develop 10 open-ended questions that could be used to guide an interview process designed to collect this type of information from clients.

2. Practice the interview process with a partner.

   a. Consider the importance of communicating well in the initial stages of the client–practitioner relationship. Remember that first impressions matter, and begin creating the foundation for your client's view of your confidence and your competence to meet his or her needs.

   b. Get feedback from your partner on how you phrased and timed questions throughout the interview process. Practice rephrasing questions to improve your approach. Did you listen carefully and project a good level of attention and involvement? Did you avoid jargon and slang?

3. After the interview with your partner, organize the information into a concise summary of the occupational performance of the person interviewed.

   a. Have your partner confirm whether the profile is congruent with the information he or she provided in the interview.

   b. Identify information that your past experiences or your value system may have led you to interpret incorrectly.

Assignment 4.2. Occupational Therapy Process for Individuals and Populations

Describe the similarities and differences in the occupational therapy process when services are directed toward individuals and populations.

When the client is a population, occupational performance analysis involves profiling participation rates using available population data or clinical information (e.g., proportion of people with disabilities who are employed).

The analysis of occupational performance focuses on environmental factors that contribute to, support, or hinder participation, such as the cultural, personal, physical, social, temporal (e.g., timing, chronology), and virtual (e.g., technology, media) contexts, as well as the social and space aspects of activity demands. Through the process of assessing the transactions among these aspects, the occupational therapist identifies target outcomes and determines priorities in collaboration with clients or their proxies. The evaluation and analysis process thus sets the stage for intervention.

Case Example 4.1 describes Josh, a 52-year-old who has had a stroke, and illustrates the transaction of occupational performance and environment factors in task analysis. Exhibit 4.1 shows Josh's Client Profile and Task Analysis Form.

INTERVENTION

The collaborative relationship between occupational therapy practitioners and clients is the foundation for intervention planning, implementation, and review.

Intervention Plan

The *intervention process* begins with a plan to maximize the fit among clients and their environments and occupations. During the evaluation, the occupational therapy practitioner has considered client factors, activity demands, and contextual determinants of occupational engagement, so the intervention can target any one or more of these aspects to facilitate participation. The *intervention plan*, which guides the actions taken, is developed in collaboration with the client. This process is referred to as *client-centered*, because the client directs the service through contribution to the planning process.

Early in the intervention process, practitioners and clients select the areas of occupation and levels of engagement in these areas that will become the expected goals and outcomes of services. Achieving successful outcomes of occupational therapy services depends on success in achieving predefined client goals and objectives. Although engagement in occupation to support participation in context (i.e., occupational performance) is the primary targeted outcome, other outcomes of service delivery include

- Client satisfaction,
- Role competence,
- Adaptation,
- Healthy lifestyles,
- Quality of life, and
- Health and wellness.

Treatment goals should be specific enough that information related to outcomes can be used to measure the effectiveness of both the intervention strategy and the model of service delivery. Although this text focuses on identifying priority client outcomes, readers who seek to better understand the measurement of occupational therapy outcomes are encouraged to review Forer (1996) and Watson (2000).

Client goals should be provided as much as possible from the client and carer, so the intervention is client centered and meaningful. Sometimes, the client requires input from the occupational therapy practitioner to understand what outcomes are possible given the client's current circumstances. For example, clients may not know that modified techniques and assistive devices and equipment can enable them to be independent in self-care activities. Or, clients may fear returning to the job they were doing at the time of injury and may inadvertently or overtly place barriers between themselves and their return to work.

In such circumstances, the occupational therapy practitioner educates the client about intervention options, positive outcomes, and potential consequences of following various action paths. In addition, it is the practitioner's responsibility to provide purposeful interventions that have meaning to the client and that help the client understand how participation in the activity will lead to achievement of his or her goals.

Intervention Implementation

Intervention implementation is the process of undertaking actions to influence, support, build, and strengthen client capacity to engage in occupations and participate in contexts. The occupational therapist selects services guided by theories, frames of reference, clinical reasoning, and research evidence on the effectiveness of specific services for certain clientele. Five occupational therapy approaches have been identified on the basis of theory and evidence (AOTA, 2014; Watson & Wilson, 2003):

1. Create, promote (health promotion; e.g., health and wellness programs),
2. Establish, restore (remediation, restoration; e.g., functional mobility),
3. Maintain (e.g., independent living skills),
4. Modify (compensation, adaptation; e.g., change in methods for task completion with or without aids), and
5. Prevent (disability prevention; e.g., ergonomic assessments and manual handling training within the workplace).

Task analysis is fundamental to determining what occupations or activities, tasks, or components are best used to enable client success at each stage of intervention.

Therapeutic use of self and occupations

The occupational therapy practitioner's tool kit includes therapeutic use of self and therapeutic use of occupations and activities (AOTA, 2014). According to Punwar and Peloquin (2000), *therapeutic use of self* is the practitioner's planned use of his or her personality, insights, perceptions, and judgments as part of the therapeutic process.

Therapeutic use of occupations and activities includes occupation-based activity, purposeful activity, and preparatory methods to help the client reach the goals of intervention. *Preparatory methods,* such as the use of exercise, range of motion, or physical agent modalities (e.g., assistive equipment and devices), prepare clients for engagement in purposeful activities or occupation-based activities. *Purposeful activity* (e.g., simulated occupations or meaningful activities) facilitates clients' engagement in goal-directed behaviors or activities within a therapeutically designed context. Intervention progresses to *occupation-based activity* that is used to enable clients to engage in actual occupations in their own contexts to address their goals (e.g., activities of daily living, paid work, leisure and social participation).

Collaborative consultation

In *collaborative consultation*, practitioners apply their knowledge and expertise to develop intervention goals in direct collaboration with the client. In this text, the term is intended to be more explicit about the concept of client-centered practice. After developing a client profile and understanding the values and beliefs of the client through direct communication, the practitioner imparts knowledge and information through instruction and to individuals and groups and through health education initiatives targeted toward communities and populations. Collaborative consultation is the first foundational step to enablement of the client (Townsend & Polatajko, 2007).

Collaborative consultation fosters *enablement,* which Townsend and Polatajko (2007) describe as

> the core competency of occupational therapy, drawing on an interwoven spectrum of key and related enablement skills which are value-based, collaborative, attentive to power inequities and diversity, and charged with visions of possibility for individual and/or social change. (p. 111)

Enablement depends on *capacity building,* which is the establishment of fundamental skills and abilities that meet clients' needs and enable them to perform better in their environments (Crisp, Swerison, & Duckett, 2000; Puska, Tuomilehto, Nissinen, & Vartiainen, 1995; Raeburn & Rootman, 1998). Capacity building is a process used by the occupational therapy practitioner. To build capacity in a person, group, or organization is to assist

them in the development of strategies with the purpose of enabling them to adapt or make changes that are meaningful, manageable, and measureable. Collaborative consultation contributes to capacity building by ensuring the client has the opportunity to engage in the intervention process, program planning, and outcome measurement.

Intervention Review

Intervention review involves measuring progress and determining necessary adjustments to the intervention plan. Progress measurement is done via both casual observation of the client and formal testing and is documented to monitor improvement, plateau, or decline. Progress measurement is conducted within each treatment session and at selected intervals of time. Its purpose is to help the practitioner and client ascertain whether the current intervention plan is achieving the desired outcomes within the appropriate time frame.

For example, if performance is not progressing, is declining, or is simply improving too slowly, then a new intervention plan and strategy must be undertaken to provide an effective service to the client. A practitioner does not have an indefinite period of time or funding to facilitate the targeted outcomes, so ongoing progress measurement in each therapy session is important. Task analysis ensures that incremental steps toward goal achievement can be measured. Instruments used to measure and track progress are selected on the basis of psychometric properties such as validity, reliability, and sensitivity to change.

SUMMARY

During the evaluation and analysis phase of intervention, practitioners develop the client's occupational profile and consider the client's abilities, needs, and targeted outcomes in the context of his or her lifestyle. Practitioners consider the environments in which various occupations or activities and tasks occur while comparing the client's current occupational performance to his or her targeted performance outcomes. A collaborative, client-centered approach and, as much as feasible, a client-directed approach help ensure client engagement, participation, goal attainment, and empowerment.

REFERENCES

American Occupational Therapy Association. (2010). Occupational therapy's perspective on the use of environments and contexts to support health and participation in occupations. *American Journal of Occupational Therapy, 64*(Suppl.), S57–S69. http://dx.doi.org/10.5014/ajot.2010.64S57

American Occupational Therapy Association. (2014). Occupational therapy practice framework: Domain and process (3rd ed.). *American Journal of Occupational Therapy, 68*(Suppl.), S1–48. http://dx.doi.org/10.5014/ajot.2014.682006

Crisp, B. R., Swerison, H., & Duckett, S. J. (2000). Four approaches to capacity building in health: Consequences for measurement and accountability. *Health Promotion International, 15*, 99–107.

Forer, S. (1996). *Outcome management and program evaluation made easy: A toolkit for occupational therapy practitioners.* Bethesda, MD: American Occupational Therapy Association.

Law, M., Cooper, B., Strong, S., Stewart, D., Rigby, P., & Letts, L. (1996). The Person–Environment–Occupation model: A transactive approach to occupational performance. *Canadian Journal of Occupational Therapy, 63*, 9–23.

Punwar, A. J., & Peloquin, S. M. (2000). *Occupational therapy principles and practice* (3rd ed.). Philadelphia: Lippincott Williams & Wilkins.

Puska, P., Tuomilehoto, J., Nissinen, A., & Vartiainen, E. (1995). *The North Korelia Project: 20-year results and experiences.* Helsinki, Finland: National Public Health Institute and Welfare.

Raeburn, J., & Rootman, I. (1998). *People-centred health promotion.* Toronto, ON: Wiley.

Skubik-Peplaski, C., Paris, C., Boyle, D. C., & Culpert, A. (Eds.). (2009). *Applying the Occupational Therapy Practice Framework: The Cardinal Hill Occupational Participation Process in client-centered care.* Bethesda, MD: AOTA Press.

Townsend, E. A., & Polatajko, H. J. (2007). *Enabling occupation II: Advancing an occupational therapy vision of health, well-being, and justice through occupation.* Ottawa, ON: CAOT Publications.

Watson, D. E. (2000). *Evaluating costs and outcomes: Demonstrating the value of rehabilitation services.* Bethesda, MD: American Occupational Therapy Association.

Watson, D. E., & Wilson, S. A. (2003). *Task analysis: An individual and population approach* (2nd ed.). Bethesda, MD: AOTA Press.

5

Occupational Therapy Service Delivery to Individuals, Groups, and Populations

An occupational therapy approach to service delivery requires the use of task analysis to evaluate and maximize the dynamic, interdependent, and transactional interaction of persons, environments, and occupations.

—Watson & Wilson (2003a, p. 28)

LEARNING OBJECTIVES

At the completion of this chapter, readers will be able to

- Describe the occupational therapy service delivery process for individuals, groups, and populations.

KEY TERMS

Aim	Long-term goals
Analysis of occupational performance	Medical models
Assessments	Objective
Assets	Occupational profile
Behavioral models	Organization
Clinical reasoning	Organization functions
Evaluation	Population health
Goal	Purposeful activities
Group-based services	Short-term aims and objectives
Intervention	Socioenvironmental models
Intervention planning	

Changes in the nature and distribution of health and risk of ill health coupled with an enhanced understanding of the determinants of health and illness have altered the nature of demand for the services that health practitioners provide. For more than three decades, *Healthy People* (U.S. Department of Health and Human Services [DHHS], 1979, 1998, 2000, 2010) has established benchmarks for health promotion and prevention. *Healthy People 2010* (DHHS, 2000) stated two goals: (1) Increase the quality and quantity of life of persons of all ages and (2) address diversity to eliminate disparities. In its most recent version, *Healthy People 2020* (DHHS, 2010) set out nationwide health improvement priorities.

Occupational therapy practitioners offer services not only to individual clients who seek to alter their levels of engagement and participation but also to groups of people who seek to alter their levels of health and well-being. In all instances, occupational therapy practitioners target evaluation and intervention to optimize the interactions among persons, environments, and occupations. Because people are members of groups, organizations, communities, and populations, the art and science of occupational therapy are applicable to all of these social entities. This chapter describes the similarities and differences in the service delivery process to individuals, groups, and populations and illustrates the use of task analysis as a clinical reasoning tool.

MODELS OF CARE

Whereas services directed toward individuals often reflect a medical or behavioral model of care, health services directed at communities and populations tend to be behavioral and socioenvironmental in nature. The *medical model* focuses on health as the absence of disease. The focus of intervention is to target high-risk or high-need individuals and manage disease and impairment through physiological means (e.g., immunization programs, pharmaceutical management). *Behavioral models* focus on individual responsibility for correcting unhealthy behaviors through positive lifestyle change. The intent is to reduce behavioral risk factors (e.g., smoking, poor nutrition,

insufficient physical activity) in individuals or among individuals in a population. *Socioenvironmental models,* also called *ecological models,* are used to focus services on broad determinants of the health of the population, including physical, social, cultural, institutional, political, and virtual environments (World Health Organization [WHO], 2001).

Occupational therapy practitioners can and should integrate medical, behavioral, and socioenvironmental models into their practice, as all of these models have had, and continue to have, a role in enabling health, engagement in occupations, and participation in contexts. Medical models are appropriate to use when the focus is on altering or minimizing impairments to reduce risk of disability. Behavioral models are appropriate to use when the focus is on changing the lifestyles of individuals or populations. Socioenvironmental models are appropriate to address the broader, contextual determinants of health. Whether services are directed toward individuals, groups, communities, or populations, occupational therapy evaluation and intervention always focus on understanding and promoting the fit among persons, environments, and occupations.

EVALUATION

Practitioners and clients collaborate during the *evaluation* process to identify client goals and priorities. Clients describe or demonstrate the meaningful occupations that they have difficulty with but would like to perform. The therapist uses task analysis, clinical observations, and formal and standardized *assessments* to evaluate the dimensions of occupational performance and structure and streamline the evaluation process. A thorough evaluation helps clients make more informed decisions regarding the need for specific modes of intervention and treatment strategies.

The first step in building a client–practitioner relationship is to establish a common purpose with the understanding that the focus is on client goals and that the practitioner sets therapeutic aims in accordance with agreed-on priorities. In a therapeutic relationship, a *goal* is the client's target or desired result, or what the client is

---

CASE EXAMPLE 5.1. INDIVIDUAL SERVICES FOR MRS. T

After a stroke, **Mrs. T, age 65 years,** identified her goal as being to live independently. She and her occupational therapist made the collaborative decision to start with cooking, because Mrs. T was independent with self-care. Given that Mrs. T had memory difficulties after her stroke, the therapeutic aim was to begin with facilitating decisions about what to cook for a simple breakfast meal, identifying and obtaining the ingredients needed, and then cooking the meal. The initial objective or strategy was to provide standby assistance for Mrs. T to measure her capacity to safely chop foods and use the stovetop. Once Mrs. T mastered planning the task over 3–4 sessions, she spent another week cooking with minimal supervision to master the use of assistive devices needed for one-handed food preparation. Once she was 100% capable of making 3 simple meals safely, she was considered independent in this area.

---

working toward within a therapeutic or problem-solving context. The *aim* is the focal point of the practitioner, an end target to keep an eye on and to measure progress toward over time.

For example, the goal of the client might be to return to independent living with competence in instrumental activities of daily living (IADLs; see Case Example 5.1). The *objective* is the task that client is trying to achieve to meet his or her desired goal (e.g., cook a meal). The practitioner would use task analysis to break down each activity into achievable components and set therapeutic aims and objectives that are realistic and measurable. Through task analysis, the practitioner also specifies objectives that include strategies, resources used, and anticipated timelines. The first aim might be to accomplish a simple task; once this aim is achieved, the next might be to master more complex tasks. The focus of the step-by-step process is always on the client's goal to have the capacity for independent living.

It is important to keep in mind the meaning of the terms *goal, aim,* and *objective* in the therapeutic process, because in other contexts, the meaning may be different (and the terms may even be used synonymously). Correct use of these terms results in greater clarity and less professional confusion and facilitates clear delineation of the roles and responsibilities of both the client and the practitioner. In addition, correctly using the terms assists with communicating intervention strategies and measuring outcomes and supports qualitative data gathering that examines the efficacy of an intervention for a single-subject or population study.

Ultimately, a clear understanding of the investment each party is to make in the outcome sets the stage for a therapeutic and respectful interaction. To help the client attain or maintain a sense of personal power or empowerment, the practitioner determines the best way to help the client build capacity. In other words, a practitioner does not retain power but rather facilitates or enables the progressive occupational empowerment of the client. This core principle in client-centered practice provides the boundaries and guidelines for communication and therapeutic interaction.

Occupational Profile

Once a referral, request, or contract is received, an occupational therapy practitioner starts the service delivery process with information gathering and development of the *occupational profile*. Information is gathered by interviewing the referral source regarding the purpose of the assessment, reviewing documents such as case records, and conducting Internet research on clients that are groups or populations.

Once this level of information gathering is completed, the occupational therapy practitioner initiates contact and conducts an interview or consultation with the client. During the interview, the practitioner asks about the client's historical, current, and desired future occupational profiles and present and future goals. This interview provides the practitioner with baseline considerations and insight into assessment measures needed to develop task steps for intervention.

CASE EXAMPLE 5.2. INDIVIDUAL OCCUPATIONAL PROFILE FOR JULIA

Julia was a resilient 22-year-old who was academically strong and whose ambition was to be a professional writer. Her vocabulary and written communication were recognized in her undergraduate studies and publication of her short stories in a small-town newspaper. Since she was age 8 years, she had taken on learning challenges, not wishing to have her diagnosis of severe spastic quadriplegic cerebral palsy impede her creative personality. As a young woman, she realized that as a person with substantial oral speech difficulties, her voice would need to be expressed in writing. Her goal was to develop a virtual support team and increased technological resources to enable her to undertake graduate studies in journalism. She was dependent in transfers, used power mobility, and could not independently toilet or feed herself. She had personal assistance through her assistive living residence. The technology she was using was 4 years old, and she needed to explore additional technology that could assist her performance in her graduate studies. What is the therapeutic aim for occupational therapy services for Julia, and what steps or task objectives are needed to enable the achievement of her goals?

The occupational profile describes the practitioner's understanding of the client (e.g., person, group, population), what the client has done and wants to do, and the context of the client's life and environment. The therapeutic aim is to gain information and insight from initial interviews, observations, and assessments to establish reasonable and realistic steps toward achievement of client goals (see Case Example 5.2).

Analysis of Occupational Performance and Task Analysis

The first phase of working with clients is identification and confirmation of the issues they face and development of the occupational profile. The next phase of the evaluation is the *analysis of occupational performance,* which "focuses on collecting and interpreting information to more specifically identify supports and barriers related to occupational performance and identify targeted outcomes (American Occupational Therapy Association [AOTA], 2014, p. S13).

Clinical reasoning, an essential ability of occupational therapy practitioners, guides task analysis relative to modalities used (i.e., any physical agent used in conjunction with or in preparation for involvement in a purposeful activity such as ergonomic equipment, braces, paraffin, cold packs) and tasks (e.g., dressing, writing, typing) to be used in treatment. Task analysis is grounded in the practitioner's understanding of activity and task demands and their fit with client abilities and limitations. Additionally, task analysis helps occupational therapy practitioners determine which occupations or activities and tasks a client must perform to achieve desired goals and how an impairment or disability influences engagement and participation.

The final product of the evaluation, the analysis of occupational performance, is built from the initial occupational profile and helps the practitioner make predictions about potential future gains in functional levels and decide how best to prioritize intervention.

Evaluation Considerations With Individuals

During the analysis of occupational performance, the *individual client* demonstrates his or her physical, mental, and sensory abilities and limitations and functional capacity through assessment of body functions, body structures, and performance skills in a customary environment or in a clinical context. The practitioner uses a variety of tools and techniques to facilitate this information gathering, including standardized assessment tools, nonstandardized assessment tools, and observation and facilitation techniques. The practitioner then reviews and analyzes the assessment information and, in consideration of the client profile and goals, identifies needs and expectations and designs an intervention plan that includes intervention aims, client goals, and short- and long-term task objectives.

For reasons of practicality, time, or financial constraints, a practitioner may not be able to conduct a task analysis of an activity in all settings in which the activity may take place. Therefore, the practitioner must use clinical reasoning to generalize the task analysis to other settings, taking into consideration the facilitators and barriers present in those settings. For example, a community-based occupational therapist must consider a person's function using a four-wheeled walker not just in navigating the kitchen but also in safely entering and leaving the home, retrieving mail at the end of the driveway, entering and exiting a taxi, and shopping for small grocery items in the community.

Evaluation Considerations With Organizations

Organizations often request occupational therapy consultation to measure how effective an approach, program, or service is in achieving specified ends or to analyze contexts or environments to determine the best fit of services or resources to a specified clientele (see Case Example 5.3). When the client is an organization, the task analysis principles remain constant, with an important difference. The practitioner collects information about the organization, such as its vision statement, code of ethics, value statements, and so forth. He or she assesses *organization functions,* including planning, organizing, coordinating, and implementing its mission, services, and productivity, as well as organization structures, including leadership, departments, ad hoc committees, job titles, performance measures, and so forth.

An important difference between work with individuals and organizations is the source of observations for the evaluation. Whereas an individual client is the source of information about factors that contribute to his or her performance in context and environments, in work with an organization the observer is the occupational therapy consultant and team or a committee designated to solve an organizational problem or develop new programs and services.

Evaluation Considerations With Populations

The primary focus of *population health* is wellness. Occupational therapy practitioners working to promote population health strive to optimize the fit among persons, environments, and occupations in a population as a whole (see Case Example 5.4). Population health practice involves influencing public policy, developing health promotion strategies, providing disease prevention services, and recommending care protocols. Population health research and population-based initiatives are a growing area of occupational therapy practice. Occupational therapy practitioners are involved in population research, work with WHO, and

---

CASE EXAMPLE 5.3. EVALUATION FOR A COMMUNITY REHABILITATION MODEL

An **occupational therapist** was recruited to assist a **community leadership organization** with the development of a rehabilitation model that would be transferable to other communities of similar cultural values and beliefs. Previous programs designed for First Nations communities were not perceived as community centered, and implementation had been unsuccessful overall. The occupational therapy practitioner worked with community members to construct an initial community profile that articulated values, beliefs, and cultural sensitivities. The next step was to develop a community-based implementing team, which was made up of nonclinical "outreach" employees of the community leadership organization, to evaluate the rehabilitation residents' needs. The practitioner used task analysis to break down the activity into manageable components that could be delegated to members of the implementing team, so collected information would be cohesive across designates, collated seamlessly, and communicated to community leaders. How might the practitioner communicate the analysis of community needs and explain the project plan to the implementing team?

CASE EXAMPLE 5.4. POPULATION HEALTH EVALUATION

An **occupational therapy consultant** was contracted by a **community health center** to coordinate a community mobilization project that was to be measured by population health researchers. The client's goal was to build the capacity of each community to develop physical or social activities that could promote community participation and healthy activities, facilitate activity implementation, and measure task components relative to community strengths and barriers. The task was to enlist one community district from each of four quadrants of a large Midwestern city. What process might the consultant use to conduct task analyses for community enlistment, community process, activity design, and achievable, time-limited aims?

---

collaborate with policymakers, extending the role of the profession beyond individuals to populations.

To begin, "enabling change within populations requires information or data-gathering to identify the occupational issues affecting a population" (Townsend & Polatajko, 2007, p. 170). The evaluation process examines population factors, including biology and behavior, and contexts, including social, physical, and cultural aspects. Occupational therapy practitioners who seek to influence the health and behaviors of populations can incorporate goals, objectives, and intervention processes such as the Healthy People in Healthy Communities Framework (DHHS, 2001). The goals and objectives articulated in the Healthy People framework focus, for example, on improving functioning, preventing disability, and enabling productive citizenry.

INTERVENTION

Occupational therapy practitioners direct *intervention* services at maximizing the fit among the person (i.e., client) and his or her environments (i.e., contexts) and occupations, and they use task analysis to determine whether to target intervention to the person (e.g., remediation, maintenance, compensation), occupation (e.g., alteration of activity demands), or context (e.g., health promotion, disability prevention). Intervention directed at enabling people to develop the foundational abilities to support performance and participation includes

- Restoring, remediating, or maintaining performance skills and client factors;

- Teaching new methods or compensation strategies through practice opportunities; and
- Promoting new performance patterns, lifestyles, or ways of living through educational approaches.

Intervention directed at the occupation includes

- Enabling clients to practice occupation-based activities to promote participation, mastery, and self-esteem;
- Helping clients engage in purposeful activities to develop or improve performance skills and client factors; and
- Altering activity demands to promote success.

When intervention must address both personal and environmental contexts, it may include modifying or altering environments and promoting healthy attitudes that foster participation, prevent injury, and minimize the disabling effects of impairments.

Intervention planning occurs after the initial evaluation and subsequent identification of the client's long-term goals and practitioner treatment aims and objectives. *Long-term goals* relate to activity limitations in areas of occupation that clients want addressed (e.g., independence in self-feeding). *Short-term aims and objectives* relate to the performance skills and patterns and client factors that must be altered, modified, or augmented and environmental parameters that must be addressed for the client to achieve the long-term goals. Task analysis may be used to divide long-term goals into smaller, measurable units of activity (e.g., independently use a rocker knife and an adaptive fork to cut food on a plate for one-handed utensil use). It is progress toward these goals that clients will monitor and therapists will measure. By measuring progress toward targeted outcomes, therapists are assessing the intervention plan and implementation to ensure that they are effective. Confirming the efficacy of a therapeutic strategy or approach ensures that there is a good fit with client needs and goals.

Purposeful activities are an intervention that translates theories, models, approaches, and strategies into concrete activities that promote skills and adaptation (Hagedorn, 1997; Trombly, 1995b). On the basis of task analysis, practitioners can design intrinsically rewarding, meaningful, and therapeutic interventions that balance situational challenges with personal skills (Csikszentmihalyi, 1990). Purposeful activities are therapeutic when they are relevant, meaningful, and goal directed; elicit coordination among sensorimotor, cognitive, psychological, and psychosocial systems; and promote mastery and feelings of self-competence (AOTA, 1993; Fidler & Fidler, 1978; Trombly, 1995a).

Practitioners who are skilled at task analysis are able to select the most appropriate activity from among those of interest to a particular client (Trombly, 1995b). Task analysis can also help practitioners determine alternative ways for clients to participate in their contexts in ways that may involve modifying activity demands, optimizing its therapeutic value. Activity has been used as a treatment modality since the early years of occupational therapy practice, and the use of therapeutic activity to improve performance skills and patterns is "based on the assumption that the activity holds within itself a healing property that will change organic or behavioral impairments" (Trombly, 1995a, p. 964). In this context, engagement in purposeful activities has the potential to restore or remediate both client factors and performance skills and patterns. "Doing" is an important therapeutic tool.

Intervention Considerations With Individuals

Individual clients are frequently referred to the practitioner through settings such as hospitals, clinics, and home care. Immediate family members, such as parents and siblings, are often involved as advocates or caregivers. Intervention is directed toward the individual at the center of this family group, and family members may or may not have some say in the client's goals, depending on the circumstances and the wishes of the individual. Family education is frequently an intervention aim.

Intervention Considerations With Groups of Individuals

When services are directed toward groups of individuals, practitioners evaluate each group member and design cohesive intervention plans to address the goals and objectives of all the individuals in the group. Interventions may be targeted toward improving participation and health among group members and reducing risk of activity limitations and participation restrictions (AOTA, 2014). *Group-based services* focus on the practitioner's use of self to create an environment that will support change among members. Purposeful activities completed within the group promote performance skills and develop or restore client factors required for enhanced engagement in occupations.

Remedial interventions used in groups, therefore, include the practitioner's therapeutic use of self, purposeful activities, and the facilitation of group process and interactions (Tomlinson & White, 2014). Although interventions are directed at the group level, it is the individuals within the group who are being served. If the group is not cohesive around goals and objectives that are driven by individual clients, the group may not facilitate individual change toward desired outcomes.

Intervention Considerations With Organizations

Organizations often request occupational therapy services as part of their wellness or health and safety programs to respond to work-related injuries, to prevent injuries, to improve the productivity of staff, to demonstrate to employees that they are valued and that their health and well-being matter to the employer, to comply with health and safety and workers' compensation laws or mandates, or to meet specific criteria required to reduce workers' compensation insurance rates. The practitioner first interviews pertinent staff to learn the needs of the organization and to learn the job descriptions of employee groups. He or she then conducts worksite assessments, including ergonomic assessments and physical demands analysis as appropriate.

Common purposes for worksite assessments are to learn the details of the job tasks via the use of task analysis. By using task analysis each activity the worker performs is broken down to a minute level. This facilitates the understanding of the job task, the purpose of the task, and the need for the task and provides information to consider appropriate intervention strategies. During the task analyses, the practitioner consults with workers to learn details beyond that of visual observations including issues and possible solutions from the perspectives of those affected by the job tasks. What might be some leading questions to stimulate sharing of perspectives?

Insurance and legal system clients may request expert opinion regarding functional capacity after injury or illness, recommendations for care needs that may include life care planning, and the cost of present and future care. Occupational therapy practitioners may face an ethical dilemma if the client is the insurance company or legal firm and the request is for assessment of or intervention for an individual. The practitioner must keep in mind that the request for expertise in occupational performance analysis is for a unique purpose that is outside of the procedures in a hospital, clinic, or other health care system. The purpose of an insurance or legal consultation is to answer a specific question, such as whether a person has the functional capacity to return to work or what a person's chronic care needs will be over the lifespan when there is a permanent disability. Although the questions are directed to the need of an insurance or legal system and this entity is the client, the occupational therapy practitioner should not be distracted from the role of expert in the field. Opinions and recommendations must focus on the abilities and needs of the individual.

Intervention Considerations With Communities and Populations

Community and population health service delivery has developed rapidly as a role for occupational therapy practitioners. Health interventions are being designed to enable communities to build and strengthen multisector partnerships to promote healthy lifestyles and improve health and social conditions in the places people live, work, and play: "Community partnerships, particularly when they reach out to non-traditional partners, can be among the most effective tools for improving health in communities" (DHHS, 2000, p. 4). The healthy communities concept, which has its origins in seminal documents published in Canada and the United States, is a strategy WHO (1980) recommended to strengthen health promotion activities in regions. This strategy integrates public health, health education, and community development.

> When considering the health of communities, it is important to understand that there is not necessarily a direct relation between disability and health; many people with disabilities rate their health as excellent. Therefore, health practitioners are shifting their focus from evaluation and intervention for clients with disabilities to the provision of services to people who have activity limitations and participation restrictions that result in undesirable states of health. Furthermore, the prevalence of disability is increasing and can be expected to accelerate in the coming decades as the population ages and medical technology advances. (Watson & Wilson, 2003b, p. 38)

Brault (2012) reported that in 2010, approximately 56.7 million people in the United States had a disability; about 38.3 million of them had a severe disability; and about 12.3 million people 6 years or older needed assistance with one or more activities of daily living (ADLs) or IADLs. As a response to the high rates of disability in the general population, health interventions are increasingly being targeted to communities and are focusing on health promotion and disability prevention.

CASE EXAMPLE 5.5. HEALTHY PEOPLE 2010:
A REAL-WORLD POPULATION HEALTH INITIATIVE

In 2000, **DHHS** outlined a comprehensive, nationwide agenda to improve the health of the U.S. population that addressed the needs of individuals as a collective. The Healthy People 2010 agenda included health goals, objectives, and indicators that were "grounded in science, built through public consensus, and designed to measure progress" (DHHS, 2000, p. 1). The underlying premise of Healthy People 2010, and subsequently Healthy People 2020, is that the health of individuals is inseparable from the health of the larger community and that it is the health of every community that determines the overall health of the nation. Likewise, the health of communities is profoundly influenced by the collective behaviors, actions, attitudes, and beliefs of the individuals who live in them. Can you identify current community projects that are designed to improve the health and well-being of the community? How will these projects have a positive impact on the nation?

Populations can be defined on the basis of geography (e.g., neighborhoods, communities) or shared characteristics (e.g., age, worker status, membership in an organization). Population-based services focus on the needs of a group of individuals rather than on the specific needs of an individual (Moyers & Dale, 2007). Case Example 5.5 describes a population-wide health initiative.

Like the plan to improve the health of the nation, occupational therapy intervention plans designed to improve the health of populations must also be grounded in science, built in collaboration with clients, and designed to address targeted outcomes. Interestingly, the dimensions of concern identified in Healthy People 2010 and 2020 as the determinants of the population's health are strikingly similar to the dimensions of concern to occupational therapy practitioners. Whereas health status is seen by the DHHS (2000) as a function of the interaction of people and environments, participation in occupations is seen by AOTA (2014) as a function of people and contexts.

When providing services to populations, practitioners first profile the needs, assets, and priorities of the people within them (i.e., develop an occupational profile). They do this by establishing collaborative relationships with individuals who serve as proxies for the collective and who are empowered to direct the course of intervention. Needs are defined on the basis of discrepancies between current and desired levels of engagement in occupations, and disparities in attainment of desired levels of participation among groups within the population must be considered when identifying needs. *Assets* are the inherent attributes and available resources of populations

that might be used in attaining target outcomes. The analysis of occupational performance of populations requires an understanding of the persons (e.g., health status indicators; prevalence, incidence, and temporal trends in impairments; health conditions and risk behaviors; performance patterns or lifestyles), environments (e.g., social, political, and cultural contexts), and occupations (e.g., activity demands).

Intervention Considerations With Policymakers

Policymakers are a unique occupational therapy client in that intervention is targeted toward environmental contexts. Occupational therapy practitioners can and do influence public policy, and they design and offer prevention and health promotion services to influence the population's level of participation in meaningful occupations. For example, occupational therapy practitioners have been involved in drafting and revising federal legislation governing the educational rights of people with disabilities. They have been involved in designing and evaluating prevention programs to enhance capacity for successful aging by using consultative and educational intervention approaches to help older adults better appreciate and engage in meaningful occupations (Clark et al., 1997, 2001; Hay et al., 2002). Whenever city councils or regional governing bodies are designing or altering local and national policies and programs that influence health, there is a role for occupational therapy practitioners. The fundamental conditions and resources for health defined by the WHO (2001), which include peace, shelter, education, food, income, a stable ecosystem, sustainable resources, social justice, and equity, are all amenable to socioenvironmental intervention with policymakers by occupational therapy practitioners.

Case Example 5.6, illustrates how occupational therapy practitioners can use task analysis in providing services to individuals, groups, and populations. The case study also demonstrates the domain and process of occupational therapy practice with different types of clients, and Exhibit 5.1 shows the Client Profile and Task Analysis Form (CPTA) for one of these clients, Camille.

(text continued on page 75)

CASE EXAMPLE 5.6. NICHOLAS: A MULTIFACETED OCCUPATIONAL THERAPY CAREER

WORK WITH INDIVIDUALS

Nicholas was an occupational therapy practitioner working at a facility providing inpatient, outpatient, and community-based services. He had extensive experience in work with clients who had had traumatic injuries, and one of his clients was **Camille,** a single mother whose dominant hand had recently been amputated at the wrist after an injury in a commercial kitchen. Her initial priorities were related to returning to her roles as a mother of 2 young boys, homemaker, worker, and sole provider. Camille was particularly concerned with her ability to help her 3-year-old son dress and undress and her ability to cook for her family, which was directly related to her capacity to return to her job as a chef.

Camille and Nicholas agreed that improvements in levels of participation in basic ADLs (e.g., dressing, personal hygiene), IADLs (e.g., meal preparation and cleanup), and social participation (interaction with family, peers, and community) were necessary for reentry into the workforce. Nicholas completed an evaluation, and he and Camille worked together to establish client goals and treatment objectives.

Camille was discouraged by the amount of time and effort required for ADLs and her lack of independence in this area. Nicholas observed Camille dressing and applying makeup and determined that she had not developed proficiency with her hook prosthesis (a motor performance skill). Furthermore, all of her blouses had buttons, her cosmetic bag had a small zipper, and her makeup containers were very small and delicate (activity demands); all required a higher level of manipulative skill than Camille was capable of performing.

Camille was awaiting insurance approval for a specialized custom prosthesis with a quick-release tool socket and modified tools such as kitchen utensils, pencil holder, hairbrush, and key holder. It would also have a posterior forearm attachment so that her smart phone would be easily accessible. The insurer stated that a decision for approval of this custom prosthesis would take at least 2 weeks. If approved, the assessment, fabrication, trials, fittings, and final product for a custom prosthesis and an initial outlay of custom tools would take approximately 4 more weeks. Even if the new prosthesis was approved, it was important for Camille to be proficient with her current prosthesis both in the immediate term and in case she needed it as a backup to her specialized prosthesis. Therefore, Nicholas and Camille needed to work with the current basic hook prosthesis, which was made shortly after her initial surgery.

Using task analysis, Nicholas determined that activity demands (e.g., small zippers and containers), contextual dimensions (e.g., recent injury, lack of spouse, not wanting her 6-year-old son to assist with her personal care), and performance skill dimensions (e.g., dexterity) were causing participation restrictions and frustrating limitations. Nicholas used his analytical skills to determine which areas of dressing to address first to ensure that Camille attained success rapidly. On the basis of ongoing task analysis and consultation with Camille, Nicholas modified and expanded the initial objectives in the area of dressing over time to ensure success in progressively more difficult activities. Once they agreed on goals, Nicholas elected to use a remedial approach to developing performance skills and a compensatory approach to modifying activity demands. He expected to use therapeutic use of self, therapeutic use of occupations and activities, consultation, and education.

Nicholas explored Camille's interest in beginning with several IADLs and leisure and professional activities, including baking, sewing, typing, and writing letters (handwriting was also a work-related activity). Camille decided to try baking cookies and handwriting. During initial baking sessions, Nicholas encouraged Camille to practice manipulating all of the ingredients and utensils (i.e., preparatory method) with and without her prosthesis as appropriate. Nicholas determined, using his task analysis skills, that Camille was easily frustrated by her inability to adjust to the lack of upper-limb sensory information (i.e., client factors) that she had relied on before the amputation. This lack of sensory information caused her to drop objects she held in her prosthesis when she directed her vision and attention elsewhere (i.e., performance skill). Camille was frustrated by her inability to work with both hands to bake. She needed to learn safe practices associated with heat when baking to prevent secondary injury. Nicholas realized he needed to enrich his intervention plan to include a prevention approach.

Nicholas used task analysis to determine that Camille's ability to control the bowl when stirring cooking ingredients was insufficient and made a clinical judgment that this task would remain difficult until she was more proficient with the prosthesis. He suggested modifying the work surface through the use of nonslip matting to keep the bowl from sliding while Camille mixed ingredients and formed cookies (i.e., alteration in activity demands). As Camille's coordination and manipulative performance skills improved (through remedial use of therapeutic occupations and activities), she progressed to practicing opening and closing containers. When she was still unable to open the package of chocolate chips, Nicholas showed her how to use modified scissors (alteration of activity demands, education as an intervention). Nicholas created a thermoplastic pencil holder to be held between the hooks, and Camille was pleased to find that she could print legibly, although her writing was larger than it had been before the injury (adaptation). Cursive writing remained extremely difficult to read.

Through the individualized therapy process, Camille eventually gained greater independence in ADLs, IADLs, and work-related activities, and she began to envision herself actively participating in the important roles in her life: mother, homemaker, and worker. Nicholas helped Camille recognize how the intervention process had prepared her to return to work. During group therapy, she discussed potential problems that might emerge at her workplace, and she was able to discuss her fear of returning to work with some of her colleagues.

WORK WITH GROUPS

Nicholas completed evaluations of 3 adults who were referred for occupational therapy services after a motor vehicle accident or workplace injury. (Camille was one of these clients.) After completing an occupational profile and analysis of occupational performance for each client, he realized that they would likely face similar challenges in returning to work. Armed with this information and insight, he approached all 3 clients to determine their interest in meeting as a group to work on workplace performance skills. Nicholas proposed several potential therapeutic activities they could do together (e.g., planning a menu and hosting a luncheon) to simultaneously address common adaptation issues and individualized goals (e.g., performance skills). For example, Camille could direct group activities using the performance skills related to the demands of her job (e.g., preparing and carrying plates of food). Nicholas relied on using the intervention approach of therapeutic use of self to guide discussions around adaptation. He used task analysis and clinical reasoning to guide decisions regarding alterations of activity demands to address the different individualized goals of the clients participating in the group.

WORK WITH POPULATIONS

Over the years, Nicholas had worked with individual clients, groups of workers, and industry organizations. In his practice with injured workers, employers and insurers often asked him to determine how best to get an individual worker back on the job and to provide recommendations for altering job demands and environmental conditions to prevent further injuries at the site. Nicholas realized that many of the recommendations he made to prevent workplace injury for an individual applied to the population of workers. These recommendations often derived from his experience working with people such as Camille who had upper-limb amputations after a workplace injury. In fact, Nicholas's clientele represented a portion of the population of people in the United States with this type of injury.

Nicholas was among a group of practitioners who were contacted by researchers to assist in an important project by collecting data about his clientele. The research goal was to describe the population of people with upper-limb amputations resulting from workplace injury, accurately estimate their occupational

(Continued)

CASE EXAMPLE 5.6. NICHOLAS: A MULTIFACETED
OCCUPATIONAL THERAPY CAREER *(Cont.)*

outcomes, and identify factors that contributed to successful recovery after injury. Before developing a return-to-work program for his clients, Nicholas reviewed the literature to evaluate evidence regarding effective intervention strategies. To his disappointment, there was no substantial body of high-quality research in this area. He hoped that by contributing to this study, the evidence generated would assist him and other practitioners in identifying the most effective approaches to workplace injury prevention and rehabilitation. This evidence would enable Nicholas and others to target prevention occupational therapy services.

Nicholas was approached by a workers' compensation insurer, who had learned about Nicholas and his work through Camille. The insurer was becoming increasingly concerned about severe workplace upper-limb injuries, and the company wanted to do something about it. When they approached Nicholas, he wondered why he had not previously thought of working with the insurer. He was enthusiastic about possibly designing health interventions with the company to reduce risk of injury and promote successful adaptation among those who were injured. After attending a meeting with the insurer, Nicholas hypothesized that most of the work injuries described were preventable. To fully understand the issues, he met with a focus group of local rehabilitation practitioners (e.g., occupational therapists, physical therapists, kinesiologists), a group of orthopedic surgeons, workplace rehabilitation personnel, and occupational health and safety experts.

Together with project officers from the insurer, Nicholas and some of his colleagues set out to determine the characteristics of the population of workers in their community and their work contexts to profile their needs and assets and establish priorities. One of the project officers was familiar with obtaining and using information from the U.S. Bureau of the Census, and Nicholas volunteered to contact the regional health department to solicit its partnership in this initiative. Nicholas and his team searched for information on the incidence of severe upper-limb workplace injuries, the incidence of mortality due to injury, the prevalence of morbidity due to injury, characteristics of those most at risk for injury, the level of knowledge among employers regarding risk factors for injury, and return-to-work statistics after severe upper-limb injuries. The team collected data on the most frequent causes of upper-limb injury among workers, current levels of engagement of employees in these activities, and contextual factors that might influence rates of injury and morbidity after injury (e.g., job site orientation, safety and maintenance of workplace equipment, injury prevention programs).

On the basis of current and relevant information and his expertise in task analysis, Nicholas recommended that the insurer engage the community and all employers in initiatives that their research findings suggested would potentially have the greatest impact on the rates of workplace injury and resulting morbidity. Knowing that the insights he gained from the population health data would be of great interest to and arouse concern among others, Nicholas worked with the group to create an intersectoral and interdisciplinary coalition of people from the community to develop an action plan that would address the full scope of factors that contributed to the prevention of severe upper-limb injury in the workplace. This coalition eventually consisted of stakeholder representatives from the profit, not-for-profit, and volunteer sectors, as well as local and state government.

Nicholas, acting as a committee member for the coalition, worked with employers and other members of the team to partner with several organizations and industries in their community to design educational materials to inform the community about the prevalence and incidence of the problem, about the economic impact and burden of illness after workplace injury, and about behaviors that put people at risk of injury while at work. The objective of the material was to stimulate individual and community action to alter risk behaviors, maximize compliance with legislation designed to reduce risk of injury (e.g., laws that require isolation guards and emergency stops on machines and alteration of physical environments that place workers at risk, such as cluttered and noisy work areas). The newly formed coalition merged health promotion initiatives with those designed to prevent injury in the workplace, such as enhancing the safety of the job sites associated with the highest rates of injury; increasing the availability of first aid, ambulance, and emergency services; ensuring that medical and rehabilitation services were directed toward minimizing activity limitations among workers with injury-related impairments; and promoting industry-supported fitness programs.

Assignment 5.1. Exploring Client Needs

1. Read Case Example 5.6, and review the CPTA form to become familiar with the dimensions of evaluation in the development of an occupational profile.
2. Using the information provided in Case Example 5.6, record Camille's short-term goals on the CPTA form. Identify the occupations or activities and related tasks that would be the focus of the intervention plan. Consider the context and environment and potential barriers to goal achievement. Retain this information for future use in Chapter 12, "Adulthood: Maintaining Meaningful Lifestyles."

EXHIBIT 5.1. CLIENT PROFILE AND TASK ANALYSIS FORM: CAMILLE

CLIENT PROFILE

Name: Camille	Birthdate:	Age at assessment: 32
Advocates: None	**Work occupation:** Chef at a commercial kitchen	
Diagnoses: Right wrist and hand amputation	**Current interventions:** 1. Occupational therapy 2. Prosthetics or orthotics 3. Orthopedic follow-up	
Referral source: Rehabilitation facility		

PERSONAL INFORMATION

Family unit	Single mother of two young sons
Caregiver(s)	n/a
Roles and responsibilities (e.g., student, spouse, parent, friend, worker)	1. Mother 2. Homemaker 3. Worker and sole provider
Home environment (e.g., home design, number of people living in the home)	Townhouse with kitchen and living areas on the main floor, bedrooms and main bathroom on the upper floor, and laundry facilities in the basement.
Community context (e.g., rural, urban, metro; single family home, residential care)	Metropolitan area with access to medical equipment suppliers

(Continued)

EXHIBIT 5.1. CLIENT PROFILE AND TASK ANALYSIS FORM: CAMILLE *(Cont.)*

School or work context (e.g., public, special, or private school; stationary or travel location for work)	n/a
Client priorities	1. Help 3-year-old son with dressing. 2. Cook for the family. 3. Increase ADL and IADL skills. 4. Reestablish social participation in the community. 5. Reenter workforce.
Values/beliefs/spirituality (e.g., principles, standards, beliefs, personal quest)	Camille's priority is to care for and provide for her family in her customary manner. She has always been self-reliant.

SUMMARY, PLAN, AND GOALS
(Fill in for Assignment 5.1, "Exploring Client Needs.")

Assessments completed (formal and observational):	
Practitioner–client plan (e.g., further formal and observational assessments, inclusion of others):	
Tasks Requiring Assessment or Intervention	
Short-term goals (Primarily client driven, measurable, global task, or activity achievements)	**Long-term objectives** (Primarily practitioner driven, measurable, incremental, stepwise, or mini achievements)
1.	1.a. 1.b.
2.	2.a. 2.b.
3.	3.a. 3.b.
4.	4.a. 4.b.

TASKS ANALYZED
(Fill in for Assignment 5.1, "Exploring Client Needs.")

Occupation or Activity	Tasks (specific activity component)	Context or Environment (external and internal)

ANALYSIS (OF PERFORMANCE SKILLS)

Performance Skills	Client Challenges (Performance qualifier)
Rating: 0 = *no restriction*, 1 = *mild limitation*, 2 = *moderate restriction*, 3 = *severe restriction*, 4 = *complete impairment*	
Motor and praxis	**Rating**
Posture	0

(Continued)

EXHIBIT 5.1. CLIENT PROFILE AND TASK ANALYSIS FORM: CAMILLE *(Cont.)*

Energy	0
Execution	2
Process skills	**Rating**
Mental energy	0
Knowledge	0
Organization	0
Adaptation	I
Social interaction skills	**Rating**
Communication posture	0
Gestures	0
Initiation	0
Information exchange	0
Acknowledging	0
Taking turns	0

ANALYSIS (OF PERFORMANCE PATTERNS)

Performance Patterns	Daily Life Activities	Client Challenges (skill deficits and context restrictions)
Habits (Automatic and integrated behaviors)	Camille wakes in the morning before her children, showers, and grooms. She then prepares breakfast before waking her children for the day.	Self-care takes an extraordinary amount of time, which has changed her regular habits. She must use new techniques and develop routines for meal preparation.
Routines (Regular activities that provide daily structure)	Camille would get ready for the day, prepare breakfast, get her children up and ready for their day, take her children to school, and then proceed to work.	Everything takes longer for Camille, and she has not reestablished a routine that works for her and her children. She has not returned to work and is eager to have a routine in place to support her return to work.
Roles (Expected behaviors and responsibilities)	Mother and chef	As noted, she is having difficulty with the roles and routines needed for her children to manage their day. She is challenged to adapt her approach to meal preparation. She has not returned to work and is the sole provider.

Rituals (Customary cultural and social activities)	Not explored at this stage of intervention	

(Fill in for Assignment 5.1, "Exploring Client Needs.")

Synopsis of performance skills and performance patterns (strengths, deficits, and challenges):

_____

_____

_____

_____

_____

_____

OCCUPATIONAL PROFILE AND ANALYSIS OF NEEDS

Functional ability (i.e., how strengths and deficits affect ability to perform activities and tasks)	Amputation of her dominant hand resulted in substantial restrictions in all activities that require the use of her hand. This includes basic ADLs, IADLs, and work.
Activity tolerance (e.g., physical and mental fatigue levels, energy to complete activities and tasks, temporal and environmental contexts)	It takes Camille significantly more time to manage all daily tasks, which has caused her frustration, because she must return to her role as a mother, her routines for her family, and work that is required for economic self-sufficiency.
Effect on occupational performance (reflect on client roles, responsibilities, and priorities)	The daily routine of the family has been disrupted, affecting not only herself but her also children. She has not returned to work, which adds to her stress levels.
Intervention needs (e.g., physical, cognitive, emotional, social)	Active occupational therapy is required to improve Camille's level of participation in basic ADLs. She must become proficient in the use of her prosthesis to achieve her goal of increasing independence and speed of performance.
Resource needs (e.g., assistive devices or equipment, technology)	Camille is waiting for insurance approval for a specialized custom prosthesis with a quick-release tool socket and modified tools. Even with provision of the specialized prosthesis, Camille needs to become proficient with her current prosthesis in the immediate term and in case she needs it as a backup to her specialized prosthesis.
Program needs (e.g., day programs, return-to-work programs, socialization)	Individualized therapy sessions for basic ADL and IADL training.
Outlook (practitioner projection of long-term needs and life care planning)	Camille will gain independence using her prosthesis but whether she will be competitively employable as a chef is questionable. Retraining for an alternate career should be discussed with Camille.

(Continued)

EXHIBIT 5.1. CLIENT PROFILE AND TASK ANALYSIS FORM: CAMILLE *(Cont.)*

GUIDELINES AND CHECKLIST FOR TASK ANALYSIS

Areas of Occupation

Activities of daily living	**Instrumental activities of daily living**
☑ Bathing and showering	☑ Care of others
☐ Bowel and bladder management	☐ Care of pets
☑ Dressing	☐ Child rearing
☑ Eating and swallowing	☐ Communication management
☐ Feeding	☐ Driving and community mobility
☐ Functional mobility	☐ Financial management
☑ Personal device care	☐ Home establishment
☑ Personal hygiene and grooming	☑ Home management and maintenance
☐ Sexual activity	☑ Meal preparation and cleanup
☑ Toileting and toilet hygiene	☐ Religious and spiritual observance
	☐ Safety and emergency maintenance
	☑ Shopping

Rest and sleep	**Play**
☐ Rest and relaxation	☐ Peer interaction
☐ Sleep participation	☐ Play exploration
☐ Sleep preparation	☐ Play participation

Leisure	**Social participation**
☑ Customary activities or hobbies	☑ Community
☑ Leisure exploration	☑ Family
☑ Leisure participation	☑ Peer or friend

Education	**Work**
☐ Access issues	☐ Employment interests and pursuits
☐ Formal education participation	☐ Employment seeking and acquisition
☐ Informal personal education or exploration	☑ Job performance
☐ Informal personal education participation	☐ Retirement preparation and adjustment
	☐ Volunteer exploration
	☐ Volunteer participation

Client Factors

Body functions and structures	**Body functions and structures**
Physical	*Sensory and pain*
☐ Cardiovascular and hematological systems	☐ Hearing functions
☐ Digestive, metabolic, and endocrine systems	☑ Pain grading and description
☐ Genitourinary and reproductive functions	☐ Seeing and related functions
☑ Movement-related functions	☑ Tactile functions
☐ Respiratory and immunological systems	☐ Taste and smell functions
☑ Skin and related structure functions	☑ Temperature and pressure reception
☐ Voice and speech functions	☐ Vestibular and proprioceptive functions

Body functions: Mental

Specific mental functions
- ☐ Attention
- ☐ Emotional
- ☐ Experience of self and time
- ☐ Higher-level cognitive
- ☑ Motor sequencing
- ☐ Memory
- ☐ Perception
- ☐ Thought

Body functions: Mental

Global mental functions
- ☐ Consciousness
- ☐ Energy and drive
- ☐ Orientation
- ☐ Sleep
- ☐ Temperament and personality

Values, Beliefs, and Spirituality

Values
- ☑ Meaningful qualities
- ☑ Principles
- ☑ Standards

Beliefs and spirituality
- ☐ Cognitive content health as true
- ☐ Guiding actions
- ☑ Life meaning and purpose

Activity and Occupational Demands

Objects and their properties
- ☑ Inherent properties (e.g., heavy, light)
- ☑ Required tools, materials, equipment

Space demands
- ☑ Size, arrangement, surface, lighting

Social demands
- ☐ Cultural context
- ☐ Social environment

Sequence and timing
- ☐ Sequence and timing
- ☐ Specific steps

Required actions and performance skills
- ☐ Cognitive
- ☐ Communication and interaction
- ☐ Emotional and social
- ☑ Motor and praxis
- ☐ Sensory–perceptual

Required body functions and structures
- ☑ Anatomical parts
- ☐ Level of consciousness
- ☑ Mobility of joints

Performance Skills

Motor skills
- ☑ Movement actions or behaviors
- ☑ Skilled purposeful movements
- ☑ Ability to carry out learned movement

Process skills
- ☐ Judgment
- ☐ Select and sequence objects or tools
- ☐ Organize and prioritize
- ☐ Create and problem solve
- ☐ Multitask

Social interaction skills
- ☐ Identify, manage, and express feelings
- ☐ On a one-to-one basis
- ☐ In groups
- ☐ Communication and interaction skills

(Continued)

EXHIBIT 5.1. CLIENT PROFILE AND TASK ANALYSIS FORM: CAMILLE *(Cont.)*

Performance Patterns

Habits	**Routines**
☑ Automatic behavior	☑ Observable patterns of behavior
☑ Repeated activities	☑ Time commitment
☑ Good, bad, or impoverished	☑ Satisfying, promoting, or damaging
Roles	**Rituals**
☑ Set of expected behaviors	☐ Symbolic actions
☑ Social or cultural	☐ Spiritual, cultural, or social
☑ Within context	☐ Link to values and beliefs

Contexts and Environments

Cultural	**Personal**
☐ Customs and beliefs	☑ Age and gender
☑ Activity patterns	☑ Socioeconomic status
☑ Expectations	☐ Educational status
Temporal	**Virtual**
☑ Location of performance in time	☐ Communication environment
☐ Experience shaped by engagement	
Physical	**Social and political**
☐ Natural environment (e.g., geography)	☑ Relationship to individuals
☐ Built environment (e.g., building, furniture)	☑ Relationship to organizations or systems

TASK ANALYSIS TEMPLATE

An individual form is required for each task that is examined.
Task: Baking

Task Demands	Action Demands (What is required of the person to do the task)	Client Challenges (Availability of required body functions and structures)
Objects used (e.g., equipment, technology)	Modified scissors for opening product bags Nonslip matting to keep the mixing bowl from sliding	Loss of use of her dominant hand and a restriction in bilateral activities makes preparation and cooking challenging for her. A specialized prosthesis will be assistive but is not yet available for her use.
Space demands (e.g., physical context)	n/a	None
Social demands (e.g., social environment and context)	n/a	n/a

Sequence and timing (e.g., process to carry out the task)	Camille must prepare meals for her family, which is often time sensitive.	Reestablishing routines around meal preparation requires Camille to learn new approaches and strategies that will be incorporated into her routines.
Required actions and performance skills (e.g., basic requirements)	Handling kitchen tools and using the stovetop and oven safely.	Handling tools and hot foods can be a safety risk if new habits and routines are not established and practiced.

Note. ADLs = activities of daily living; IADLs = instrumental activities of daily living; UE = upper extremity.

SUMMARY

Collaborative relationships with clients and their proxies, client-directed services, and partnerships with stakeholders who are interested in similar target outcomes remain the constant foundation of the occupational therapy process. Practice with individuals, groups, organizations, and populations has provided evidence for the robust ability of the profession's theories, knowledge base, practice models, and intervention approaches to enable clients to engage in occupations and participate in contexts. By reflecting on the interventions they have used in their practice with individual clients, practitioners can learn more about what interventions can enable groups and populations to engage in occupations and participate in contexts.

REFERENCES

American Occupational Therapy Association. (1993). Position paper: Purposeful activity. *American Journal of Occupational Therapy, 47*, 1081–1082. http://dx.doi.org/10.5014/ajot.47.12.1081

American Occupational Therapy Association. (2014). Occupational therapy practice framework: Domain and process (3rd ed.). *American Journal of Occupational Therapy, 68*(Suppl.), S1–48. http://dx.doi.org/10.5014/ajot.2014.682006

Brault, M. W. (2012). *Americans with disabilities: 2010 household economic studies.* Retrieved from www.census.gov/prod/2012pubs/p70-131.pdf

Clark, F., Azen, S. P., Carlson, M., Mandel, D., La-Bree, L., Hay, J., . . . Lipson, L. (2001). Embedding health-promoting changes into the daily lives of independent living older adults: Long-term follow-up

of occupational therapy intervention. *Journals of Gerontology, Series B: Psychological Sciences and Social Sciences, 56*, 60–63.

Clark, F., Azen, S. P., Zemke, R., Jackson, J., Carlson, M., Mandel, D., . . . Lipson, L. (1997). Occupational therapy for independent living older adults. *JAMA, 278*, 1321–1326.

Csikszentmihalyi, M. (1990). *Flow: The psychology of optimal experience.* New York: Harper & Row.

Fidler, G. S., & Fidler, J. (1978). Doing and becoming: Purposeful action and self-actualization. *American Journal of Occupational Therapy, 32*, 305–310.

Hagedorn, R. (1997). *Foundations for practice in occupational therapy.* New York: Churchill Livingstone.

Hay, J., Labree, L., Luo, R., Clark, F., Carlson, M., Mandel, D., . . . Azen, S. P. (2002). Cost-effectiveness of preventive occupational therapy for independent living older adults. *Journal of the American Geriatrics Society, 50*, 1381–1387.

Moyers, P., & Dale, L. M. (2007). *The guide to occupational therapy practice* (2nd ed.). Bethesda, MD: AOTA Press.

Tomlinson, J., & White, S. (2014). Group activities occupations. In J. Hinojosa & M.-L. Blount (Eds.), *The texture of life: Purposeful activities in the context of occupation* (4th ed., pp. 209–232). Bethesda, MD: AOTA Press.

Townsend, E. A., & Polatajko, H. J. (2007). *Enabling occupation II: Advancing an occupational therapy vision of health, well-being, and justice through occupation.* Ottawa, ON: CAOT Publications.

Trombly, C. A. (1995a). Occupation: Purposefulness and meaningfulness as therapeutic mechanisms [Eleanor Clark Slagle Lecture]. *American Journal of Occupational Therapy, 49*, 960–972. http://dx.doi.org/10.5014/ajot.49.10.960

Trombly, C. A. (1995b). Purposeful activity. In C. A. Trombly (Ed.), *Occupational therapy for physical dysfunction* (pp. 237–253). Baltimore: Williams & Wilkins.

U.S. Department of Health and Human Services. (1979). *Healthy People: The Surgeon General's report on health promotion and disease prevention.* Washington, DC: U.S. Government Printing Office.

U.S. Department of Health and Human Services. (1998). *Healthy People 2010 objectives: Draft for public comment.* Washington, DC: Author.

U.S. Department of Health and Human Services. (2000). *Healthy People 2010: Understanding and improving health.* Washington, DC: Author. Available from www.health.gov/healthypeople

U.S. Department of Health and Human Services. (2001). *Healthy people in healthy communities: A community planning guide using Healthy People 2010.* Rockville, MD: Author. Retrieved from www.health.gov/healthypeople/Publications/ Healthy Communities2001/default.htm

U.S. Department of Health and Human Services. (2010). *Healthy People 2020.* Washington, DC: Author. Retrieved from www.healthypeople.gov/2020/ about/default.aspx

Watson, D. E., & Wilson, S. A. (2003a). Process of occupational therapy. In *Task analysis: An individual and population approach* (2nd ed., pp. 28–32). Bethesda, MD: AOTA Press.

Watson, D. E., & Wilson, S. A. (2003b). Serving individuals and populations. In *Task analysis: An individual and population approach* (2nd ed., pp. 34–42). Bethesda, MD: AOTA Press.

World Health Organization. (1980). *International classification of impairments, disabilities, and handicaps: A manual of classification relating to the consequences of disease.* Geneva: Author.

World Health Organization. (2001). *International classification of functioning, disability and health.* Geneva: Author.

6

Care Planning: Needs Analysis and Use in Consultation

Transitions can be evolutionary with relatively smooth, planned, controlled, and gradual adjustments, or they can be violent shifts, creating a tidal wave of crisis management and life-altering change.

—Gregg Landry

CHAPTER OBJECTIVES

At the completion of this chapter, readers will be able to

- Understand the fundamentals of care planning, including needs analysis;
- Describe how occupational therapy practitioners use task analysis skills to inform third-party clients, such as the legal system and insurance industry; and
- Market occupational therapy task analysis skills as an asset that has cross-sectoral value.

KEY TERMS

Activity–action fit
Activity demands
Analysis of impairment
Beliefs
Body functions and structures
Care planning
Client factors
Cost-of-care analysis
Direct costs
Disability profile

Impairment
Indirect cost
Injury management advisors
Medical legal consultant
Needs analysis
Return-to-work rehabilitation
Spirituality
Task demands
Values

Occupational therapy practitioners are important players in developing a life care plan. *Care planning* is a means of assessing future care needs and associated costs to make informed decisions about the client's abilities and needs. The practitioner then outlines, plans, advises on, and implements interventions as appropriate to meet the client's needs. Common interventions include adaptive equipment; home or vehicle modifications; and physical, psychological, or return-to-work rehabilitation. Interventions may also include support services for the home, community, or workplace.

Clinical evidence is the basis for care planning and is a testimony to the truth for the courts, insurance companies, and workplaces. The occupational therapy practitioner produces evidence using task analysis in assessing a client's activity limitations and performance restrictions.

Care planning is not the application of generic formulas to a diagnostic category but rather a process of describing client-specific needs relative to activity limitations and participation restrictions. Needs, rather than funding sources, drive the care planning process. The method of analysis should remain the same from case to case.

NEEDS ANALYSIS AND CARE PLANNING

The care planning process includes the occupational therapy assessment (e.g., observation, testing, outcomes), the analysis of impairment, the disability profile, a needs analysis, and the determination of resources. To engage in care planning, it is essential first to delineate the needs that resulted directly from the illness, catastrophic impairment, or injury (Katz & Delaney, 2002) and then to determine the severity of the residual deficits that will affect a client and his or her family across all areas of occupational performance.

The occupational therapy practitioner conducts a *needs analysis* that includes assessment of the client and synthesis of information provided in cross-disciplinary reports. The needs analysis is part of care planning that uses task analysis to determine what assistive devices, community resources, and chronic therapeutic intervention are required to optimize the fit of the person, in customary environments, across occupations and activities and aims to restore the client as close as possible to a without-injury lifestyle.

Occupational Therapy Assessment

The core component of a needs analysis is the occupational therapy assessment of limitations, restrictions, and associated needs, which, unique to the field, enables a thorough analysis of limitations and restrictions relative to occupational performance. The occupational therapy assessment addresses both client factors and task demands. A task analysis approach is used in the assessment. The therapist includes any recommendations made by other disciplines in the needs analysis.

Client factors

Client factors are "specific capacities, characteristics, or beliefs that reside within the person and that influence performance in occupations" (American Occupational Therapy Association [AOTA], 2014, p. S7). They include values, beliefs, and spirituality; body functions; and body structures. An understanding of these factors is important in developing a care plan or cost-of-care determination.

Values are the "principles, standards, or qualities considered worthwhile by the client who holds them" (AOTA, 2014, p. S7). *Beliefs* are "cognitive content held to be true" (e.g., sense of power over a situation or circumstance; AOTA, 2014, p. S7). Values and beliefs encompass emotion, perception of purpose, and sociocultural perspectives.

Spirituality refers to how a client looks beyond the material world for the meaning of existence and of life changes, such as a greater awareness of mortality after injury (McColl, 2011). Values, beliefs, and spirituality coexist within a person, provide meaning to life, and interconnect with what a person considers to be meaningful goals, activities, and tasks.

Occupational therapy practitioners must be fully aware of how a disability affects the client, his or her family, and the community. As articulated in the Canadian Model of Client-Centered Enablement, occupational therapy practitioners use a value-based interview that focuses on a client-centered approach (Townsend & Polatajko, 2007). Understanding is derived through a conversational interview that explores these client factors. After injury and disability, the principles, standards, and qualities a person upholds in life direct how the person's life can be restored as closely as possible to his or her customary lifestyle.

In conversational interviews, the practitioner adjusts his or her language to ensure understanding and, given the often personal nature of the information sought, seeks to build the client's sense of confidence in revealing information (e.g., in line with expectations of the client's culture group). A conversational interview improves response accuracy compared with a linear question-and-answer approach, which can overlook critical information given that all clients' circumstances are unique and some may be atypical. Although the conversational approach requires more time than a question-and-answer approach, the time spent yields greater and often optimal needs assessment information.

Client factors also include *body functions* and *body structures* (AOTA, 2014). Along with ascertaining the client's perception of the impairment and disability, the practitioner must collect information about the following:

- *Mental functions:* Specific mental functions include higher-level cognition, memory, attention, and perception; global mental functions include consciousness, orientation, temperament and personality, energy and drive, and sleep.
- *Sensory functions and pain:* Sensory functions include visual and related functions, hearing, vestibular, taste, smell, proprioceptive, touch, temperature, and pressure and pain.
- *Neuromuscular and movement-related functions:* Functions of the joints and bones include joint mobility, joint stability, muscle power, muscle endurance, motor reflexes, involuntary and voluntary movement, and gait patterns.

- *Muscle functions:* Muscle functions include muscle power, tone, and endurance.
- *Cardiovascular, hematological, immunological, and respiratory system functions.*
- *Voice and speech functions:* Voice and speech functions include fluency and rhythm and alternative vocalization functions (e.g., assistive technology).
- *Digestive, metabolic, and endocrine system functions.*
- *Genitourinary and reproductive functions.*
- *Physiological functions:* Physiological functions include cardiovascular, hematological, immunological, respiratory, digestive, metabolic, endocrine, genitourinary, and reproductive functions.
- *Skin and related-structure functions:* Skin and related-structure functions pertain to the skin, hair, and nails.

The *Occupational Therapy Practice Framework: Domain and Process* (3rd ed., hereinafter referred to as the *Framework*) provides a useful guide to enable practitioners to record information about impairments in body functions and body structures (AOTA, 2014). In addition, the practitioner conducts specific standardized or clinical testing to acquire any necessary information and adds information available from interdisciplinary sources.

Task demands

A fundamental requirement for engaging independently in occupations and activities is the ability to perform related tasks or task components. The occupational therapy practitioner uses various measurement strategies such as clinical observation of task performance and administration of standardized tests.

To fully understand the impact of impairment on performance, the occupational therapy practitioner must analyze all aspects of an occupation or activity and task and use this information to determine how specific task demands challenge a client. This analysis allows for full exploration of potential needs for assistive devices, augmentative technology, mobility aids, and so forth. *Task demands* include the properties of an object and the sequencing and timing of required actions or skills (AOTA, 2014). The following are elements of *task–action fit*:

- Required body functions and structures to accomplish the occupation, activity, or task independently or semi-independently;
- Required performance skills such as motor and praxis skills, sensory–perceptual skills, emotional regulation skills, cognitive skills, and communication and social skills; and
- Required performance patterns, including habits, routines, rituals, and roles.

Analysis of Impairment

An understanding of the client's impairment and its lifelong impact on health and well-being is essential to care planning. *Analysis of impairment* is a synthesis of medical, psychological, and rehabilitation information that is available before conducting an interview and assessment. Medical documentation provides important diagnostic information and highlights precautions that may be needed in assessment (e.g., cannot lift heavy loads in a functional capacity evaluation because of a disc compromise); psychological information provides diagnostics and information about an individual's mental and emotional status; and rehabilitation information provides an overview of what interventions have been provided to date and the outcome of these interventions.

Impairment inherently imposes restrictions on body functions, both physical and psychological.

For example, the extent of a spinal cord injury dictates the motor options available to a client, and the severity of a brain injury dictates a client's cognitive and emotional capacity.

The occupational therapy practitioner first poses questions about the client's residual capacity. Physician opinion on diagnosis and causation is paramount as baseline evidence. Additional understanding may be obtained from a review of multidisciplinary medical records and neuropsychological reports. If necessary, the practitioner seeks further understanding of the impact of impairment on physiological or psychological functions through direct assessment.

The *Framework* provides guidelines on aspects of impairment that practitioners need to examine thoroughly as part of care planning (AOTA, 2014). One aspect is mental functions, which the practitioner considers in addressing specific limitations and restrictions to the client's ability to perform cognitive activities within the range considered normal. Likewise, medical diagnosis provides substantial insight into motor expectations for neuromusculoskeletal and movement-related functions in conditions such as spinal cord injury and muscular dystrophy. Understanding the presenting patterns of movement, such as those occurring with cerebral palsy, is obtained through clinical observation. Impairment of body structures may be interwoven with movement-related impairments or may be specific to an injury. Case Example 6.1 provides an opportunity analyze impairment.

The aim of impairment analysis is to understand and describe any impairment that restricts normal function. The practitioner seeks to address

---

CASE EXAMPLE 6.1. CLIENT WITH TRAUMATIC BRAIN INJURY

Carrie was age 18 years when she was in a motor vehicle collision resulting in a traumatic brain injury (TBI) that manifested in memory loss, attention problems, language deficits, fatigue, and decreased processing speed. She also sustained fractures of the mandible with severe dental injury, right ankle fracture, and back and left shoulder musculoskeletal strain. Two years later, Carrie's impairment symptoms have not resolved. What assumptions can you make to design an occupational therapy evaluation approach? Do your analysis using the framework provided in Exhibit 6.1. Use the Client Profile and Task Analysis Form's (CPTA; Appendix A) "Guidelines and Checklist for Task Analysis" section to guide your considerations and then the "Occupational Profile and Analysis of Needs" section to consider how the impairment affected ability, tolerance, and occupational performance. Explore literature related to TBI for more insight into what assumptions can be made about the impairment's impact.

EXHIBIT 6.1. FRAMEWORK FOR DESIGNING AN APPROACH TO CARE PLANNING	
Physical or Cognitive Impairment	**Predicted Functional Impact**

all impairment-related needs in a care plan, including both needs the practitioner has assessed directly and those identified through document review across disciplines, which may include impairments in cardiovascular, hematological, immunological, and respiratory system functions; voice and speech functions; digestive, metabolic, and endocrine system functions; genitourinary and reproductive functions; and skin and related structure functions.

Disability Profile

A *disability profile* provides evidence of limitations and restrictions that are linked to the impairment or condition suffered by the individual. It is developed using task analysis and is a gold standard of evidence of need; therefore, the disability profile is an essential evaluation component in life care planning. Complex information about functional limitations and restrictions is best managed with a checklist that is evidence based and provides salient information about the client. The *Framework* provides a useful structure for categorizing client factors, areas of occupation, and context and environment based on the Person–Environment–Occupation model (AOTA, 2014). It is readily understood across sectors, including the legal system, the insurance industry, and the public. Performance aspects are further delineated through assessment of activity demands, performance skills, and performance patterns.

To develop a disability profile, the occupational therapy practitioner uses available cross-disciplinary information and an understanding of the power of interdisciplinary evidence. Incorporating the findings and opinions of all rehabilitation practitioners ensures a holistic disability profile.

Key informants are physiatrists, psychiatrists, occupational therapy practitioners, physical therapists, chiropractic practitioners, massage therapists, and any others involved in the client's care.

On completing a disability profile, the practitioner reviews all clinical reports and creates a summary of the impairment and disability information that is consistently presented in these reports. It is useful to create a spreadsheet that identifies information of interest; examples of categories for a spreadsheet include body structure and physical and cognitive conditions, unique postinjury outcomes, pain and pain situations, range of motion and quality of movement, grip strength and manual handling, functional tolerances, ability to perform activities of daily living, and social conditions.

Determination of Resources

An occupational therapy practitioner conducting a needs assessment must have full knowledge of the resources available to meet the client's identified needs. The practitioner applies specific assessment batteries and observational skills to develop the occupational therapy opinion of need. A needs analysis adds to the profile developed by the occupational therapy practitioner by examining the evidence provided across discipline (e.g., speech–language recommendations).

A *cost-of-care analysis* is an in-depth report on the allocation of costs of the needs recommended in care planning. This requires an understanding of both *direct costs* (e.g., cost of a wheelchair) and *indirect costs* (e.g., home floor maintenance with use of a wheelchair in the home).

The practitioner may work with an economist if the analysis is requested by a community

---

CASE EXAMPLE 6.2. CARE PLANNING FOR A SEVERELY INJURED CLIENT

Christopher, a 40-year-old electrician who was married and had 3 school-age children, was injured in an industrial accident. He suffered a comminuted fracture of the right humerus that required surgical fixation; he was right dominant. His left radius and ulna were also fractured and his left wrist dislocated. His left hand, mangled by multiple fractures and muscle degloving, required amputation. Christopher also had an open fracture of the left femur that required surgical fixation, and significant bone loss resulted in shortening of the left lower extremity compared with the right. Christopher was concerned about his ability to carry out full-time job duties so that he could continue to support himself and his family.

What is needed to ameliorate Christopher's condition and situation? Identify at least 3 essential needs in the areas of self-care, housekeeping, and work, and explore resources in your geographic area that might fit his needs. Using the CPTA form (Appendix A), build a disability profile using an understanding of the impairment and potential activity limitations and performance restrictions for this client.

(e.g., examination of access barriers and solutions) or an organization (e.g., determining cost drivers for care delivery in assisted living environments).

Resources may be available at the local (e.g., mental health programs), national (e.g., funding sources), and international (e.g., unique assistive equipment) level. Resources come with a cost. For example, specialized equipment or state-of-art prosthetic solutions are typically very expensive. The client has a right to the best resources available. Of course, options depend on the context and issue. If the resource is assisted living accommodations, then local options are best recommended. If a client with an upper-limb amputation is to be restored as closely as possible to his or her customary lifestyle, a specialized prosthetic team might be recommended (i.e., direct cost) along with travel costs to attend a specialized clinic (i.e., indirect cost).

An occupational therapy practitioner involved in care planning and cost-of-care determination must stay abreast of information about assistive devices and equipment, barrier-free design providers, alternative living arrangements, housekeeping services, educational resources, back-to-work resources, and leisure and social participation options. Creating and continuously updating a spreadsheet and then summarizing this information as a clinical resource enables the occupational therapy practitioner to retrieve information quickly.

When engaging in care planning and cost-of-care analysis, the occupational therapy practitioner must determine the client's both short- and

Assignment 6.1. Identifying Care Needs, Resources, and Cost

1. A 21-year-old man experienced a moderate TBI. At the time of the injury, he was attending a university with the goal to become a physician. Predict how the brain injury will affect this client's long-term career planning and economic self-sufficiency. What might his needs be relative to his training and work capacity? It may be helpful to start your exploration using the articles "A Review of Outcome After Moderate and Severe Closed Head Injury With an Introduction to Life Care Planning" by Sherer, Madison, and Hannay (2000) and "Life Care Planning After Traumatic Brain Injury" by Zasler, Ameis, and Ridick-Grisham.

2. Using the information in this chapter about the components of care planning, develop a reporting framework for the evidence necessary to support your recommendation to address needs and the determination of the cost of these recommendations. To accomplish this assignment, use the *Occupational Therapy Practice Framework,* (AOTA, 2014), the Cardinal Hill Occupational Participation Process (Skubik-Peplaski, Paris, Boyle, & Culpert, 2009), or the Client Profile and Task Analysis Form (Appendix A) in this volume. Use one of the cases presented in this volume to frame salient aspects of the analysis and reporting.

long-term needs. The practitioner must also determine how often a resource must be replaced because cost will accumulate over time on the basis of the estimated lifespan of the client or the nature of the impairment (e.g., mortality statistics associated with a disease, illness, or injury). For simple assistive devices and mobility equipment, the stated warranty specifies the replacement expectation. For many resources, accumulating costs over time can be determined by an economist, actuary, or specialist accountant, typically commissioned by the funder. Case Example 6.2 presents a client who needs a plan of care.

CONSULTATION WITH THIRD-PARTY CLIENTS

Occupational therapy practitioners are established leaders in the medical–legal consulting arena, in insurance claims management, and in the return-to-work rehabilitation field.

Medical–Legal Consultation

The *medical–legal consultant* is viewed as an expert in the field of needs analysis, care planning, and cost of care. Occupational therapy is the go-to profession for medical–legal cases in which cost-of-care issues are being decided. Typically, plaintiff and defense lawyers hire occupational therapy practitioners to evaluate the past, present, and future abilities of and past, present, and future costs of providing care to clients who have had injuries. Attorneys and insurance companies want a detailed outline of needs and future expenses that they can use in negotiation (Harris, 2011; Katz & Delaney, 2002). Judges understand the complexity of life care planning reflected in a cost-of-care analysis and expect both the plaintiff and defense lawyers to provide details.

Occupational therapy practitioners use their expertise to answer the following questions: How does an impairment affect the client's function now? What are the predicted future issues related to impairment and its limitations? An occupational therapy expert's analysis is conducted in the same manner for either the plaintiff or the defense: It aims to represent the truth.

The required expertise includes medical, clinical, and lifespan development knowledge; analytical skills, including task analysis; access to updated scientific information and the capacity to interpret research findings; understanding of the role and expertise of other disciplines; and current information about resources such as services and assistive devices. An occupational therapy expert consultant is considered an expert witness in the courts. When testifying in court, the occupational therapy expert presents his or her qualifications, which provide proof of expertise. The expert also presents the framework of occupational therapy as a gold standard of disability analysis. The plaintiff and defense lawyers ask questions to further establish the expert's expertise.

The occupational therapist conducts the appropriate assessments and research information as needed and then completes a highly detailed report that may be used in court proceedings. The occupational therapist may engage an occupational therapy assistant in collecting evidence, but the occupational therapy assistant would not qualify as a court expert. Occupational therapists must anticipate the possibility of being called into court to act as an expert witness and to defend the information in their report. Assessment and documentation are expected to reflect an unbiased professional opinion on the client's abilities and needs. In addition to the ethical implications of providing biased reports, purposefully or unintentionally biased reports are damaging to the individual practitioner because a judge can disqualify him or her from being an expert witness. Once an expert is disqualified, his or her usefulness to lawyers ends, and the medical–legal and cost-of-care report the expert provided is dismissed, highlighting the need for occupational therapy practitioners to use consistent, coherent, and accurate evidence to support their recommendations and cost-of-care determinations.

Occupational therapy science supports the development of a disability profile. The frame of reference of a medical–legal analysis is *impairment*, which is any loss or abnormality of psychological, physiological, or anatomical structure or function (World Health Organization, 2001). The occupational therapy expert reviews all medical and rehabilitation reports, which provide interdisciplinary information

(Lacerte & Johnson, 2013; Weed & Berens, 2010). Physician opinion answers questions about the diagnosis and causation and serves as baseline evidence. Review of the current scientific literature about an impairment provides the expert with up-to-date knowledge about health and functional outcomes.

After completing the needs analysis, the occupational therapy expert's first presentation of evidence to the court is in written form. A medical–legal report includes the expert's opinion of the impact of the impairment and resulting disability on occupational performance and quality of life. The action demand in the report must be clear, concise, and compelling. The report must speak to the audience, in this case lawyers and judges. The report must be neither too dense nor too simple; the goal is to educate the audience in a succinct way, providing evidence to inform decision making.

Needs in a medical–legal report must be accompanied by costs. The occupational therapy expert must have extensive knowledge about resources such as services, assistive devices, mobility aids, and so forth to prescribe the required items. The expert must also be able to predict at what points over the lifespan a client will need resources. Some future resource needs must be predicted from experiential or scientific evidence. The cost of the items must be included, along with replacement intervals (e.g., a manual wheelchair under warranty is expected to last 4–5 years, depending on the environment in which the wheelchair is used). The needs and cost schedule are typically presented as the final section of a report in table form. An economist then takes this information and extrapolates the settlement amount over the lifespan of the client consistent with current life expectancy statistics.

Insurance Industry Consultation

A niche area for occupational therapy is insurance claims management, in which the practitioner manages the entirety of insurance claims and may or may not acquire the services of occupational therapy practitioners. Occupational therapists are also employed as *injury management advisors (IMAs),* who are internal consultants for insurers. Their role is to advise insurance claims managers on client needs and timing of services for injury

recovery from the time of injury through return to work. These roles require knowledge of and a process for care planning. The occupational therapy team may include an occupational therapy assistant who gathers requested information under the guidance of the occupational therapist. Because insurers can be brought to court during litigation, it is advisable that the work for the insurer is guided and reported by the occupational therapist.

Some occupational therapy practitioners are employed in positions commonly referred to as *injury claims manager, insurance case manager, insurance adjuster, claims manager,* or *claims adjuster.* Often these practitioners work directly for insurance companies and make most or all decisions on insurance claims. In these roles, occupational therapy practitioners are not working under the title of *occupational therapist* but use their skills to manage injury claims. The unique occupational therapy skill sets are particularly useful to workers' compensation insurance boards and private insurers that manage workers' compensation claims. This area has employment potential for occupational therapy assistants because their intervention skills and knowledge support their ability to manage injured workers' insurance claims. Occupational therapy practitioners use task analysis to determine the cause of injury related to consideration for claim acceptance. Moreover, they use task analysis in conjunction with their own clinical understanding of the stages of recovery to help prioritize client needs and timing of services.

Insurance companies also employ occupational therapy practitioners as IMAs. The role of IMAs is to provide expertise on client needs to insurance case managers, who typically lack clinical knowledge. The IMA is the internal adviser for expectations regarding recovery times, physical and psychological rehabilitation needs, home care and home modification needs, and return-to-work planning. Traditional IMA professionals include medical doctors and rehabilitation nurses, who have knowledge pertaining to medical management, including medications. Some insurers now hire medical doctors to act as medical advisers and hire occupational therapy practitioners as IMAs. Occupational therapy practitioners are recruited because of their broad knowledge of physical and cognitive injury management and return-to-work rehabilitation skills, which set them apart from others in the industry. The IMA uses task analysis to determine the client's current status and work role and then advises the case manager on strategy options to facilitate recovery and return to work.

Return-to-Work Rehabilitation

In the *return-to-work rehabilitation* market, occupational therapy practitioners provide a holistic approach to interventions, skills to manage both the physical and the psychological impact of injuries, and tools to measure readiness to return to work.

The occupational therapy approach to return to work is unique compared with the approaches used by ergonomists, exercise physiologists, kinesiologists, nurses, physical therapists, psychologists, vocational counselors, and other professionals because the occupational therapy domain of practice is supporting health and participation in life through engagement in occupation (AOTA, 2014).

Occupational therapy practitioners use task analysis to learn a worker's preinjury job tasks and current task tolerances and determine methods to bridge the gap between the client's current status and his or her needs to achieve a successful return to work. In addition, practitioners use task analysis to assess the impact of any direct psychological injury or side effects of the impairment so that measures can be taken to appropriately address those issues.

SUMMARY

Occupation and task analysis are the art of occupational therapy practitioners, along with the ability to make recommendations that close the gap between disability and ability through resources that either resolve the client's issues or enable the client to adapt to a permanent disability. The premise is to restore a client as closely as possible to his or her customary lifestyle.

The interview is paramount because of the importance of the client's values and beliefs, sociocultural environment, and role expectations. Although the occupational therapy evaluation process requires clinical information, the practitioner must first initiate a conversational approach and remain open and adaptive to the information the client communicates. By hearing the client's story, the practitioner develops a stronger understanding of the person, including his or her values, beliefs, and priorities. This approach allows spontaneous generation of questions that probe for salient information in a natural flow of interaction. An open and adaptable interviewer facilitates openness and trust in the client.

REFERENCES

American Occupational Therapy Association. (2014). Occupational therapy practice framework: Domain and process (3rd ed.). *American Journal of Occupational Therapy, 68*(Suppl. 1), S1–48. http://dx.doi.org/10.5014/ajot.2014.682006

Harris, C. (2011, February/March). Unraveling the complexity of future care costs and life care plans. *Claims Canada*, pp. 13–18.

Katz, R. T., & Delaney, G. A. (2002). Life care planning. *Physical Medicine and Rehabilitation Clinics of North America, 13*, 387–303.

Lacerte, M., & Johnson, C. B. (2013). Life care planning. *Physical Medicine and Rehabilitation Clinics, 24*(3), xv–xvi.

McColl, M. A. (2011). *Spirituality and occupational therapy.* Ottawa, ON: CAOT Publications.

Sherer, M., Madison, C. F., & Hannay, J. (2000). A review of outcome after moderate and severe closed head injury with an introduction to life care planning. *Journal of Head Trauma Rehabilitation, 15*, 767–782.

Skubik-Peplaski, C., Paris, C., Boyle, D. C., & Culpert, A. (Eds.). (2009). *Applying the Occupational Therapy Practice Framework: The Cardinal Hill Occupational Participation Process in client-centered care.* Bethesda, MD: AOTA Press.

Townsend, E. A., & Polatajko, H. J. (2007). *Enabling occupation II: Advancing an occupational therapy vision of health, well-being, and justice through occupation.* Ottawa, ON: CAOT Publications.

Weed, R. O., & Berens, D. E. (Eds.). (2010). *Life care planning and case management handbook.* Boca Raton, FL: CRC Press.

World Health Organization. (2001). *International classification of functioning, disability and health.* Geneva: Author.

Zasler, N. D., Ameis, A., & Ridick-Grisham, S. N. (2013). Life Care planning after traumatic brain injury. *Physical Medicine and Rehabilitation Clinics of North America, 24*, 445–465.

Part II. Occupation and Intervention Strategies

Occupations Across the Lifespan

7

Occupational therapists have the knowledge and skills in the biological, physical, social and behavioral sciences to evaluate and intervene with individuals across the life course.

—American Occupational Therapy Association (2011, p. S46)

LEARNING OBJECTIVES

At the completion of this chapter, readers will be able to

- Understand the lifespan transitions that influence engagement in occupations and participation in contexts and
- Describe how the dynamic interaction among persons, environments, and occupations is consistent across the lifespan.

KEY TERMS

Adolescence
Adolescent occupations
Adulthood
Adult occupations
Childhood
Childhood occupations

Family
Older adulthood
Older adult occupations
Stigma
Therapeutic play

Lifespan transitions influence engagement in occupations and participation in contexts. Newborns begin to develop performance skills (e.g., feeding) and patterns (e.g., routines) during the first few days after their birth, and young infants engage in increasingly complex occupations through participation in activities of daily living (ADLs), social interactions, and play. Daily life occupations provide tremendous opportunities for learning during the early years; these experiences lay the foundation for further refinement of performance skills and patterns during the preschool years and for acquisition of knowledge and application of skills during the school years.

Engagement in occupations during childhood leads to the development of identity, social skills, emotional well-being, and prevocational pursuits in adolescence and, later, to the vocational pursuits and expanded diversity of social interactions in adulthood. Because the maintenance of health and well-being during older adulthood seems to be predicated on developmental and occupational history, among other things, occupational therapy practitioners require an understanding of lifespan trajectories and transitions.

CHILDHOOD OCCUPATIONS

Childhood encompasses ages birth to 11 years and is the period of life in which they are prepared for adulthood (Segal, 2014). Case-Smith (2010) described childhood as "hopeful, joyful, and ever new" (p. 1). The role of occupational therapy practitioners who work with children and collaborate with parents, caregivers, and other stakeholders is to enhance children's engagement in their occupations and participation in their contexts.

> Occupational therapists are responsible for formal evaluation and also are accountable for the safety and effectiveness of the service delivery process, including intervention planning, implementation, outcome review, and dismissal/discharge. The occupational therapy assistant implements the intervention plan under the supervision of and in partnership with the therapist. (American Occupational Therapy Association [AOTA], 2011, p. S52)

Practitioners seek to support *childhood occupations*, which include ADLs, play, education, social participation, and leisure. Occupational therapy practitioners first evaluate individual children or the status of a population of children to identify underlying performance skills and patterns, as well as contexts, activity demands, and client factors (both internal and external to the client) that support or hinder participation in areas of occupation. The purposes of the evaluation process are to profile occupational history and identify interests, values, and needs; analyze activity demands

and contextual characteristics; and understand the concerns of the family, school, and community.

For an individual child, primary sources of information for an occupational profile are interviews with parents, teachers, the child, and caregivers. The occupational therapy practitioner also observes actual performance in the child's customary environments to identify the contextual components that support or hinder engagement in occupations. Finally, standardized and informal evaluation tools can help occupational therapists confirm their hypotheses regarding performance skills and patterns and client factors that contribute to or hinder engagement and participation (see Case Example 7.1 and Exhibit 7.1).

In collaboration with parents; day care, preschool, and school staff members; the child; and other stakeholders, practitioners then develop intervention plans to address target outcomes for their pediatric clients. The practitioner must consider whether the intervention should focus on acquiring or restoring physical, cognitive, or behavioral function; bridging performance skills via adaptation through modified techniques or equipment; or focusing on adaptation as a long-term solution to performance skills issues.

The primary therapeutic medium used in remedial or restorative approaches to intervention with children is *therapeutic play*. When a child needs to develop particular performance skills and patterns, occupational therapy practitioners identify purposeful and therapeutic activities and artfully blend these activities into the typical daily routine of the child and family. Play delights a child and has added purpose other than entertainment and exercise; purposeful play activities are therapeutic when they are relevant, meaningful, and goal directed; elicit coordination among sensorimotor, cognitive, perceptual, and psychosocial systems; and promote mastery and feelings of self-competence (AOTA, 1993, 2014; Fidler & Fidler, 1978).

(text continues on page 98)

CASE EXAMPLE 7.1. JONESY AS A CHILD: DEVELOPMENTAL DELAY

Jonesy is a 3-year-old child with generalized developmental delay of fine motor and language skills and has been assessed by a team at the Children's Hospital. The family expressed the desire to have an occupational therapy practitioner engage with Jonesy in their home and develop therapeutic strategies that could be incorporated into daily life and to receive training to carry out the home program.

EXHIBIT 7.1. CLIENT PROFILE AND TASK ANALYSIS FORM: JONESY (AGE 3 YEARS)

CLIENT PROFILE

Name: Jonesy	Birthdate:	Age at assessment: 3
Advocates:	**Education:** n/a **Work occupation:** n/a	
Diagnoses: Developmental delay	**Current interventions:** 1. Occupational therapy 2. Speech–language therapy 3. Early intervention home program	

Referral source: Children's Hospital. Jonesy has a generalized developmental delay. The family is eager to incorporate therapeutic strategies into Jonesy's day-to-day activities to enhance his learning.

PERSONAL INFORMATION

Family unit	Father: age 26 years (accountant) Mother: age 25 years (stays home; trained as nurse) Brother: age 11 months
Caregiver(s)	Stay-at-home mother and live-in grandparents
Roles and responsibilities (e.g., student, spouse, parent, friend, worker)	1. Son 2. Big brother 3. Grandson
Home environment (e.g., home design, number of people living in the home)	Suburban townhouse; 6 people live in the home. Grandparents are temporarily living in the home to assist with child care (their home is 200 miles away).
Community context (e.g., rural, urban, metro; single-family home, residential care)	A small close-knit community that is supportive of each other and offers play date opportunities for Jonesy.
School or work context (e.g., public, special, or private school; stationary or travel location for work)	n/a
Client priorities (Jonesy's parents are the proxy for his priorities.)	1. Develop fine motor skills to the 2-year-old level. 2. Develop balance for better walking and play. 3. Communicate in simple sentences with others. 4. Develop eating skills using a spoon and cup by himself.
Values/beliefs/spirituality (e.g., principles, standards, beliefs, personal quest)	All children deserve a chance. Parents are fully prepared to give time and effort to developing both of their children, with one parent staying home until the youngest child is in 3rd grade.

(Continued)

EXHIBIT 7.1. CLIENT PROFILE AND TASK ANALYSIS FORM: JONESY (AGE 3 YEARS) *(Cont.)*

SUMMARY, PLAN, AND GOALS

Assessments completed (formal and observational):
Practitioner–client plan (e.g., further formal and observational assessments, inclusion of others): Determine which pediatric assessments will be most applicable to the case. Development of a home program, goals, and reevaluation plan.

Tasks Requiring Assessment or Intervention	
Short-term goals (Primarily client driven, measurable, global task, or activity achievements)	**Long-term objectives** (Primarily practitioner driven, measurable, incremental, stepwise, or mini achievements)
1. Fine motor skills in free play and formal assessment of developmental stage	1.a. Make recognizable play dough figures. 1.b. Be able to put together and take apart objects using large, plastic, interlocking brick set.
2. Gross motor skills in free play and formal assessment of developmental stage	2.a. Learn to push himself with his legs while seated on his push car. 2.b. Learn to peddle his wide, seated plastic tractor.
3. Feeding assessment and provision of a home program with reevaluation plan	3.a. Feed self with built-up handled fork and spoon. 3.b. Feed self with age-appropriate fork and spoon.
4. Coordination of program planning with the speech therapist and early intervention worker who is available to work in the home	4.a. A case coordinator is in place to assist the family with acquiring the needed interventions and resources for Jonesy. 4.b. Funding is in place for the home-based services through application to organizations that support the needs of children in the community (e.g., Easter Seals).

TASKS ANALYZED

Occupation or Activity	Tasks (specific activity component)	Context or Environment (external and internal)
Activities of daily living	Eating Bathing Toilet training	Observed at mealtime at his home Parent description of challenges Review of attempts made
Play	Playing with toys Playing with others	Observed in free play at home. Observed on a play date.

ANALYSIS (OF PERFORMANCE SKILLS)

Performance Skills	Client Challenges (Performance qualifier)
Rating: 0 = *no restriction,* 1 = *mild limitation,* 2 = *moderate restriction,* 3 = *severe restriction,* 4 = *complete impairment*	

Motor and praxis	Rating
Posture	1
Mobility	2
Coordination	2
Strength	2
Effort	1
Energy	1
Execution	3
Process skills	**Rating**
Mental energy	3
Knowledge	3
Organization	3
Adaptation	3
Social interaction skills	**Rating**
Communication posture	0
Gestures	1
Initiation	2
Information exchange	3
Acknowledging	3
Taking turns	3

ANALYSIS (OF PERFORMANCE PATTERNS)

Performance Patterns	Daily Life Activities	Client Challenges (skill deficits and context restrictions)
Habits (Automatic and integrated behaviors)	Morning washing and brushing teeth	Jonesy is dependent on others to initiate and execute these tasks.
Routines (Regular activities that provide daily structure)	Jonesy wakes in the morning to wash his hands and face before eating. Breakfast occurs with the family. After breakfast, he washes his hands and face, brushes his teeth, and gets dressed for the day.	Jonesy is dependent on others to initiate and execute all these tasks. He requires one-on-one assistance with eating, as he must be cued to scoop with a spoon and to use two hands on his cup when drinking. He becomes distracted and will not progress with eating unless he is cued.

(Continued)

EXHIBIT 7.1. CLIENT PROFILE AND TASK ANALYSIS FORM: JONESY (AGE 3 YEARS) *(Cont.)*

Roles (Expected behaviors and responsibilities)	Jonesy is a member of his family and expected to listen to his parents and grandparents and interact with his brother.	Jonesy is often distracted from cuing that is provided by his parents and grandparents. This results in an extraordinary amount of time to get through his daily routines. He is somewhat more attentive to the cues from his brother.
Rituals (Customary cultural and social activities)	On a regular basis his parents and grandparents take him to the park and other preschool activities in the community.	Jonesy needs assistance with physical play on the playground equipment. He also needs encouragement to play cooperatively with children his age but is drawn to toddlers who enjoy parallel play.

Synopsis of performance skills and performance patterns (strengths, deficits, and challenges): Jonesy understands his daily routines, but he requires direct supervision and ongoing cuing to participate in and execute self-care activities. He has not developed adequate gross motor coordination and skills to independently play on playground equipment and thus needs direct assistance from an adult. He enjoys other children but fits best with toddler play.

OCCUPATIONAL PROFILE AND ANALYSIS OF NEEDS

Functional ability (i.e., how strengths and deficits affect ability to perform activities and tasks)	Jonesy enjoys gross motor play at the level of a toddler. He does not have the necessary foundational gross motor abilities to use preschool-level play equipment, such as trikes and swings. His fine motor skills are also delayed, and he requires continued direct intervention. His communication is delayed at the toddler level, and direct treatment is indicated.
Activity tolerance (e.g., physical and mental fatigue levels, energy to complete activities and tasks, temporal and environmental contexts)	Because he does not engage in spontaneous and active physical play, he has not developed the endurance expected at his age. He tires easily and needs to have quiet time after about 10 minutes of active play.
Effect on occupational performance (reflect on client roles, responsibilities, and priorities)	Without age-appropriate gross motor, fine motor, and speech and language skills, he is unable to play alongside his peers. He requires supervision, assistance, and cuing from an adult to participate in self-care and play tasks.
Intervention needs (e.g., physical, cognitive, emotional, social)	Physical therapy, occupational therapy, speech and language therapy, and integrated home program
Resource needs (e.g., assistive devices or equipment, technology)	Utensils with built-up handles to assist with grip
Program needs (e.g., day programs, return-to-work programs, socialization)	Specialized play program that includes interventions and strategies

Outlook (practitioner projection of long-term needs and life care planning)	Jonesy's prognosis for closing his developmental gaps is poor. The aim of interventions must be to advance him as far as possible in his development. Initially, this means developing basic ADLs and participation in integrated peer play with children as close as possible to his age level.

GUIDELINES AND CHECKLIST FOR TASK ANALYSIS

Areas of Occupation

Activities of daily living	**Instrumental activities of daily living**
☑ Bathing and showering	☐ Care of others
☑ Bowel and bladder management	☐ Care of pets
☑ Dressing	☐ Child rearing
☑ Eating and swallowing	☐ Communication management
☑ Feeding	☐ Driving and community mobility
☑ Functional mobility	☐ Financial management
☐ Personal device care	☐ Home establishment
☑ Personal hygiene and grooming	☐ Home management and maintenance
☐ Sexual activity	☐ Meal preparation and cleanup
☐ Toileting and toilet hygiene	☐ Religious and spiritual observance
	☐ Safety and emergency maintenance
	☐ Shopping

Rest and sleep	**Play**
☐ Rest and relaxation	☑ Peer interaction
☐ Sleep participation	☑ Play exploration
☐ Sleep preparation	☑ Play participation

Leisure	**Social participation**
☐ Customary activities or hobbies	☐ Community
☐ Leisure exploration	☐ Family
☐ Leisure participation	☑ Peer or friend

Education	**Work**
☐ Access issues	☐ Employment interests and pursuits
☐ Formal education participation	☐ Employment seeking and acquisition
☐ Informal personal education or exploration	☐ Job performance
☐ Informal personal education participation	☐ Retirement preparation and adjustment
	☐ Volunteer exploration
	☐ Volunteer participation

Client Factors

Body functions and structures *Physical*	**Body functions and structures** *Sensory and pain*
☐ Cardiovascular and hematological systems	☐ Hearing functions
☐ Digestive, metabolic, and endocrine systems	☐ Pain grading and description
☐ Genitourinary and reproductive functions	☐ Seeing and related functions

(Continued)

**EXHIBIT 7.1. CLIENT PROFILE AND TASK
ANALYSIS FORM: JONESY (AGE 3 YEARS)** *(Cont.)*

☑ Movement-related functions	☐ Tactile functions
☐ Respiratory and immunological systems	☐ Taste and smell functions
☐ Skin and related structure functions	☐ Temperature and pressure reception
☑ Voice and speech functions	☑ Vestibular and proprioceptive functions

Body functions: Mental	**Body functions: Mental**
Specific mental functions	*Global mental functions*
☑ Attention	☐ Consciousness
☐ Emotional	☐ Energy and drive
☐ Experience of self and time	☐ Orientation
☐ Higher-level cognitive	☐ Sleep
☑ Motor sequencing	☐ Temperament and personality
☐ Memory	
☐ Perception	
☐ Thought	

Values, Beliefs, and Spirituality

Values	**Beliefs and spirituality**
☐ Meaningful qualities	☐ Cognitive content health as true
☐ Principles	☐ Guiding actions
☐ Standards	☐ Life meaning and purpose

Activity and Occupational Demands

Objects and their properties	**Space demands**
☑ Inherent properties (e.g., heavy, light)	☐ Size, arrangement, surface, lighting
☑ Required tools, materials, equipment	

Social demands	**Sequence and timing**
☐ Cultural context	☑ Sequence and timing
☑ Social environment	☑ Specific steps

Required actions and performance skills	**Required body functions and structures**
☑ Cognitive	☐ Anatomical parts
☑ Communication and interaction	☐ Level of consciousness
☑ Emotional and social	☐ Mobility of joints
☑ Motor and praxis	
☑ Sensory–perceptual	

Performance Skills

Motor skills	**Process skills**
☑ Movement actions or behaviors	☐ Judgment
☑ Skilled purposeful movements	☐ Select and sequence objects or tools
☑ Ability to carry out learned movement	☐ Organize and prioritize
	☐ Create and problem solve
	☐ Multitask

Social interaction skills
- ☐ Identify, manage, and express feelings
- ☐ On a one-to-one basis
- ☐ In groups
- ☑ Communication and interaction skills

Performance Patterns

Habits	**Routines**
☑ Automatic behavior	☑ Observable patterns of behavior
☑ Repeated activities	☑ Time commitment
☐ Good, bad, or impoverished	☐ Satisfying, promoting, or damaging
Roles	**Rituals**
☑ Set of expected behaviors	☐ Symbolic actions
☑ Social or cultural	☐ Spiritual, cultural, or social
☑ Within context	☐ Link to values and beliefs

Contexts and Environments

Cultural	**Personal**
☐ Customs and beliefs	☐ Age and gender
☑ Activity patterns	☐ Socioeconomic status
☑ Expectations	☐ Educational status
Temporal	**Virtual**
☐ Location of performance in time	☐ Communication environment
☑ Experience shaped by engagement	
Physical	**Social and political**
☑ Natural environment (e.g., geography)	☑ Relationship to individuals
☐ Built environment (e.g., building, furniture)	☐ Relationship to organizations or systems

TASK ANALYSIS TEMPLATE

An individual form is required for each task that is examined.
Task:

Task Demands	**Action Demands** (What is required of the person to do the task)	**Client Challenges** (Availability of required body functions and structures)
Objects used (e.g., equipment, technology)	Builtup handles on utensils	To sustain a grasp on a utensil to support self-feeding
Space demands (e.g., physical context)	Supportive playground equipment for his yard to enhance his opportunities for semi-independent play	The playground equipment in the local park does not provide the support Jonesy needs for semi-independent play.

(Continued)

EXHIBIT 7.1. CLIENT PROFILE AND TASK ANALYSIS FORM: JONESY (AGE 3 YEARS) *(Cont.)*

Social demands (e.g., social environment and context)	A suitable play group is needed for Jonesy.	Jonesy continues to parallel play with toddlers. He has not learned to actively and cooperatively play with his peer group.
Sequence and timing (e.g., process to carry out the task)	Jonesy requires one-to-one assistance and cuing for all basic ADLs.	Jonesy is functioning at less than a 2-year level in his basic ADLs.
Required actions and performance skills (e.g., basic requirements)	Self-feeding, toilet training, active motor play, and language development are needed for Jonesy to progress to a preschool program.	Jonesy has a global delay across performance areas (delay of more than 1 year).

Note. ADLs = activities of daily living.

Occupational therapy practitioners also use compensation and adaptation approaches to intervention to revise current contexts or activity demands and give children the opportunity to learn and practice new methods that support their engagement in occupations.

ADOLESCENT OCCUPATIONS

The decade of *adolescence* (ages 11–18 years) is a time of rapid change. Adolescents undergo a transition from their childhood roles of dependency and reliance on parents and others to adult roles that are marked by emotional independence from parents and self-regulation. Adolescence is also a time for further development of performance skills and patterns and alteration in body structures and functions. *Adolescent occupations* undergo a transition from childhood roles of dependency and reliance on parents to greater self-reliance and development of self-identity. Adolescents continue to establish their self-identity, develop an enhanced interest in sexuality, move toward self-sufficiency, and increase their competence and maturity.

Social obstacles and social *stigma* play a dominant role during the adolescent period. Gray and Hahn (1997) defined *stigma* as "an undesirable difference that becomes a basis for separating an individual bearing such traits from the rest of society" (p. 395). Others impose stigma, and adolescents instinctively know and are acutely aware of any deviation in their appearance or traits that separate them from their peer group. For adolescents, the struggle to reconcile reality with a desired image is constant, and any dissonance can compromise self-image and self-esteem. Living with a disability intensifies the challenges adolescents confront in their efforts to adapt to social and cultural norms.

Issues for families and parents change as children progress through developmental periods, with adolescence marking a critical evolution in the roles of both child and parent. Relationships with parents and families are often strained during this phase of life for adolescents with special needs as they seek to overcome isolation from their peers and stigma related to their activity limitations and participation restrictions. The family, whose physical and emotional resources may already be depleted or exhausted, often faces increased concern about the child's potential for isolation and vulnerability as he or she begins to move away from the familiar structures of the educational system to the community at large. Such concerns do not end when the child reaches adulthood; families of people who have disabilities often continue to experience anxiety about future options for independent living and the aging and eventual death of the parents.

Adolescents must develop skills for basic and instrumental activities of daily living (IADLs), education, work, leisure, and social participation to optimize their potential for a successful transition to the roles they will assume in their adult years. Because performance contexts—educational systems and workplaces—are so important to successful entry into adulthood, occupational therapy intervention can be targeted to these contexts to ensure that they are welcoming and accommodating. Education and work opportunities are dramatically reduced for people with physical,

mental, and communication and interaction disabilities (McNeil, 1997). For some adolescents, the challenge is to match abilities with an appropriate vocational training, sheltered workshop, or community placement that will prepare them for and sustain them through adulthood. In Case Example 7.2 and Exhibit 7.2, Jonesy is now an adolescent, moving rapidly toward young adulthood.

(text continues on page 107)

CASE EXAMPLE 7.2. JONESY AS AN ADOLESCENT: DEVELOPMENTAL DELAY

Jonesy participates in a special education program and is seen for follow-up by the Children's Hospital. Because he requires resource room help at school and an individualized education program, he is pulled out of the regular classrooms for a half a day. Although not intended, this segregates him from many of his peers, and he has not developed friendships within the larger student body, who frequently exclude him from activities. Jonesy's family requests that an occupational therapy consultant work with the school and the community to develop strategies for increased inclusion with his peers.

As Jonesy moves toward young adulthood, his parents are concerned that he has not developed the skills needed to live independently as an adult. They request that the occupational therapy practitioner analyze Jonesy's capacities and develop strategies for developing IADLs to support his transition toward independent functioning at school. The long-term goal is to build adequate skills for greater independence in adulthood by the time he is age 20 years.

EXHIBIT 7.2. CLIENT PROFILE AND TASK ANALYSIS FORM: JONESY (ADOLESCENT)

CLIENT PROFILE

Name: Jonesy	Birthdate:		Age at assessment: 14
Advocates:	Work occupation: Student		
Diagnoses: Developmental delay Emotional disturbance	Current interventions: 1. Occupational therapy 2. Special education 3. Boys and Girls Club		
Referral source: Children's Hospital. This family has requested occupational therapy intervention to find ways to help Jonesy better integrate with his peer group and in the community as well as to increase his skills for future independent living.			

PERSONAL INFORMATION

Family unit	Father: age 37 years (accountant) Mother: age 36 years (stays home [never returned to the workforce]; trained as nurse) Sister: age 11 years
Caregiver(s)	Stay-at-home mother and shared evenings and weekend care from father

(Continued)

EXHIBIT 7.2. CLIENT PROFILE AND TASK ANALYSIS FORM: JONESY (ADOLESCENT) *(Cont.)*

Roles and responsibilities (e.g., student, spouse, parent, friend, worker)	1. Son 2. Brother 3. Student
Home environment (e.g., home design, number of people living in the home)	Suburban townhouse; 4 people live in the home.
Community context (e.g., rural, urban, metro; single-family home, residential care)	The small, close-knit community is supportive of each other. However, Jonesy has no close friends who spend time with him out of school, so his parents enrolled him in the Boys and Girls Club to give him a social venue.
School or work context (e.g., public, special, or private school; stationary or travel location for work)	Jonesy goes to a special resource classroom in the morning. He reintegrates in the afternoon for social studies, art, music, and physical education. The other kids have grown up with him and are very accepting but often exclude him from their group work or conversations.
Client priorities Jonesy states what he wants, and his parents help him with priority setting.	1. Stay in the classroom for the full day. 2. Develop friends who will go to the movies with him. 3. Join a swim club to compete. 4. Learn to take public transit to the Boys and Girls Club.
Values/beliefs/spirituality (e.g., principles, standards, beliefs, personal quest)	Jonesy wants to be more independent but does not have the skills. His parents would like to work on these skills for greater independence, so he has more options for independent living as an adult.

SUMMARY, PLAN, AND GOALS

Assessments completed (formal and observational):
Practitioner–client plan (e.g., further formal and observational assessments, inclusion of others): Determine which adolescent assessments will be most applicable to the case to add formal assessment to information gathered through observation and informal assessment. Establish a working relationship with Jonesy's parents, school personnel, and facilitators at the Boys and Girls Club to integrate his goals into his everyday environments and to measure and update intervention goals every 3 months.

Tasks Requiring Assessment or Intervention

Short-term goals (Primarily client driven, measurable, global task, or activity achievements)	**Long-term objectives** (Primarily practitioner driven, measurable, incremental, stepwise, or mini achievements)
1. Develop a skills training program that can initially be implemented with the occupational therapy assistant and then by his parents.	1.a. Learn to navigate in the community by bus and on foot while focusing on signage and landmarks for reference. 1.b. Learn to navigate in the community by bus and on foot via map applications on smartphone and tablet.
2. Meet with the special educator and teacher to determine what IADL skills can be taught and practiced within the school program (e.g., money handling).	2.a. Learn how to make wise purchase decisions when buying from the school cafeteria and bookshop. 2.b. Learn how to make wise purchase decisions when on monthly school outings in the community.

3. Observation of Jonesy at the Boys and Girls Club by the occupational therapist to determine whether and how he is approaching social situations with his peers outside of the school environment.	3.a. Attend movies twice monthly with a small group of club friends during club nights. 3.b. Join swim club that supports lower tiered competitions, as he does not have the stamina and power to compete at the upper tiers. Club friend to attend 2 of the 3 weekly sessions.
4. Observation of Jonesy in his classroom by the occupational therapist to determine whether and how he is integrating with his school peers and to identify any social barriers.	4.a. Classrooms to have assigned seating vs. free seating. Jonesy will be placed at tables and desks with students considered most open to interact with him. 4.b. The teachers will require Jonesy to answer verbal questions at an equal rate to his classmates. *Note.* He will typically require more teacher guidance with finding the correct answer.

TASKS ANALYZED

Occupation or Activity	Tasks (specific activity component)	Context or Environment (external and internal)
Instrumental activities of daily living	Navigation in familiar setting	Observed in hallways walking to classes and making his way to the school bus.
	Navigation in unfamiliar setting	Observed suburb map reading, bus route map reading, and bus time schedules in a life skills class session in the special education classroom.
	Money management	Observed paying for school lunch with meal ticket and practicing buying and selling in a life skills class session in the special education classroom.
Leisure and social participation	Socializing	Observed at lunch in school, in hallways walking between classes, in physical education class, and in the special education classroom.
	Playing sports	Observed in physical education class playing volleyball.

ANALYSIS (OF PERFORMANCE SKILLS)

Performance Skills	Client Challenges (Performance qualifier)
Rating: 0 = *no restriction,* 1 = *mild limitation,* 2 = *moderate restriction,* 3 = *severe restriction,* 4 = *complete impairment*	
Motor and praxis	**Rating**
Posture	1
Mobility	1

(Continued)

**EXHIBIT 7.2. CLIENT PROFILE AND TASK
ANALYSIS FORM: JONESY (ADOLESCENT)** *(Cont.)*

Coordination	I
Strength	I
Effort	I
Energy	I
Execution	I
Process skills	**Rating**
Mental energy	I
Knowledge	2
Organization	2
Adaptation	2
Social interaction skills	**Rating**
Communication posture	I
Gestures	I
Initiation	2
Information exchange	2
Acknowledging	I
Taking turns	I

ANALYSIS (OF PERFORMANCE PATTERNS)

Performance Patterns	Daily Life Activities	Client Challenges (skill deficits and context restrictions)
Habits (Automatic and integrated behaviors)	• Polite to others. • Quiet and does not disrupt class setting. • Kind toward others and always willing to lend a hand if asked.	His demeanor has helped him to be accepted in the integrated class by his peers, but without assistance from others, he can become a bit invisible and socially isolated. This is the case in his special education and integrated classrooms.
Routines (Regular activities that provide daily structure)	• Attends school 5 days per week. • Attends Boys and Girls Club every Tuesday. • Completes homework as needed Sunday, Monday, and Thursday. • Attends swimming stroke improvement lessons at same pool as his sister on Saturdays and Sundays.	• Social isolation as previously described. • Social as previously described. • Requires increased time to complete tasks that have been modified compared with peers'. • Diminished coordination and strength results in poorer execution of strokes, quicker fatigue, and slower lap speeds.

	• Parents are teaching him how to do laundry and stove cooking safely. • Cleans his bedroom and bathroom on Saturday.	• Requires direct supervision for accuracy and or safety. • Requires direct supervision using safer bathroom cleaning agents.
Roles (Expected behaviors and responsibilities)	• Student • Swimmer • Budding home manager • Club friend • Family member	• As described.
Rituals (Customary cultural and social activities)	• Attend school. • Attend swim school. • Attend Boys and Girls Club.	• Difficulty with independent navigation and transportation to community activities. • Decreased independence making purchases.

Synopsis of performance skills and performance patterns (strengths, deficits, and challenges): Jonesy has a kind and warm disposition; he is quiet and obliging almost to a fault regarding social interactions. His coordination and strength are somewhat diminished, which is demonstrated in reduced pen-and-paper and fine motor art applications. In addition, they result in his experiencing fatigue during swimming and other sport activities. He has cognitive deficits resulting in difficulty attaining and managing certain life skills necessary for independent community access and participation.

OCCUPATIONAL PROFILE AND ANALYSIS OF NEEDS

Functional ability (i.e., how strengths and deficits affect ability to perform activities and tasks)	He is kind and treated respectfully in the classroom but has difficulty making meaningful friendships. He is aware of this isolation and wants to change it. He also enjoys swimming regularly and seeks to improve his stroke and strength. He wants to compete, which shows drive, initiative, and resiliency, because he knows he may not always win.
Activity tolerance (e.g., physical and mental fatigue levels, energy to complete activities and tasks, temporal and environmental contexts)	He physically fatigues, likely in part because of his diminished coordination and strength. However, he continues to participate in sports. He mentally fatigues when challenged to work outside of his comfort zone or usual capacity.
Effect on occupational performance (reflect on client roles, responsibilities, and priorities)	He is socially isolated. He lacks independence in home management activities. He lacks independence in community access and activities.
Intervention needs (e.g., physical, cognitive, emotional, social)	Social and cognitive: He requires increased structure by classroom teachers to facilitate integration with peers. He requires life skills training to increase independence in community. He requires club friends to increase socialization into the community. He requires family assistance to increase home management skills.

(Continued)

**EXHIBIT 7.2. CLIENT PROFILE AND TASK
ANALYSIS FORM: JONESY (ADOLESCENT)** *(Cont.)*

Resource needs (e.g., assistive devices or equipment, technology)	• Smartphone and tablet technology for community independence and safety. • Bus passes and taxi vouchers to facilitate transport independence and safety.
Program needs (e.g., day programs, return-to-work programs, socialization)	• Boys and Girls Club participation for movies and swim classes. • Life skills training in special education. • Home management skills training at home.
Outlook (practitioner projection of long-term needs and life care planning)	He will likely need ongoing assistance for independent community living. Family should start exploring community options now to focus life skills training toward that aim.

GUIDELINES AND CHECKLIST FOR TASK ANALYSIS

Occupation

Activities of daily living	**Instrumental activities of daily living**
☐ Bathing and showering	☐ Care of others
☐ Bowel and bladder management	☐ Care of pets
☐ Dressing	☐ Child rearing
☐ Eating and swallowing	☐ Communication management
☐ Feeding	☑ Driving and community mobility
☐ Functional mobility	☑ Financial management
☐ Personal device care	☐ Home establishment
☐ Personal hygiene and grooming	☑ Home management and maintenance
☐ Sexual activity	☐ Meal preparation and cleanup
☐ Toileting and toilet hygiene	☐ Religious and spiritual observance
	☐ Safety and emergency maintenance
	☐ Shopping

Rest and sleep	**Play**
☐ Rest and relaxation	☑ Peer interaction
☐ Sleep participation	☐ Play exploration
☐ Sleep preparation	☑ Play participation

Leisure	**Social participation**
☐ Customary activities or hobbies	☑ Community
☑ Leisure exploration	☐ Family
☑ Leisure participation	☑ Peer or friend

Education	**Work**
☐ Access issues	☐ Employment interests and pursuits
☑ Formal education participation	☐ Employment seeking and acquisition
☐ Informal personal education or exploration	☐ Job performance
☐ Informal personal education participation	☐ Retirement preparation and adjustment
	☐ Volunteer exploration
	☐ Volunteer participation

Client Factors

Body functions and structures
Physical
- ☐ Cardiovascular and hematological systems
- ☐ Digestive, metabolic, and endocrine systems
- ☐ Genitourinary and reproductive functions
- ☐ Movement-related functions
- ☐ Respiratory and immunological systems
- ☐ Skin and related structure functions
- ☐ Voice and speech functions

Body functions and structures
Sensory and pain
- ☐ Hearing functions
- ☐ Pain grading and description
- ☐ Seeing and related functions
- ☐ Tactile functions
- ☐ Taste and smell functions
- ☐ Temperature and pressure reception
- ☐ Vestibular and proprioceptive functions

Body functions: Mental
Specific mental functions
- ☐ Attention
- ☐ Emotional
- ☐ Experience of self and time
- ☑ Higher-level cognitive
- ☐ Motor sequencing
- ☐ Memory
- ☐ Perception
- ☑ Thought

Body functions: Mental
Global mental functions
- ☐ Consciousness
- ☐ Energy and drive
- ☐ Orientation
- ☐ Sleep
- ☐ Temperament and personality

Values, Beliefs, and Spirituality

Values
- ☐ Meaningful qualities
- ☐ Principles
- ☐ Standards

Beliefs and spirituality
- ☐ Cognitive content health as true
- ☐ Guiding actions
- ☐ Life meaning and purpose

Activity and Occupational Demands

Objects and their properties
- ☐ Inherent properties (e.g., heavy, light)
- ☐ Required tools, materials, equipment

Space demands
- ☐ Size, arrangement, surface, lighting

Social demands
- ☐ Cultural context
- ☑ Social environment

Sequence and timing
- ☐ Sequence and timing
- ☑ Specific steps

Required actions and performance skills
- ☑ Cognitive
- ☑ Communication and interaction
- ☑ Emotional and social
- ☐ Motor and praxis
- ☐ Sensory–perceptual

Required body functions and structures
- ☐ Anatomical parts
- ☐ Level of consciousness
- ☐ Mobility of joints

Performance Skills

Motor skills
- ☐ Movement actions or behaviors
- ☐ Skilled purposeful movements

Process skills
- ☐ Judgment
- ☐ Select and sequence objects or tools

(Continued)

**EXHIBIT 7.2. CLIENT PROFILE AND TASK
ANALYSIS FORM: JONESY (ADOLESCENT)** *(Cont.)*

☐ Ability to carry out learned movement	☐ Organize and prioritize ☑ Create and problem solve ☑ Multitask

Social interaction skills
☐ Identify, manage, and express feelings
☑ On a one-to-one basis
☑ In groups
☑ Communication and interaction skills

Performance Patterns

Habits ☐ Automatic behavior ☐ Repeated activities ☐ Good, bad, or impoverished	**Routines** ☐ Observable patterns of behavior ☐ Time commitment ☐ Satisfying, promoting, or damaging
Roles ☐ Set of expected behaviors ☐ Social or cultural ☐ Within context	**Rituals** ☐ Symbolic actions ☐ Spiritual, cultural, or social ☐ Link to values and beliefs

Contexts and Environments

Cultural ☐ Customs and beliefs ☐ Activity patterns ☐ Expectations	**Personal** ☐ Age and gender ☐ Socioeconomic status ☐ Educational status
Temporal ☐ Location of performance in time ☐ Experience shaped by engagement	**Virtual** ☐ Communication environment
Physical ☐ Natural environment (e.g., geography) ☐ Built environment (e.g., building, furniture)	**Social and political** ☐ Relationship to individuals ☐ Relationship to organizations or systems

TASK ANALYSIS TEMPLATE

An individual form is required for each task that is examined.
Task: Taking the bus to the movies

Task Demands	**Action Demands** (What is required of the person to do the task)	**Client Challenges** (Availability of required body functions and structures)
Objects used (e.g., equipment, technology)	A smartphone and tablet with navigation applications and bus schedule applications will assist Jonesy with community access.	Jonesy will require repetitive training at home and in actual usage to learn to use these tools.

Space demands (e.g., physical context)	In the community and on the bus	New learning is difficult for Jonesy. This is especially the case in an unstructured environment such as when navigating in the community.
Social demands (e.g., social environment and context)	Jonesy feels isolated and wants friends and group interaction.	He is quiet and does not always understand the depth of discussions.
Sequence and timing (e.g., process to carry out the task)	He has to learn when to get to the bus stops and when to get off the bus.	He will have to develop an understanding of timetables on technology devices, as well as reading the timetables at bus stops.
Required actions and performance skills (e.g., basic requirements)	Ability to enter and exit the bus and walk on a moving bus	He rides the school bus daily. This is not a challenge for him.

Note. IADL = instrumental activities of daily living.

YOUNG AND MIDDLE ADULT OCCUPATIONS

Adulthood as a phase of development begins with enhanced personal freedom, choice, and responsibility as young adults begin to separate from parents and siblings. It is a time of increased responsibility as one learns to care for oneself and others emotionally, spiritually, physically, and financially. *Adult occupations* develop through the emerging adult stage of developing career roles and personal partnerships to the midlife stage of maintaining established roles in the community and society.

Many cultures celebrate a person's transition to adulthood, because it represents the achievement of a state of maturity. For example, among North American cultures, many people celebrate their transition to adulthood through high school graduation ceremonies and proms. Although these occasions do not specifically acknowledge a coming of age, they serve to recognize significant changes in life roles. Distinct events in the adult years mark transitions from adolescence to early, middle, and older adulthood. In young adulthood one chooses a lifestyle and assumes new and complex roles: friend, lover, spouse, student, colleague, boss, worker, breadwinner, volunteer, parent, and citizen, among others. The events considered most important at this stage are developing a vocational path to establish economic self-sufficiency, becoming a partner through cohabitation or marriage, and starting a family. One's identity as an adult is often shaped by the roles one assumes in society, and these roles are influenced by environmental and personal contexts. Indeed, competency as a worker is a primary social and cultural expectation of adults in most societies.

Adulthood can be turbulent yet stable, demanding yet straightforward, difficult yet rewarding. However, it is always a time of personal growth and transitions in performance patterns and lifestyles. Adults continue to experience physiological, psychological, and sociological changes after the transitions of young adulthood are over. Many of these changes reflect the societal roles of worker and provider, partner, parent, grandparent, and retiree (Matuska & Barrett, 2014). During the middle years of adulthood, adults refine their vocational choices and skills through experience in the workforce and eventually anticipate and prepare for the transition to retirement. During these years, social participation is crucial to role competency and adaptation as relationships are established and maintained with friends, lovers, spouses, partners, children, colleagues, neighbors, and others.

Although children and adolescents contribute to their communities, it is more common for adults to assume civic responsibilities and community leadership roles. Adults are paid workers, employers, organizational leaders, and volunteers. They hold responsibility for maintaining households, nurturing families, and building communities. Family units predominate in the social and cultural structure of society. *Family* is an operational term, not a categorical one; the family itself constitutes a complex and dynamic social unit (Donovan & McIntyre, 1985).

For example, the sociocultural demand of Western societies on adults to maintain highly productive career roles may become maladaptive as the family struggles to accommodate a plethora of roles and responsibilities that challenge value and belief systems around work and family roles and routines. Traumatic injury or disease may interrupt adult roles, and people challenged with resulting physical, mental, or communication and interaction disabilities must reestablish meaningful roles and patterns to resume engagement and participation.

OLDER ADULT OCCUPATIONS

The roles that people assume change across the lifespan. Children become students when they enter school, adolescents become employees when they start their first job, adults become parents when they have their first child, and older adults become retirees when they leave the workforce. Just as other stages in the lifespan require people to adapt, so too does *older adulthood,* which typically is considered the period ages 65 years or older. Older adulthood involves changes in roles and occupations due to physiological, psychological, and life circumstances that occur with aging (Segal, 2014).

Older adult occupations involve a substantial transition to new roles and activities as older adults leave the workforce and find new ways to occupy their time. People are living longer than ever before, and society and everyday life are changing so rapidly that the process of aging is much different now than in the past. Older adults have been forced to create new guidelines

for the "proper way to age" (Jackson, Mandel, Zemke, & Clark, 2001, p. 5).

Many older adults relinquish or experience a progressive loss of roles and occupations as they age. Indeed, older adults experience many life changes that place them at risk for social isolation and for loss of self-esteem and a sense of meaning in life. Changes in roles and performance patterns brought about by retirement, fixed and diminished income, loss of spouse and friends, or a decline in health can affect the breadth and depth of social participation. Conversely, occupations that older adults celebrate and that produce a sense of self-worth often seem mundane to others (e.g., going to movies, reading). These occupations have developed either over time or to adapt to a changing lifestyle and have intrinsic meaning and substantial importance to quality of life. The challenge to society and communities, therefore, is to find ways to enable older adults to age successfully.

People differ in the ways they respond to growing older. This variability may be due to personal experiences, societal expectations of appropriate roles, cohort effects, or personality factors that influence attitudes toward aging, among other factors (Bonder, 1994). Increases in the population of older adults and in life expectancy have led to an increase in the prevalence of chronic disease. The population of older adults will continue to burgeon as the Baby Boom generation ages, suggesting that the size of the population with disabilities will increase in coming years. The World Health Organization and National Institute on Aging (2011) have pointed out that the aging population is increasing in almost every country.

> The world is on the brink of a demographic milestone. Since the beginning of recorded history, young children have outnumbered their elders. In about five years time, however, the number of people aged 65 and older will outnumber children under age 5....The number of people aged 65 or older is projected to grow from an estimated 524 million in 2010 to nearly 1.5 billion in 2050, with most of the increase in developing countries. (p. 2)

According to the U.S. Bureau of the Census (2012), 13.7% of the U.S. population is ages 65 years or older. Two factors that come into play for the occupational therapy practitioner in light of these statistics are (1) disability prevention and (2) the possibility of an extended need for life care planning.

Occupational therapy practitioners providing services to older adults who have or are at risk for activity limitations and participation restrictions can use task analysis and the Client Profile and Task Analysis (CPTA) form (Appendix A) to identify performance restrictions and limitations, activity demands, and contextual variables that limit engagement. The CPTA form can then be used to gather information about the older client's supports, values, roles, and goals. This information can facilitate client and practitioner decision making concerning intervention strategies to address barriers and risks to health, safety, dignity, and independence.

SUMMARY

Individuals' occupations are in a perpetual stage of transition. The occupations of children include basic ADLs, play, education, leisure, and social participation. As children move into adolescence, occupations shift from roles of dependency and reliance on parents toward greater self-reliance and development of self-identity. In adulthood, occupations become largely related to career roles, personal partnerships, child rearing, and maintaining established roles in the community and society. Typically, the occupations of older adults transition again when they leave the workforce.

Assignment 7.1. Meaningful Occupations Across the Lifespan

1. Track the trajectory of your life through infancy, preschool, school, and work. List the occupations at each stage that had primary and secondary influences on your life and development. Identify tasks and activities associated with these occupations. What prerequisite performance skills and patterns were required of you to enable you to engage in these occupations and participate in your customary contexts during each phase of development?

2. List tasks that were meaningful during your childhood because the "choice or control of the activity" was yours (Law, 2002, p. 642). Consider when a lack of choice or control rendered a task less meaningful. Describe the value of engagement in meaningful tasks.

3. Consider the social and cultural contexts of your own adolescence. What social obstacles and cultural expectations had a significant positive or negative impact on you as an adolescent? Recall the impact of social and cultural contexts you observed over time on peers who have a disability.

4. Discuss the social and cultural expectations that influence an adult's choice of work occupations. What social and cultural expectations influenced your decision to become an occupational therapy practitioner? Share this information with others who have chosen the same career path. Describe the variability in social and cultural contexts that influenced this group of people.

5. Reflect on discussions you have had with an older adult about his or her occupational history. Consider the array of roles, occupations, tasks, and activities he or she engaged in over his or her lifespan. How might you structure an interview with an older client to establish an occupational profile during the evaluation phase of service delivery? How could this information be used during the course of intervention to ensure that occupational therapy services are meaningful?

REFERENCES

American Occupational Therapy Association. (1993). Position paper: Purposeful activity. *American Journal of Occupational Therapy, 47,* 1081–1082. http://dx.doi.org/10.5014/ajot.47.12.1081

American Occupational Therapy Association. (2011). Occupational therapy services in early childhood and school-based settings. *American Journal of Occupational Therapy, 65*(Suppl.), S46–S54. http://dx.doi.org/ajot.2011.65S46

American Occupational Therapy Association. (2014). Occupational therapy practice framework: Domain and process (3rd ed.). *American Journal of Occupational Therapy, 68*(Suppl. 1) S1–48. http://dx.doi.org/10.5014/ajot.2014.682006

Bonder, B. R. (1994). The psychosocial meaning of activity. In B. R. Bonder & M. B. Wagner (Eds.), *Functional performance in older adults* (pp. 28–40). Philadelphia: F. A. Davis.

Case-Smith, J. (2010). Foundational knowledge for occupational therapy for children. In J. Case-Smith & J. C. O'Brien (Eds.), *Occupational therapy for children* (6th ed., pp. 1–21). Maryland Heights, MO: Mosby/Elsevier.

Donovan, D. M., & McIntyre, D. (1985). *Healing the hurt child: A developmental–contextual approach.* New York: Norton.

Fidler, G. S., & Fidler, J. (1978). Doing and becoming: Purposeful action and self-actualization. *American Journal of Occupational Therapy, 32,* 305–310.

Gray, D. B., & Hahn, H. (1997). Achieving occupational goals. In C. H. Christiansen & C. M. Baum (Eds.), *Occupational therapy: Enabling function and well-being* (2nd ed., pp. 392–409). Thorofare, NJ: Slack.

Jackson, J., Mandel, D. R., Zemke, R., & Clark, F. A. (2001). Promoting quality of life in elders: An occupation-based occupational therapy program. *World Federation of Occupational Therapists Bul-letin, 43,* 5–12.

Law, M. (2002). Participation in the occupations of everyday life. *American Journal of Occupational Therapy, 56,* 640–649. http://dx.doi.org/10.5014/ajot.56.6.640

Matuska, K., & Barrett, K. (2014). Patterns of occupation. In B. A. B. Schell, G. Gillen, & M. E. Scaffa (Eds.), *Willard and Spackman's occupational therapy* (12th ed., pp. 163–172). Philadelphia: Lippincott Williams & Wilkins.

McNeil, J. M. (1997). *Americans with disabilities: 1994–95* (U.S. Bureau of the Census, Current Population Reports, P70-61). Washington, DC: U.S. Department of Commerce.

Segal, R. (2014). Dimensions of occupation across the lifespan. In J. Hinojosa & M.-L. Blount (Eds.), *The texture of life: Occupations and related activities* (4th ed., pp. 37–53). Bethesda, MD: AOTA Press.

U.S. Bureau of the Census. (2012). *U.S. Census Bureau projections show a slower growing, older, more diverse nation a half century from now.* Retrieved from https://www.census.gov/newsroom/releases/archives/population/cb12-243.html

World Health Organization, & National Institure on Aging, National Institutes of Health. (2011). *Global health and aging.* Retrieved from www.who.int/ageing/publications/global_health/en/

Play as Occupation

8

Play, especially social play with children, serves a variety of developmental functions, all of which promote children's mental health.

—Gray (2011, p. 458)

LEARNING OBJECTIVES

At the completion of this chapter, readers will be able to

- Describe the features, characteristics, and utility of purposeful play activities and
- Describe the use of task analysis in defining the motor performance skills, sensory functions, and performance contexts that are challenged during participation in play.

KEY TERMS

Activity	Performance contexts
Activity demands	Performance patterns
Free play	Physical environment
Fun	Play
Object play	Sensory impairments
Peer play	Spirit
Perceptual contexts	Spiritual context
Perceptual impairments	Temporal context
Perceptual learning	Virtual context

According to Vandenberg and Kielhofner (1982), evolutionary evidence suggests that *play* is an important factor in the evolution of humans, enabling them to learn adaptive responses. What is known from watching children is that play is internally controlled and intrinsically motivating. It focuses attention but suspends reality, stimulates behavior, requires participation, and allows freedom from externally imposed rules (Bundy, 1993).

Play consists of both action and attitude, teaches symbolic meaning, leads to the pleasure of doing, and promotes skill acquisition (Ferland, 1992; Reilly, 1974). Indeed, play is a way to rehearse for life and to assimilate learning within a cultural context (Sabonis-Chafee &

Hussey, 1998; Vandenberg & Kielhofner, 1982; Zemke & Clark, 1996). Play as a primary occupation of children is a precursor to the productive work habits, roles, and routines of adults (Reilly, 1974). To provide a broad view of play and its influence on learning, task analysis can be a valuable evaluation tool.

Psychologist Jean Piaget (1950) was among the first to document practice as a function of play and the pleasure of finding meaning in novel activities as an inherent purpose of play; to this day, this outlook on play is the overarching premise of scholars. In an overview of the nature of play, Henricks (2008) described scholars' difficulty in identifying and deciphering the activities that constitute play, which has led to the development of its many definitions. It is generally agreed, however, that play is an important aspect of human life and therefore significant in understanding human nature. Henricks (2008) noted that scholars consistently believe that "play contributes in some fashion to broader patterns of individual and social behavior or to idealized version of those behaviors" (p. 158).

Is play an action, activity, or interaction? Henricks (2008) suggested that "focusing on what individuals do and experience while they are playing—and calling those patterns 'play'—is clearly an appropriate way of defining that phenomenon" (p. 162). Thus, play can be seen as social or cultural action that includes activity and interaction.

In the *Occupational Therapy Practice Framework: Domain and Process*, (3rd ed., hereinafter, *Framework*; American Occupational Therapy Association [AOTA], 2014), play is generally viewed as an occupation—the doing or action of a child. The type of play a child engages in is the *activity*. The *Framework* defines *performance patterns* as "the habits, routines, roles, and rituals used in the process of engaging in occupations or activities; these patterns can support or hinder occupational performance" (p. S27).

Similarly, Henricks (2008) stated that play can be seen as "a pattern of individual action" (p. 176). Repetitive play can be viewed as the routine the child adopts to learn a new concept or skill through play (e.g., number games). Routines provide stability within a social structure.

PLAY AND DEVELOPMENT

Play positively influences human development. Many theories of play support "a belief that play provides more numerous opportunities for personally controlled expression than can be found in other domains of human experience" (Henricks, 2008, p. 169). Occupational therapy practitioners who use play as a health intervention infuse play experiences, playfulness, and imaginative activities into the intervention process. Play is an occupation or activity that is meaningful and valued by a child. Participation in play promotes development, and therefore, it can be used as an intervention. To use play activity in intervention, the occupational therapy practitioner first conducts a task analysis that examines the action demands of the play activity while simultaneously considering client factors and the child's performance skills.

For example, playing ball is an activity that typically starts in infancy. Balls are different sizes, which dictates whether one can be held in one hand or must be held with two hands. A ball may have different textures or weight, and a child may be sensitive to certain textures or too weak to hold a certain weight. Different performance skills are needed for the actions of rolling a ball, throwing a ball with two hands, or tossing a ball to another person. For treatment to be effective, the ball must have a size, weight, and texture that the child can manage. The action demands required for a planned game need to fit the child's functional abilities while providing a supported learning opportunity for improving ability and developing a skill.

Infants and Toddlers (Ages 0–2 Years)

The drive to play first appears in infants as they adapt the physical world to their needs (Elkind, 2008). Anything an infant grasps becomes an object on which to suck. Infants first learn about themselves and others through stretching and kicking their limbs to explore their personal space (e.g., motor play). Slightly older infants begin to differentiate themselves from others using visual and tactile information (e.g., looking at and touching a parent's face). Older infants may do mirror play, recognizing themselves as the image. For example, showing a 1-year-old child his or her dirty face in a mirror can excite and delight the child. Exploration of movement, visual information, and language represent the development of intrapersonal and interpersonal intelligence. Play "exercises and expresses intelligence" (Eberle, 2011, p. 31). A child learns to engage others in play when, for example, he or she deliberately drops a rattle for a parent to retrieve.

Preschool-Age Children (Ages 3–5 Years)

A preschooler's imagination and imaginative play arise from playful associations between objects (Elkind, 2008). Food can be quickly transformed into a face, a butterfly, and many other things. Imaginative and creative play contributes to the development of autonomy and the quest for freedom to make decisions and take action. Elkind (2008) identified another important aspect of play—love—that represents the need to express desires, feelings and emotions, although "preschoolers center their love largely on themselves" (p. 3).

Preschoolers do not like to share, not because they are selfish, but because they feel that the toy is part of them. Although preschoolers may be affectionate toward a parent or sibling, generally this affection represents their own emotional need rather than their recognition of the emotional needs of others. Preschoolers enjoy dramatic play to act out roles such as mother, father, doctor, and so forth as they experiment with and practice observed roles. In dramatic play, children's capacity for learning is limited by their social situation, their emotional condition, and their physical and intellectual development.

Young School-Age Children (Ages 6–8 Years)

Young school-age children develop higher-order skills, such as initiative, and gain a sense of independence when they begin to venture away from home to play in their neighborhoods. It is through playful experiences and engagement in play as an occupation that children develop skills, such as taking turns and using manipulative tools (e.g., pencils, scissors), and demonstrate social competency, which includes learning social rules. *Peer play* is connection or engagement in social interaction between children through play. Peer play begins with the isolated play of infants in the presence of their peers and develops into reciprocal friendships and cooperative play in the late preschool and early school years. Communication is a key component of the development of peer interactions as a child matures and can be a specific limitation for children with language deficits (e.g., autism spectrum disorder).

Elkind (2008) aptly noted that although children learn through play, learning may be limited by the social situation, emotional condition, and physical and intellectual development. Games with rules assist with the development of social understanding, emotional maturity, and physical and intellectual development. Children learn to develop strategies through games while observing others.

Older School-Age Children (Ages 9–11 Years)

As children grow and learn, play becomes more complex, with increasing levels of rules, moral judgment, and language development (Kool & Lawver, 2010). Language use has developed from infancy through the preschool years and continues to develop throughout the school years. Language acquisition becomes increasingly important for regulating emotions and bridging action with thought, which are necessary in peer play. Typically, adults guide younger children to regulate their emotions in different situations, but by age 9 years, children are expected to have learned social rules (e.g., turn taking, respect for others) and to control their emotions (e.g., anger). Understanding this concept assists practitioners in using play and play therapy as modalities for facilitating cognitive and emotional growth. Often play and play therapy for children this age is conducted in groups, which provides a coached opportunity to use communication and practice social rules that are fundamentally necessary for development into adolescence and young adulthood.

In the absence of this learning, children often face situations in social environments with which they cannot cope. This deficit may illustrate unhealthy psychological development and may lead to anxiety, unhappiness, and even depression (Gray, 2011).

Miller and Kuhaneck (2008) conducted an interesting qualitative study that examined children's perceptions of play experiences and play preferences. The 10 participants were ages 7–11 years, had typical development, spoke English, and had no medical diagnosis. Each child participated in a one-on-one semistructured interview consisting of open-ended questions focused on play choices and preferences. Children identified *fun* as the reason to continue a play activity and identified the opposite of *fun* as *boring*. It did not matter to them what the activity was, as long as it was fun and made them happy. The level of activity and amount of participation were important to the child participants. Fun was also related to movement, such as running around, and participants showed a definite preference for outdoor play. Children identified enjoyment of challenges tempered by a need to succeed. All children interviewed preferred to play with children rather than adults.

Adolescents (Ages 12–18 Years)

Adolescents often no longer wish to engage in play that resembles childhood play, but they continue to play. Adolescents engage in play activities including music appreciation, dancing, and engagement in a plethora of social and pleasure activities. Activities and tasks for adolescents must be constructed to provide them healthy opportunities to learn to get along with a broader group, solve problems, inhibit their impulses, and regulate their emotions (Gray, 2011). Practitioners guiding adolescent play should remember that meaningful play must be structured by the adolescent. In analyzing an adolescent's decrease in healthy play occupations, a practitioner must consider the adolescent's contexts or environments. For example, increased time and weight are given to schooling and to other adult-directed, school-like activities, such as homework, tutoring, and lessons (Gray, 2011). Gray's (2011) work indicates that over the past half-century, play has declined, and the mental health of children and adolescents has declined simultaneously.

DIMENSIONS OF PLAY

All of the dimensions of occupational performance influence a child's participation in the occupation of play, including performance skills and patterns, contexts, activity demands, and client factors. Conversely, play provides a vehicle for the development of performance patterns and motor, process, communication, and interaction performance skills. As Henricks (2008) aptly put it, "Play has different qualities and aspects, and it is not surprising that different scholars choose to focus on one or more of these aspects in their studies" (p. 164).

This chapter focuses on the sensory and perceptual body functions and motor performance skills and the performance contexts that are challenged during participation in the occupation of play. Task analysis of these dimensions reflects Henricks's (2008) analysis of play, in which Piaget's (1962) work was reviewed. Henricks described *play* as "a project of personal control and self-direction, a way of building needed skills and acquiring the confidence to use those skills for wider situations" (p. 161).

Assignment 8.1. The Activity of Play

1. What gross motor play and leisure activities did you participate in and enjoy during early childhood? What characteristics and qualities of these activities influenced the activity demands required of you? *Activity demands* are the aspects of an activity (e.g., required equipment and space, process used to carry out the activity, required actions) and the required underlying body functions and structures needed to carry out the activity.

2. Read "Position Paper: Purposeful Activity" (AOTA, 1993) in Appendix B. What are the features or characteristics of a purposeful activity? Does the occupation of play qualify as a purposeful activity? Is riding a tricycle a purposeful activity? Reflect on how riding a tricycle enhanced your performance skills and the functional integrity of your client factors during your childhood. How did riding a tricycle allow you to participate in your play occupations?

Sensory and Perceptual Body Functions and Motor Performance Skills

Participation in play contributes to the maturation and condition of body functions (i.e., client factors), and integrity of these functions enables children to participate in play. Through play and engagement in other occupations, children receive and process sensory information and produce motor responses, which require both motor and process performance skills. Learning to ride a two-wheeled bike illustrates how sensory information obtained through hearing, vision, and proprioception; perceptual functions, such as spatial orientation; and motor responses, such as joint mobility and stability, muscle tone, and endurance work together in developing a skill.

Initially, children may use training wheels on a bicycle to modify the demands of the activity. Training wheels help children practice riding as they develop proprioception, balance, and other skills necessary for riding without training wheels. When children have gained confidence, those extra wheels are removed. To compensate for the greater difficulty and extra balance challenge, children typically sit on the seat and propel the bike with their feet on the ground. With practice, they can lift their feet and coast without falling. As their confidence increases, so does their willingness to try propelling with the pedals. As their postural stability and coordination improve, so do their chances for success. The self-confidence they gain through riding a bike prepares children to participate in neighborhood bicycle races and to venture long distances on errands. In this way, enhanced sensorimotor performance promotes children's engagement in community activities, social participation, and self-concept.

Sensory impairments affect people's ability to receive, process, and integrate incoming information. *Perceptual impairments* affect the ability to interpret this information, and motor impairments affect the production or expression of a desired response. Occupational therapy practitioners are trained in determining whether activity limitations are based on underlying sensory, perceptual, or motor functions. They use task analysis to evaluate the interaction of the child, his or her play tasks, and the performance contexts and to design intervention that modifies activity demands, alters environments, or both to facilitate the child's adaptation. Practitioners use remedial and restorative approaches to intervention to promote development or recovery of central nervous system functioning.

Several evaluation methods are available for measuring the integrity of specific sensory, perceptual, and motor functions, but performance is used to determine the impact of impairments on engagement in occupation. Through observation of clients' engagement in play and task analysis, occupational therapy practitioners create and test hypotheses regarding the performance skills, client factors, and activity demands that facilitate or hinder participation.

Performance Contexts

The *performance contexts* of children, including environmental factors (e.g., physical play areas, social context of day care) and personal factors (e.g., age, gender), must be considered in developing an occupational profile; performance contexts "represent the complete background of the individual's life and living" (World Health Organization, 2001, p. 21). As they play, children both influence and are influenced by their environment. The *physical environment* includes accessibility and expectations for the function of the area (e.g., safe playground equipment, placement of furniture and activity centers). For the occupational therapy practitioner, the primary concern is with "how physical settings shape naturally occurring activity and social interaction and with the symbolic meanings attached to places" (Spencer, 1998, p. 297).

Cultural, social, personal, spiritual, temporal, and virtual contextual factors all influence engagement in play (AOTA, 2014). Culture and society place different developmental expectations on children of different ages, and the gender role expectations placed on boys and girls vary across sociocultural contexts. The socioeconomic status of people and their communities is considered to be one of the most significant determinants of health. This sociocultural contextual factor influences access to other important determinants of health, such as cohesive and nurturing communities, quality housing and play and leisure facilities, education and literacy, community resources, familial resources, and economic opportunity (Graham-Berman, Coupet, Egler, Mattis, & Banyard, 1996).

A child's *personal context* includes his or her age, gender, socioeconomic status, and educational stage. Obviously, the chronological age of the child contributes to his or her ability to acquire motor and process performance skills. The *spiritual context* refers to the fundamental orientation of the child's life and includes whatever inspires or motivates him or her. *Spirit* represents the essence of the person and influences his or her selection of important occupations. *Temporal context* comes into play when stages of life, time of day, time of year, and so on are considered. The *virtual context* refers to media environments such as radio, television, and the Internet through which people communicate without physical contact. The virtual context of television has had a significant effect, both positive and negative, on child development (e.g., increased access to information, decreased physical activity).

LEARNING FROM PLAY

The value of play in the development and learning of young children is widely accepted across education and therapeutic disciplines. An international study conducted by the Organization for Economic Cooperation and Development (2004) highlighted the issue of learning through play. The key is to establish what play means in the context of children's learning and to link play to learning. For the occupational therapy practitioner, acquisition of a knowledge base in the neurology of play and learning is an important focus given that play is an intervention modality.

A significant body of evidence in the psychological literature supports the role of play in learning. Whitebread, Coltman, Jameson, and Lander (2009) explored the literature about particular aspects of play. They cited evidence that play, and particularly symbolic play, is particularly significant in its contribution to the development of children as "metacognitively skillful, self-regulated learners" (p. 40). Their finding

echoes the insightful work of Vygotsky (1978), who surmised that in play children can set their own level of challenge. Play is important to developing problem-solving skills and creativity.

The first 5 years of life are the most critical years for brain development (Eliot, 1999). Indeed, it has been hypothesized that the number of dendrite connections formed in the first 5 years of growth is more than 100 billion (Miller & Cummings, 2007). Intense neurological growth is needed for developing language, learning to motor plan, understanding social expectations, and so much more. This rapid growth in the minds of young children inspires them to play and explore and to assimilate what they learn through a spiral of learning and practice. Environments offer the opportunity for this learning but may also restrict learning.

Gray (2011) reflected on the historical change in attitude toward *free play*, or play structured by children themselves. Early in the 20th century, "sentimentality about childhood fostered a positive attitude toward children's free play and the development of parks and other play spaces to promote it" (p. 444). Free play has declined as adults exert more control over children's activities. The greatest decline is in outdoor play, often blamed on television, computer games, and Internet activities (Gray, 2011). In addition, the emphasis on academic excellence in the form of homework extends a child's workday. Gray cited the findings of a University of Michigan study (Hofferth & Sandberg, 2000) that time spent doing schoolwork at home increased 145% from 1981 to 1997. Structured lessons such as ballet, hockey, musical instruments, and so forth also increase the performance challenges a child faces in the context of home and school.

Play Exploration and Participation

In the *Framework,* play is viewed as the occupation of children, with the tasks being play exploration and play participation (AOTA, 2014). As an infant, oral and manual exploration provides information about objects in the environment (i.e., *object play*). Using task analysis to break down what a child must do to explore the environment, the occupational therapy practitioner observes grasping, banging, sliding, and rolling of objects and takes into account whether limitations for the child include such factors as the weight, shape, and surface texture of the object. This observation leads the practitioner to alter the environment to fit the child and allow for motor success.

With motor success, the child can explore and learn from the characteristics of the object. Over time, object exploration becomes multimodal, including visual, tactile, proprioceptive, and auditory information (Soska, Adolph, & Johnson, 2010). Visual exploration couples with manual actions that evolve to visual–manual or visual–motor exploration using kinetic information. Postural control and balance are also integrated into more sophisticated exploration.

Peer Play

Peer play is a central aspect of childhood play because it contributes to learning: "At play with others, we negotiate our place in the world and sort out our sense of ourselves as we take stock of our capabilities" (Eberle, 2011, p. 19). Preschoolers learn to play cooperatively with others. They learn to play along with others in creating a story through actions—for example, by acting out the activities perceived as appropriate for a princess and a pony. They also learn to play against others—for example, in a game of tag. Through peer play, they develop interpersonal intelligence (Eberle, 2011, p. 27).

A study by Tanta, Deitz, White, and Billingsley (2005) found that "for preschoolers with developmental play skill delays, play with familiar peers who had higher-level skills generally resulted in higher levels of both initiation and response" (pp. 442–443). This research suggests that in intervention planning, pairing a child with delayed play development with typically functioning peers can facilitate better performance. Case Example 8.1 depicts children's play on the playground, and Exhibit 8.1 provides the Client Profile and Task Analysis (CPTA) form for this group.

Perceptual Learning

Perceptual learning is a large part of play. Perceptual skills enable children to evaluate and predict the environment and their own performance. Significant development of perceptual processes such as understanding space and quantity and symbolic representation (e.g., drawing and other forms of visual art) are practiced in play. Developing perceptual skills enables children to problem solve and to be creative. With practice, perceptual concepts become increasingly automated and integrated into the child's cognitive processes (Whitebread et al., 2009). As development advances, children move from playing with objects to learning how to use objects in several ways, increasing their problem-solving capacity.

(text continues on page 124)

CASE EXAMPLE 8.1. PLAYGROUND LEARNING

A group of children on a playground was engaged in a variety of insular and connected activities. **Johnny, who was 2 years old**, dipped his thumb repeatedly into the sand and promptly reinserted it into his mouth. This exploration of the texture of sand stopped when his mother interrupted the activity. Johnny started crying because he could not finish what he was learning. When his mother redirected him to rub the sand between his hands to explore the texture, he happily stopped the thumb dip–suck approach. If this option had not been introduced, Johnny might have appeared to have a behavior problem as he continued to communicate his frustration through crying.

Nearby, **two 3-year-old children** were squabbling over a swing. They pulled and pushed each other to see who would let go of the swing first. The strategy was not successful, and they next began biting and scratching. Their fathers intervened with the solution of taking turns. The first in line smiled in victory. The second pouted while waiting to see if she would actually get a turn, and when she did, she learned a lesson in negotiation that would follow her to the boardroom. What did the first child in line for the swing learn, given the strategy? Would redirecting both children to other separate or cooperative activities result in greater learning?

EXHIBIT 8.1. CLIENT PROFILE AND TASK ANALYSIS FORM: PLAY GROUP

CLIENT PROFILE

Name: Play group	Birthdate:	Age at assessment: ages 2–3 years
Advocates:	Education: Preschool Work occupation: n/a	
Diagnoses: n/a	Current interventions: 1. Parenting strategies	
Referral source: Observational study of parenting of preschoolers.		

PERSONAL INFORMATION

Family unit	Parents accompanying children to the playground
Caregiver(s)	Parents
Roles and responsibilities (e.g., student, spouse, parent, friend, worker)	1. Preschool learners 2. Exploring play environment 3. Learning to take turns and cooperative play
Home environment (e.g., home design, number of people living in the home)	n/a
Community context (e.g., rural, urban, metro; single-family home, residential care)	The playground is actively used by these families. They typically use the playground at the same time, and their children are learning together.
School or work context (e.g., public, special, or private school; stationary or travel location for work)	n/a
Client priorities	1. The 2-year-old is learning about the environment. 2. The 3-year-olds are learning about turn taking.
Values/beliefs/spirituality (e.g., principles, standards, beliefs, personal quest)	Children value play for learning and enjoyment.

SUMMARY, PLAN, AND GOALS

Assessments completed (formal and observational): Observation
Practitioner–client plan (e.g., further formal and observational assessments, inclusion of others): The practitioner is available to provide the parents with strategies to cue their children.

Tasks Requiring Assessment or Intervention	
Short-term goals (Primarily client driven, measurable, global task, or activity achievements)	**Long-term objectives** (Primarily practitioner driven, measurable, incremental, stepwise, or mini achievements)
1. 2-year-old Johnny's next developmental step is to increase exploration using his hands and to transition from mouthing all objects and materials.	1.a. Johnny will play with sand toys by loading and dumping them. 1.b. Johnny will transition from one play activity to another without getting upset by the transition.
2. The 3-year-old children need to learn to use their words to negotiate turn taking and understand how to wait for their turn and relinquish their turn.	2.a. After 1 month of playing together, cooperative play among the children is observable. 2.b. By the end of summer, children will use their words to organize play projects and games.

TASKS ANALYZED

Occupation or Activity	**Tasks** (specific activity component)	**Context or Environment** (external and internal)
Play (2-year-old)	Sand play	*External:* playground sandbox *Internal:* exploring with his mouth
Play (3-year-olds)	Playground swing play	*External:* 1 swing for 2 children *Internal:* wants swing for oneself

ANALYSIS (OF PERFORMANCE SKILLS)

Performance Skills	**Client Challenges** (Performance qualifier)
Rating: *0 = no restriction, 1 = mild limitation, 2 = moderate restriction, 3 = severe restriction, 4 = complete impairment*	
Motor and praxis	**Rating**
Posture	0
Mobility	0
Coordination	0
Strength	0
Effort	0
Energy	0
Execution *3-year-old learning level*	2

(Continued)

EXHIBIT 8.1. CLIENT PROFILE AND TASK ANALYSIS FORM: PLAY GROUP *(Cont.)*

Process skills		Rating
Mental energy		0
Knowledge	*As per developmental levels*	2
Organization	*3-year-old learning level*	2
Adaptation	*2-year-old developmental level*	2
Social interaction skills		**Rating**
Communication posture		2
Gestures		2
Initiation		2
Information exchange		2
Acknowledging		2
Taking turns		2

ANALYSIS (OF PERFORMANCE PATTERNS)

Performance Patterns	Daily Life Activities	Client Challenges (skill deficits and context restrictions)
Habits (Automatic and integrated behaviors)		2-year-old: Learning to decrease use of the mouth to explore the qualities of sand.
Routines (Regular activities that provide daily structure)		3-year-olds: Need to learn how to take turns in a free-play context.
Roles (Expected behaviors and responsibilities)		3-year-olds: Need to integrate turn-taking social rules into free-play environments.
Rituals (Customary cultural and social activities)		n/a

Synopsis of performance skills and performance patterns (strengths, deficits, and challenges): Both age groups have reached a stage at which their parents are developing strategies to cue the children on play expectations within the social context of a playground. The parent of the 2-year-old cued her son in an age-appropriate and functional way. The parents of the 3-year-olds are challenged to guide the children in such a way as to achieve their children's understanding and a mutually successful outcome for them.

OCCUPATIONAL PROFILE AND ANALYSIS OF NEEDS

Functional ability (i.e., how strengths and deficits affect ability to perform activities and tasks)	All these children have the necessary functional abilities for the new learning.
Activity tolerance (e.g., physical and mental fatigue levels, energy to complete activities and tasks, temporal and environmental contexts)	All these children have necessary activity tolerance for playground activity.
Effect on occupational performance (reflect on client roles, responsibilities, and priorities)	All the children are at a stage of new learning. The 2-year-old is at a health risk if he does not learn to move from mouthing everything as he explores. The 3-year-olds are at a behavioral risk if they do not learn to deal with taking turns in social situations.
Intervention needs (e.g., physical, cognitive, emotional, social)	The parents of the 3-year-olds would benefit from ideas on how to build communication between their children during turn-taking situations. Initially, the parents may need to set out the rules of engagement (e.g., 3 minutes each, with each child getting equal turns).
Resource needs (e.g., assistive devices or equipment, technology)	None
Program needs (e.g., day programs, return-to-work programs, socialization)	None
Outlook (practitioner projection of long-term needs and life care planning)	The parent of the 2-year-old is on target with her approach. The parents of the 3-year-olds could use parenting materials on approaches for teaching children how to take turns.

GUIDELINES AND CHECKLIST FOR TASK ANALYSIS

Areas of Occupation

Activities of daily living	Instrumental activities of daily living
☐ Bathing and showering	☐ Care of others
☐ Bowel and bladder management	☐ Care of pets
☐ Dressing	☐ Child rearing
☐ Eating and swallowing	☐ Communication management
☐ Feeding	☐ Driving and community mobility
☐ Functional mobility	☐ Financial management
☐ Personal device care	☐ Home establishment
☐ Personal hygiene and grooming	☐ Home management and maintenance
☐ Sexual activity	☐ Meal preparation and cleanup
☐ Toileting and toilet hygiene	☐ Religious and spiritual observance
	☐ Safety and emergency maintenance
	☐ Shopping

(Continued)

EXHIBIT 8.1. CLIENT PROFILE AND TASK ANALYSIS FORM: PLAY GROUP *(Cont.)*

Rest and sleep
☐ Rest and relaxation
☐ Sleep participation
☐ Sleep preparation

Play
☑ Peer interaction
☑ Play exploration
☑ Play participation

Leisure
☐ Customary activities or hobbies
☐ Leisure exploration
☐ Leisure participation

Social participation
☐ Community
☐ Family
☐ Peer or friend

Education
☐ Access issues
☐ Formal education participation
☐ Informal personal education or exploration
☐ Informal personal education participation

Work
☐ Employment interests and pursuits
☐ Employment seeking and acquisition
☐ Job performance
☐ Retirement preparation and adjustment
☐ Volunteer exploration
☐ Volunteer participation

Client Factors

Body functions and structures
Physical
☐ Cardiovascular and hematological systems
☐ Digestive, metabolic, and endocrine systems
☐ Genitourinary and reproductive functions
☑ Movement-related functions
☐ Respiratory and immunological systems
☐ Skin and related structure functions
☑ Voice and speech functions

Body functions and structures
Sensory and pain
☐ Hearing functions
☐ Pain grading and description
☐ Seeing and related functions
☑ Tactile functions
☑ Taste and smell functions
☐ Temperature and pressure reception
☐ Vestibular and proprioceptive functions

Body functions: Mental
Specific mental functions
☐ Attention
☑ Emotional
☐ Experience of self and time
☐ Higher-level cognitive
☐ Motor sequencing
☐ Memory
☑ Perception
☐ Thought

Body functions: Mental
Global mental functions
☐ Consciousness
☐ Energy and drive
☐ Orientation
☐ Sleep
☑ Temperament and personality

Values, Beliefs, and Spirituality

Values
☑ Meaningful qualities
☐ Principles
☑ Standards

Beliefs and spirituality
☐ Cognitive content health as true
☐ Guiding actions
☐ Life meaning and purpose

Activity and Occupational Demands

Objects and their properties	Space demands
☑ Inherent properties (e.g., heavy, light) ☐ Required tools, materials, equipment	☐ Size, arrangement, surface, lighting

Social demands	Sequence and timing
☐ Cultural context ☑ Social environment	☐ Sequence and timing ☐ Specific steps

Required actions and performance skills	Required body functions and structures
☐ Cognitive ☑ Communication and interaction ☑ Emotional and social ☑ Motor and praxis ☑ Sensory–perceptual	☑ Anatomical parts ☐ Level of consciousness ☐ Mobility of joints

Performance Skills

Motor skills	Process skills
☑ Movement actions or behaviors ☑ Skilled purposeful movements ☐ Ability to carry out learned movement	☐ Judgment ☐ Select and sequence objects or tools ☐ Organize and prioritize ☐ Create and problem solve ☐ Multitask

Social interaction skills	
☑ Identify, manage, and express feelings ☑ On a one-to-one basis ☑ In groups ☑ Communication and interaction skills	

Performance Patterns

Habits	Routines
☐ Automatic behavior ☐ Repeated activities ☐ Good, bad, or impoverished	☐ Observable patterns of behavior ☐ Time commitment ☐ Satisfying, promoting, or damaging

Roles	Rituals
☐ Set of expected behaviors ☐ Social or cultural ☐ Within context	☐ Symbolic actions ☐ Spiritual, cultural, or social ☐ Link to values and beliefs

Contexts and Environments

Cultural	Personal
☐ Customs and beliefs ☐ Activity patterns ☐ Expectations	☑ Age and gender ☐ Socioeconomic status ☐ Educational status

(Continued)

EXHIBIT 8.1. CLIENT PROFILE AND TASK ANALYSIS FORM: PLAY GROUP (Cont.)

Temporal ☐ Location of performance in time ☐ Experience shaped by engagement	Virtual ☐ Communication environment
Physical ☑ Natural environment (e.g., geography) ☑ Built environment (e.g., building, furniture)	**Social and political** ☑ Relationship to individuals ☐ Relationship to organizations or systems

TASK ANALYSIS TEMPLATE

An individual form is required for each task that is examined.
Task:

Task Demands	Action Demands (What is required of the person to do the task)	Client Challenges (Availability of required body functions and structures)
Objects used (e.g., equipment, technology)	Accessing the equipment by climbing on to, sliding down, and so forth	The children must learn to use the equipment safely and do so only with needed assistance from their parents.
Space demands (e.g., physical context)	There is not enough equipment for the all the children to use at once.	The children must learn to share equipment and to create imaginative play in the sand when it is not their turn on the equipment.
Social demands (e.g., social environment and context)	Parents must guide their children according to developmental expectations.	Some of the parents are learning developmental strategies from each other and from the observing practitioner.
Sequence and timing (e.g., process to carry out the task)	Children must leave the playground at the direction of their parents.	Children must learn to leave play without resistance against their parents (e.g., fussing, crying, not listening).
Required actions and performance skills (e.g., basic requirements)	Children learn about physical, proprioceptive, vestibular, and other experiences.	The children function within a spectrum of normal development with some having more motor skills and confidence in motor play than others.

Language Development

Vocabulary is in part learned through imaginative and pretend play (Han, Moore, Vukelich, & Buell, 2010). Researchers have found that children entering school with poor vocabularies often experience difficulties learning to read and write (Eberle, 2011). As children develop and learn, play acquires more complex rules and moral judgment and increased symbolism, requiring more sophisticated language to communicate (Kool & Lawver, 2010).

Motor Skills Learning

Motor skills acquisition leads to the development of visual, tactile, proprioceptive, and auditory learning (Soska et al., 2010). Elkind (2008) observed that in play, a child's behavior adapts to the demands of the physical and social environment (p. 3). Learning to crawl, walk, and then run allows the child to explore and learn from the environment (e.g., climbing cupboards, riding a bike, navigating challenging terrain).

Manual dexterity supports further exploration and learning, whether for a toddler using a spoon, a preschooler creating block structures, or a school-age child throwing snowballs or building sand castles.

Development of motor capacity through play contributes to broader patterns of individual and social behavior. For example, learning that climbing on a certain structure leads to a fall, that putting a rock in a snowball inflicts harm, and that using a pencil or computer can allow development of a creative story all affect the child's behavior. Case Examples 8.2 and 8.3, and Exhibits 8.2 and 8.3 show the role of task analysis in developing motor development through play.

(text continues on page 139)

CASE EXAMPLE 8.2. MOTOR DEVELOPMENT THROUGH PLAY

Oliver has loved his monkey rattle since he was 4 months old. He mouthed it, then banged it against his crib, and finally learned to throw it to get his father to fetch it. The first time Oliver threw the rattle while standing, he fell over, much to his surprise. After bending to pick up the toy while holding onto the crib rail a few times, he discovered that he could also keep his balance when throwing the rattle if he held on to the rail. He learned how to control the game to keep his father engaged in play, and he had his first experiences with turn taking.

By the time he was age 3 years, Oliver could initiate ball play with a friend and no longer had to hold on to keep his balance. What steps toward developing balance and equilibrium likely occurred for Oliver between infancy and age 3 years, and what play activities might he have chosen to move his own development forward?

EXHIBIT 8.2. CLIENT PROFILE AND TASK ANALYSIS FORM: OLIVER

CLIENT PROFILE

Name: Oliver	**Birthdate:**	**Age at assessment:** 3
Advocates:	**Education:** Preschooler **Work occupation:** n/a	
Diagnoses:	**Current interventions:** None	
Referral source: Observational study by a practitioner		

PERSONAL INFORMATION

Family unit	Two parents
Caregiver(s)	Parents
Roles and responsibilities (e.g., student, spouse, parent, friend, worker)	Using play to develop skills
Home environment (e.g., home design, number of people living in the home)	Stay-at-home father and working mother

(Continued)

EXHIBIT 8.2. CLIENT PROFILE AND TASK ANALYSIS FORM: OLIVER *(Cont.)*

Community context (e.g., rural, urban, metro; single-family home, residential care)	Middle-class neighborhood with a playground, day care, and preschool program within walking distance
School or work context (e.g., public, special, or private school; stationary or travel location for work)	Neighborhood preschool program
Client priorities	1. Playing ball with peers
Values/beliefs/spirituality (e.g., principles, standards, beliefs, personal quest)	Oliver's parents want to facilitate his development, so he can succeed with all new learning and develop confidence in himself and in his play with peers.

SUMMARY, PLAN, AND GOALS

Assessments completed (formal and observational):
Practitioner–client plan (e.g., further formal and observational assessments, inclusion of others): Continued opportunities to play ball with his peers, with incorporation of specific ball games to keep Oliver's interest.
Tasks Requiring Assessment or Intervention

Short-term goals (Primarily client driven, measurable, global task, or activity achievements)	**Long-term objectives** (Primarily practitioner driven, measurable, incremental, stepwise, or mini achievements)
1. Oliver will develop skills from standing and holding on to a support, to where he can maintain his balance while throwing a ball to a friend.	1. Oliver will develop his ball-throwing skills, improving from inaccurate aim in throwing the ball to another person to an accurate throw.

TASKS ANALYZED

Occupation or Activity	**Tasks** (specific activity component)	**Context or Environment** (external and internal)
Play development: Ball play from infancy to age 3 years	Holding a ball while maintaining balance	*External:* Needs placement of the ball *Internal:* Needs to balance while holding on to the crib rail
	Throwing the ball to parent	*External:* View of parent *Internal:* Ability to release
	Rolling ball between two people	*External:* Play partner *Internal:* Interest in game
	Tossing the ball to another person	*External:* Play partner *Internal:* Interest in the game

ANALYSIS (OF PERFORMANCE SKILLS)

Performance Skills	Client Challenges (Performance qualifier)
Rating: 0 = *no restriction,* 1 = *mild limitation,* 2 = *moderate restriction,* 3 = *severe restriction,* 4 = *complete impairment*	
Motor and praxis	**Rating**
Posture (as an infant)	2
Mobility	0
Coordination	2
Strength	0
Effort	0
Energy	0
Execution (as an infant)	2
Execution (as a 3-year-old)	0
Process skills	**Rating**
Mental energy	0
Knowledge	1
Organization	2
Adaptation	1
Social interaction skills	**Rating**
Communication posture	0
Gestures	0
Initiation	0
Information exchange	1
Acknowledging	0
Taking turns	2

ANALYSIS (OF PERFORMANCE PATTERNS)

Performance Patterns	Daily Life Activities	Client Challenges (skill deficits and context restrictions)
Habits (Automatic and integrated behaviors)	Oliver and his father take care of their early morning routine and prepare to leave the house to go to preschool or the playground, after which they return for lunch.	Oliver has difficulty leaving the playground and often resists his father's request to leave.

(Continued)

EXHIBIT 8.2. CLIENT PROFILE AND TASK ANALYSIS FORM: OLIVER *(Cont.)*

Routines (Regular activities that provide daily structure)	Oliver wakes, dresses, and has breakfast before leaving the house. He returns for lunch and takes a nap.	Oliver has difficulty transitioning from play and resists resting after lunch.
Roles (Expected behaviors and responsibilities)	Son, preschool student, and play-mate.	Oliver is developing his ability to play catch with another child and often loses interest if the other child fails to catch the ball.
Rituals (Customary cultural and social activities)	n/a	

Synopsis of performance skills and performance patterns (strengths, deficits, and challenges): Oliver is showing normal development.

OCCUPATIONAL PROFILE AND ANALYSIS OF NEEDS

Functional ability (i.e., how strengths and deficits affect ability to perform activities and tasks)	Oliver is interested in playing catch with his friend and has practiced with his father, so he has slightly better skills than his friend. Because of his better skill, he can be impatient with his friend.
Activity tolerance (e.g., physical and mental fatigue levels, energy to complete activities and tasks, temporal and environmental contexts)	Oliver has good physical stamina but can get distracted by other options if ball play does not move as fast as his expectations.
Effect on occupational performance (reflect on client roles, responsibilities, and priorities)	Oliver is performing within age expectation.
Intervention needs (e.g., physical, cognitive, emotional, social)	Oliver's father might encourage him to be more patient with his friend through transitioning the boys together to other games using the ball and taking breaks to do other activities together.
Resource needs (e.g., assistive devices or equipment, technology)	None
Program needs (e.g., day programs, return-to-work programs, socialization)	n/a
Outlook (practitioner projection of long-term needs and life care planning)	Oliver is developing within normal limits and with regular peer play will learn to adapt to the strengths and limitations of others.

GUIDELINES AND CHECKLIST FOR TASK ANALYSIS

Areas of Occupation

Activities of daily living
- ☐ Bathing and showering
- ☐ Bowel and bladder management
- ☐ Dressing
- ☐ Eating and swallowing
- ☐ Feeding
- ☐ Functional mobility

- ☐ Personal device care
- ☐ Personal hygiene and grooming
- ☐ Sexual activity
- ☐ Toileting and toilet hygiene

Instrumental activities of daily living
- ☐ Care of others
- ☐ Care of pets
- ☐ Child rearing
- ☐ Communication management
- ☐ Driving and community mobility
- ☐ Financial management

- ☐ Home establishment
- ☐ Home management and maintenance
- ☐ Meal preparation and cleanup
- ☐ Religious and spiritual observance
- ☐ Safety and emergency maintenance
- ☐ Shopping

Rest and sleep
- ☐ Rest and relaxation
- ☐ Sleep participation
- ☐ Sleep preparation

Play
- ☑ Peer interaction
- ☑ Play exploration
- ☑ Play participation

Leisure
- ☐ Customary activities or hobbies
- ☐ Leisure exploration
- ☐ Leisure participation

Social participation
- ☐ Community
- ☐ Family
- ☑ Peer or friend

Education
- ☐ Access issues
- ☐ Formal education participation
- ☐ Informal personal education or exploration
- ☐ Informal personal education participation

Work
- ☐ Employment interests and pursuits
- ☐ Employment seeking and acquisition
- ☐ Job performance
- ☐ Retirement preparation and adjustment
- ☐ Volunteer exploration
- ☐ Volunteer participation

Client Factors

Body functions and structures
Physical
- ☐ Cardiovascular and hematological systems
- ☐ Digestive, metabolic, and endocrine systems
- ☐ Genitourinary and reproductive functions
- ☑ Movement-related functions
- ☐ Respiratory and immunological systems
- ☐ Skin and related structure functions
- ☐ Voice and speech functions

Body functions: Mental
Specific mental functions
- ☑ Attention
- ☐ Emotional

Body functions and structures
Sensory and pain
- ☐ Hearing functions
- ☐ Pain grading and description
- ☐ Seeing and related functions
- ☐ Tactile functions
- ☐ Taste and smell functions
- ☐ Temperature and pressure reception
- ☑ Vestibular and proprioceptive functions

Body functions: Mental
Global mental functions
- ☐ Consciousness
- ☑ Energy and drive

(Continued)

EXHIBIT 8.2. CLIENT PROFILE AND TASK ANALYSIS FORM: OLIVER *(Cont.)*

☐ Experience of self and time	☐ Orientation
☐ Higher-level cognitive	☐ Sleep
☑ Motor sequencing	☑ Temperament and personality
☐ Memory	
☑ Perception	
☐ Thought	

Values, Beliefs, and Spirituality

Values	**Beliefs and spirituality**
☐ Meaningful qualities	☐ Cognitive content health as true
☐ Principles	☐ Guiding actions
☐ Standards	☐ Life meaning and purpose

Activity and Occupational Demands

Objects and their properties	**Space demands**
☑ Inherent properties (e.g., heavy, light)	☐ Size, arrangement, surface, lighting
☑ Required tools, materials, equipment	

Social demands	**Sequence and timing**
☐ Cultural context	☑ Sequence and timing
☐ Social environment	☐ Specific steps

Required actions and performance skills	**Required body functions and structures**
☑ Cognitive	☑ Anatomical parts
☑ Communication and interaction	☐ Level of consciousness
☑ Emotional and social	☑ Mobility of joints
☑ Motor and praxis	
☑ Sensory–perceptual	

Performance Skills

Motor skills	**Process skills**
☑ Movement actions or behaviors	☐ Judgment
☑ Skilled purposeful movements	☐ Select and sequence objects or tools
☑ Ability to carry out learned movement	☐ Organize and prioritize
	☑ Create and problem solve
	☐ Multitask

Social interaction skills	
☑ Identify, manage, and express feelings	
☐ On a one-to-one basis	
☐ In groups	
☐ Communication and interaction skills	

Performance Patterns

Habits	**Routines**
☑ Automatic behavior	☑ Observable patterns of behavior
☑ Repeated activities	☑ Time commitment
☐ Good, bad, or impoverished	☐ Satisfying, promoting, or damaging

Roles	Rituals
☐ Set of expected behaviors ☐ Social or cultural ☐ Within context	☐ Symbolic actions ☐ Spiritual, cultural, or social ☐ Link to values and beliefs

Contexts and Environments

Cultural	Personal
☐ Customs and beliefs ☑ Activity patterns ☑ Expectations	☑ Age and gender ☐ Socioeconomic status ☐ Educational status

Temporal	Virtual
☐ Location of performance in time ☐ Experience shaped by engagement	☐ Communication environment

Physical	Social and political
☑ Natural environment (e.g., geography) ☑ Built environment (e.g., building, furniture)	☑ Relationship to individuals ☐ Relationship to organizations or systems

TASK ANALYSIS TEMPLATE

An individual form is required for each task that is examined.
Task: Rolling and throwing a ball

Task Demands	Action Demands (What is required of the person to do the task)	Client Challenges (Availability of required body functions and structures)
Objects used (e.g., equipment, technology)	To throw a ball with one hand, the ball must fit in the palm of his hand (3-inch-diameter ball).	Oliver is learning to maintain a grip on a ball until planned release.
Space demands (e.g., physical context)	Ball play can happen in an indoor play environment or outdoors.	None
Social demands (e.g., social environment and context)	Playing cooperatively with another person is required in playing ball.	Oliver is learning to take a turn at rolling or throwing and catching.
Sequence and timing (e.g., process to carry out the task)	The sequence includes positioning oneself, feeling balanced when standing, holding on if necessary, gripping the ball, and releasing it in the right direction.	Oliver is age 3 years and spontaneous in his approach to most play tasks. He is just learning how a game is structured between two people and the action steps needed.
Required actions and performance skills (e.g., basic requirements)	The performance skills necessary are age-appropriate motor and praxis skills, perceptual skills, cognitive skills, and emotional regulation.	Oliver is developing his motor skills so that he can carry out the sequences of ball play with another person. His balance while throwing a ball is somewhat less than average for his age.

CASE EXAMPLE 8.3. CHILD WITH FINE MOTOR DIFFICULTIES

An occupational therapy practitioner began evaluating a **girl in kindergarten, Gabby,** who had reported fine motor difficulties, gross motor challenges, and extreme reluctance to play with other children. The broad interpretation of the kindergarten teacher was that Gabby appeared to have delayed play skills. The practitioner approached the evaluation using task analysis to examine the motor, cognitive, and psychosocial aspects that were Gabby's strengths and weaknesses.

Motor development testing indicated that Gabby was performing in the average range. Gabby's concept development was within normal range, as were her perceptual skills. Gabby failed to demonstrate her abilities within the classroom setting, however. In the classroom, the practitioner observed as Gabby withdrew from the activities presented but played one-on-one with another child in a quiet location. The interview with Gabby's parents revealed that the parents were overprotective and that Gabby had little early experience outside the home with other adults or children. She was by nature a shy child, and decreased exposure limited her social development.

EXHIBIT 8.3. CLIENT PROFILE AND TASK ANALYSIS FORM: GABBY

CLIENT PROFILE

Name: Gabby	Birthdate:	Age at assessment: 5
Advocates: Teacher, parents	Education: Kindergarten Work occupation: n/a	
Diagnoses: Undiagnosed. The school is concerned about Gabby's motor performance.	Current interventions: None	
Referral source: Teacher		

PERSONAL INFORMATION

Family unit	2 parents, no siblings
Caregiver(s)	Parents
Roles and responsibilities (e.g., student, spouse, parent, friend, worker)	Attending kindergarten to learn in a semistructured environment
Home environment (e.g., home design, number of people living in the home)	n/a
Community context (e.g., rural, urban, metro; single-family home, residential care)	n/a
School or work context (e.g., public, special, or private school; stationary or travel location for work)	The kindergarten is part of the public school system. An occupational therapist is available for consultation.

Client priorities (proxy by teacher)	1. Demonstrate age-appropriate fine motor and gross motor skills within the classroom. 2. Develop socialization skills.
Values/beliefs/spirituality (e.g., principles, standards, beliefs, personal quest)	n/a

SUMMARY, PLAN, AND GOALS

Assessments completed (formal and observational): Peabody Developmental Motor Scales (Folio & Fewell, 2000) and classroom observation
Practitioner–client plan (e.g., further formal and observational assessments, inclusion of others): Gabby is functioning within normal limits in all fine motor and gross motor areas. Her perceptual skills are also developing normally. She is a very shy child who is having difficulty integrating into the classroom and with the other children. Referred for play therapy to be conducted individually and in the classroom by the occupational therapy assistant under the supervision of the occupational therapist and school psychologist.

Tasks Requiring Assessment or Intervention

Short-term goals (Primarily client driven, measurable, global task, or activity achievements)	**Long-term objectives** (Primarily practitioner driven, measurable, incremental, stepwise, or mini achievements)
1. By teacher proxy: Gabby will demonstrate fine motor and gross motor skills in the classroom.	1.a. Gabby will transition from one-to-one peer play to joining small group activities through direct encouragement from the teacher within the school term. 1.b. Concurrently, Gabby's parents will learn about child development of peer play and engage Gabby in community play with other children.
2. By teacher proxy: Gabby will interact in groups within the classroom and on the playground.	2.a. By the end of the school term, Gabby will independently engage with other children on the playground. 2.b. By the end of kindergarten, Gabby will have developed the confidence to initiate group play on the playground.

TASKS ANALYZED

Occupation or Activity	**Tasks** (specific activity component)	**Context or Environment** (external and internal)
Education	Fine motor skills Gross motor skills	*External:* 15 children in the class *Internal:* Reluctance to play with others
	Play interaction skills	*External:* Gabby lacks experience with peer play in her community. *Internal:* Shyness limits her confidence in group play.

(Continued)

EXHIBIT 8.3. CLIENT PROFILE AND TASK ANALYSIS FORM: GABBY *(Cont.)*

ANALYSIS (OF PERFORMANCE SKILLS)

Performance Skills	Client Challenges (Performance qualifier)
Rating: 0 = *no restriction,* 1 = *mild limitation,* 2 = *moderate restriction,* 3 = *severe restriction,* 4 = *complete impairment*	
Motor and praxis	**Rating**
Posture	0
Mobility	0
Coordination	0
Strength	0
Effort	0
Energy	0
Execution	0
Process skills	**Rating**
Mental energy	1
Knowledge	0
Organization	0
Adaptation	3
Social interaction skills	**Rating**
Communication posture	0
Gestures	0
Initiation	3
Information exchange	2
Acknowledging	3
Taking turns	2

ANALYSIS (OF PERFORMANCE PATTERNS)

Performance Patterns	Daily Life Activities	Client Challenges (skill deficits and context restrictions)
Habits (Automatic and integrated behaviors)	Gabby arrives at school with one of her parents.	She has difficulty separating from her parent to enter the classroom.

Routines (Regular activities that provide daily structure)	The kindergarten class has a regular routine of activities that starts with a group gathering, followed by engagement in activity centers, going out for a recess break, story time, and gross motor play in the gym.	Gabby avoids group play, especially gross motor play.
Roles (Expected behaviors and responsibilities)	Daughter and kindergarten student	Gabby is overprotected by her parents and has decreased social integration skills that affect her adaptation in the classroom.
Rituals (Customary cultural and social activities)	n/a	

Synopsis of performance skills and performance patterns (strengths, deficits, and challenges):
Gabby has age-appropriate motor skills but is immature in her social integration skills. Performance expectations need to be implemented with Gabby to enable further development and emotional maturity.

OCCUPATIONAL PROFILE AND ANALYSIS OF NEEDS

Functional ability (i.e., how strengths and deficits affect ability to perform activities and tasks)	Gabby has age-appropriate motor abilities. She is emotionally immature and reticent to engage in group play.
Activity tolerance (e.g., physical and mental fatigue levels, energy to complete activities and tasks, temporal and environmental contexts)	Gabby has no limitations.
Effect on occupational performance (reflect on client roles, responsibilities, and priorities)	Delayed emotional maturity and shyness has resulted in Gabby avoiding motor play with her peer group. This created an impression that she has a motor development delay when in fact she does not.
Intervention needs (e.g., physical, cognitive, emotional, social)	Gabby needs to understand performance expectations in the classroom and gradually be encouraged to develop group play skills. Concurrently, the practitioner needs to work with her parents to decrease Gabby's reliance on their emotional support and to guide them in how to engage Gabby in community activities that will help her emotional development.
Resource needs (e.g., assistive devices or equipment, technology)	None
Program needs (e.g., day programs, return-to-work programs, socialization)	Community group play program
Outlook (practitioner projection of long-term needs and life care planning)	Gabby has the capacity to progress developmentally by the end of the school year.

(Continued)

EXHIBIT 8.3. CLIENT PROFILE AND TASK ANALYSIS FORM: GABBY *(Cont.)*

GUIDELINES AND CHECKLIST FOR TASK ANALYSIS

Areas of Occupation

Activities of daily living	Instrumental activities of daily living
☐ Bathing and showering	☐ Care of others
☐ Bowel and bladder management	☐ Care of pets
☐ Dressing	☐ Child rearing
☐ Eating and swallowing	☐ Communication management
☐ Feeding	☐ Driving and community mobility
☐ Functional mobility	☐ Financial management
☐ Personal device care	☐ Home establishment
☐ Personal hygiene and grooming	☐ Home management and maintenance
☐ Sexual activity	☐ Meal preparation and cleanup
☐ Toileting and toilet hygiene	☐ Religious and spiritual observance
	☐ Safety and emergency maintenance
	☐ Shopping

Rest and sleep	Play
☐ Rest and relaxation	☑ Peer interaction
☐ Sleep participation	☐ Play exploration
☐ Sleep preparation	☑ Play participation

Leisure	Social participation
☐ Customary activities or hobbies	☑ Community
☐ Leisure exploration	☐ Family
☐ Leisure participation	☑ Peer or friend

Education	Work
☐ Access issues	☐ Employment interests and pursuits
☑ Formal education participation	☐ Employment seeking and acquisition
☑ Informal personal education or exploration	☐ Job performance
☐ Informal personal education participation	☐ Retirement preparation and adjustment
	☐ Volunteer exploration
	☐ Volunteer participation

Client Factors

Body functions and structures	Body functions and structures
Physical	*Sensory and pain*
☐ Cardiovascular and hematological systems	☐ Hearing functions
☐ Digestive, metabolic, and endocrine systems	☐ Pain grading and description

☐ Genitourinary and reproductive functions	☐ Seeing and related functions
☑ Movement-related functions	☐ Tactile functions
☐ Respiratory and immunological systems	☐ Taste and smell functions
☐ Skin and related structure functions	☐ Temperature and pressure reception
☐ Voice and speech functions	☐ Vestibular and proprioceptive functions

Body functions: Mental
Specific mental functions
- ☐ Attention
- ☑ Emotional
- ☐ Experience of self and time
- ☐ Higher-level cognitive
- ☑ Motor sequencing
- ☐ Memory
- ☑ Perception
- ☐ Thought

Body functions: Mental
Global mental functions
- ☐ Consciousness
- ☑ Energy and drive
- ☐ Orientation
- ☐ Sleep
- ☑ Temperament and personality

Values, Beliefs, and Spirituality

Values
- ☑ Meaningful qualities
- ☐ Principles
- ☐ Standards

Beliefs and spirituality
- ☐ Cognitive content health as true
- ☐ Guiding actions
- ☐ Life meaning and purpose

Activity and Occupational Demands

Objects and their properties
- ☐ Inherent properties (e.g., heavy, light)
- ☐ Required tools, materials, equipment

Space demands
- ☐ Size, arrangement, surface, lighting

Social demands
- ☐ Cultural context
- ☑ Social environment

Sequence and timing
- ☐ Sequence and timing
- ☐ Specific steps

Required actions and performance skills
- ☐ Cognitive
- ☑ Communication and interaction
- ☑ Emotional and social
- ☑ Motor and praxis
- ☑ Sensory–perceptual

Required body functions and structures
- ☐ Anatomical parts
- ☐ Level of consciousness
- ☐ Mobility of joints

Performance Skills

Motor skills
- ☑ Movement actions or behaviors
- ☐ Skilled purposeful movements
- ☐ Ability to carry out learned movement

Process skills
- ☐ Judgment
- ☐ Select and sequence objects or tools
- ☐ Organize and prioritize
- ☐ Create and problem solve
- ☐ Multitask

Social interaction skills
- ☐ Identify, manage, and express feelings
- ☐ On a one-to-one basis
- ☑ In groups
- ☑ Communication and interaction skills

(Continued)

EXHIBIT 8.3. CLIENT PROFILE AND TASK ANALYSIS FORM: GABBY *(Cont.)*

Performance Patterns

Habits	**Routines**
☐ Automatic behavior	☑ Observable patterns of behavior
☐ Repeated activities	☐ Time commitment
☐ Good, bad, or impoverished	☐ Satisfying, promoting, or damaging

Roles	**Rituals**
☑ Set of expected behaviors	☐ Symbolic actions
☑ Social or cultural	☐ Spiritual, cultural, or social
☑ Within context	☐ Link to values and beliefs

Contexts and Environments

Cultural	**Personal**
☐ Customs and beliefs	☑ Age and gender
☑ Activity patterns	☑ Socioeconomic status
☑ Expectations	☐ Educational status

Temporal	**Virtual**
☐ Location of performance in time	☐ Communication environment
☑ Experience shaped by engagement	

Physical	**Social and political**
☐ Natural environment (e.g., geography)	☑ Relationship to individuals
☑ Built environment (e.g., building, furniture)	☐ Relationship to organizations or systems

TASK ANALYSIS TEMPLATE

An individual form is required for each task that is examined.
Task:

Task Demands	Action Demands (What is required of the person to do the task)	Client Challenges (Availability of required body functions and structures)
Objects used (e.g., equipment, technology)	School classroom, school gym, and playground	Decreased engagement in motor play with peers
Space demands (e.g., physical context)	School and playground	No issues
Social demands (e.g., social environment and context)	Integration with peers in kindergarten activities	Decreased interaction in a group
Sequence and timing (e.g., process to carry out the task)	n/a	n/a
Required actions and performance skills (e.g., basic requirements)	Age-appropriate motor and social skills	Query motor developmental delays and social maturity

INTERVENTION THROUGH PLAY

Play is an occupation, and the role of the occupational therapy practitioner is to collaborate with parents, caregivers, and other stakeholders to enhance a child's engagement in play and participation in the social context of play. Recognizing the power of play in promoting progress and growth in the motor, cognitive, perceptual, and emotional development of children and adolescents, the practitioner assesses what is meaningful for each child or adolescent to focus on use of specific activities that can be therapeutic. Task analysis that examines the fit of a play activity and its action demands with the challenges of the individual child allows practitioners to engage in modification and progression of skills for play. To foster engagement and participation in play, practitioners promote competency and facilitate adaptation by designing therapeutic activities, modifying activity demands, and altering environments.

Practitioners, parents, and other caregivers encourage a child to master challenges by supporting the different ways the child adapts to new tasks. Repetition and practice foster the child's confidence and self-esteem and promote success and satisfaction in engaging in occupations. Successful engagement, in turn, boosts the child's self-concept and confidence and supports his or her participation in contexts. Most pediatric intervention programs designed by occupational therapy practitioners aim, either directly or indirectly, to enable children to enhance their self-esteem (Mayberry, 1990; Willoughby, King, & Polatajko, 1996).

In Case Example 8.4, a child must develop several performance skills to fully participate with her peers on the playground and engage in play occupations. In Questions 4–6 of Assignment 8.1, readers can use the CPTA form to establish an occupational profile and an analysis of Carina's occupational performance. Using task analysis, readers can evaluate performance skills and patterns, contexts, activity demands, and client factors that affect Carina's participation in specific play tasks and activities. This information provides the foundation to plan a purposeful activity to challenge Carina's sensorimotor development, boost her confidence, and increase her self-esteem. The aim of intervention is to enhance Carina's engagement in the occupation of play.

CASE EXAMPLE 8.4. CARINA: DEVELOPMENTAL DELAYS

Carina was a 5-year-old girl assigned to an occupational therapy practitioner's caseload after an evaluation by a registered occupational therapist. Carina lived with her parents on a large property on the outskirts of a rural town. The family ate vegetables, fruit, meat, eggs, and dairy products they produced themselves. They had a few pigs, about a dozen chickens and ducks, 5 lambs, and a milk cow. Carina enjoyed helping her parents take care of the animals and gather eggs and fresh vegetables. She learned from her parents that tending the land and the animals is important and caring work. She was proud of her knowledge about caring for animals and growing food and of the praise she received from her parents for her hard work.

Carina's parents were worried about her confidence and increasing social isolation; Carina avoided activities that she did not think she could immediately master. Carina's parents were concerned about her lack of understanding of basic academic concepts, her inability to participate more fully in activities of daily living (ADLs), and her fear of the climbing equipment at the school playground. Carina could not identify letters, shapes, or colors, and she was unable to sort objects into same and different categories. She could not put on or remove her overcoat or manage her coat zipper and often placed her shoes on the wrong feet. Carina was so afraid of the slide, swing set, and merry-go-round that she refused to play on her own. Carina rode a tricycle short distances, but she could not ride with the speed, agility, and precision of her friends. Some of her older friends had graduated to two-wheel bikes. Unfortunately, several children teased Carina because of her clumsiness, and her parents were concerned that her fear of playgrounds limited her opportunities for social participation.

The occupational therapy report indicated that Carina's participation in ADLs, education, play, and leisure occupations was delayed compared with her peers. She had mild impairments in bilateral coordination, strength, and endurance and moderate impairments in trunk control, sequencing, and navigational skills. Sensory function testing also suggested mild impairments in proprioceptive, tactile, and vestibular function.

Assignment 8.2. Demands of Play

Note. Review Questions 1–3 before completing portions of the CPTA form (Appendix A), as you will use the form for Carina for each of remaining questions.

1. Read the case example of Carina, and complete portions of the CPTA by summarizing the activity demands of playing on a slide, swing set, and merry-go-round and riding a tricycle with speed, agility, and precision.

2. Profile Carina's performance patterns, and rate her motor performance skills using the qualifiers listed in the appropriate section of CPTA. Use the information available in the case study to profile Carina's abilities and the extent of any impairments in her sensory functions using the following qualifiers: 0 = *no impairment*, 1 = *mild impairment*, 2 = *moderate impairment*, 3 = *severe impairment*, 4 = *complete impairment*, 8 = *not specified*, and 9 = *not applicable*. This impairment scale is used in the *International Classification of Functioning, Disability and Health* (ICF; World Health Organization, 2001).

3. Rate the level of challenge of each activity demand, and compare these ratings with ratings of Carina's sensory functions. Use the following *ICF* activity demand qualifiers to rate the degree of challenge to each sensory function: 1 = *mild challenge*, 2 = *moderate challenge*, 3 = *maximum challenge*, and 9 = *not applicable*.

   a. To complete the analysis of Carina's motor performance skills and sensory functions, answer the following questions. Notice that you will be creating and, over the course of therapy, will have the opportunity to test hypotheses regarding the performance skills, activity demands, and client factors that support or hinder Carina's participation in play.

   b. Why do you think Carina is fearful of the slide, swing set, and merry-go-round? What motor performance skills are required for success in using these pieces of equipment (i.e., activity demands)? Does the case study indicate that Carina has activity limitations in these dimensions? Does she have impairments in sensory functions that might compromise the development of these performance skill competencies?

   c. Why do you think Carina has difficulty riding her tricycle with speed, agility, and precision? What motor performance skills are required to ride a tricycle in this manner? Does the case study indicate that Carina has difficulty with these performance skills as a result of sensory impairments?

   d. Why do you think Carina is unable to put on or remove her overcoat, manage her zipper, and place her shoes on the proper feet? What motor skills are required to complete these activities? Does the case study indicate that Carina has difficulty in these performance skills because of sensory impairments?

4. Use the information you have compiled to list Carina's client goals in Table 8.1, which has been started for you. Ensure that the goals are written in a way that communicates the intent to maintain or promote performance and prevent dysfunction and that fits the concerns, priorities, and resources of the family. In the clinical setting, you would establish these goals in collaboration with Carina's parents. *Note.* Long-term goals define target outcomes in occupational performance areas. Short-term objectives relate to the skills and patterns that are small units of performance, impairments and client factors that must be addressed, or the activity or environmental domains that require change if the long-term goal is to be achieved. Goals must be specific, objective, and measurable.

5. During an intervention session, the occupational therapy practitioner used therapeutic use of self to create a playful and imaginative context in which to facilitate Carina's development in the areas specified in Goals

(Continued)

Assignment 8.2. Demands of Play *(Cont.)*

1 and 3 (see Table 8.1). Carina participated in a purposeful activity. The practitioner worked with Carina to select and design an obstacle course using a farm theme. The obstacle course was designed to augment Carina's confidence and performance skills on the playground. Carina cut out a yellow paper star (sheriff's badge), wore a weighted vest (cowboy jacket) to walk across a balance beam (barnyard fence), threw red and blue beanbags (hay bales) into separate baskets, and bounced on a small trampoline (horse). Considering the therapeutic activity designed for Carina, answer the following questions:

a. Why was Carina asked to cut out a paper star? What are the activity demands in this activity?

b. Why did Carina wear a weighted vest? How does this relate to the client factors noted in the case study and the challenge of the task?

c. What activity demands are challenges for Carina when she walks across the balance beam, sorts and throws beanbags, and bounces on a trampoline?

d. How could academic skills be incorporated into this activity so that learning occurs in a fun context?

6. Reconstruct and perform this obstacle course. Assume that Carina has mastered this activity. How could you increase the activity demands to enhance the challenges and continue to develop Carina's motor skills and sensory functions?

7. Design and construct an additional activity for Carina to do while engaging in this

TABLE 8.1
Client Goals for Carina

SHORT-TERM GOAL	LONG-TERM OBJECTIVE
1. Carina will independently play on a swing set and slide for 3 minutes with confidence.	1.a. Carina will improve her vestibular and proprioceptive processing, trunk control, and bilateral coordination to climb the ladder of the slide independently by the end of the school year.
	1.b. Carina will increase her confidence with vestibular movement by first using a toddler swing seat, then progressing to an open sling seat within 2 months with daily play opportunities.
2. Carina will develop her understanding of the academic concepts of color and numbers from early preschool levels to a 4-year-old level by the end of the school year.	2.a. Carina will separate red and blue objects into color categories during activity time at school and generalize this skill across activities by the next school term.
	2.b.
3. Carina will ride her tricycle through an obstacle course with improved speed and agility as demonstrated by ease of performance and increased participation within 6 weeks with daily opportunity to practice.	3.a.
	3.b.
4.	4.a.
	4.b.

(Continued)

Assignment 8.2. Demands of Play (Cont.)

obstacle course. The activity should challenge and promote the development of areas identified in the short-term objectives. Use balls, mats, balance beams, barrels, beanbags, hoops, foam blocks, swings, and any other available objects. Be sure to create a meaningful context for this play activity.

8. Carina has mastered this new activity. Continue to provide Carina with challenges that are achievable by altering the activity to make it slightly more difficult. Explain why purposeful activities should balance achievement with challenge.

9. Take turns with another person role-playing as Carina and her occupational therapy practitioner. Explore the different frames of reference (e.g., sensory integration) a practitioner might use to guide practice. Role-playing will increase the accuracy of your task and activity analysis and enable you to practice interacting with a young child. The verbal and nonverbal interactive relationship between therapist and client provides encouragement, motivation, and feedback to reinforce and facilitate learning.

10. How might a community support the occupation of play and the subsequent developmental benefits that accrue to children who have play-based experiences? Consider how a community could influence activities in day care centers, preschool programs, and schools. How might a community get together to collaboratively define goals, objectives, and an implementation plan to contribute to a healthy future for children?

SUMMARY

The dimensions of occupational performance influence a child's participation in the occupation of play. Through play, children process sensory and perceptual body functions and in turn produce motor responses. They develop performance patterns including communication, motor, socialization, and environmental interaction performance skills. Because play is a meaningful occupation for children, occupational therapy practitioners use play both to assess abilities and performance and as an intervention that is valued by the child. Using task analysis to develop a client profile and understand what aspects of a play activity can be sequenced to enhance development is necessary for outlining and measuring an intervention plan.

REFERENCES

American Occupational Therapy Association. (1993). Position paper: Purposeful activity. *American Journal of Occupational Therapy, 47,* 1081–1082. http://dx.doi.org/10.5014/ajot.47.12.1081

American Occupational Therapy Association. (2014). Occupational therapy practice framework: Domain and process (3rd ed.). *American Journal of Occupational Therapy, 68*(Suppl. 1), S1–48. http://dx.doi.org/10.5014/ajot.2014.682006

Bundy, A. (1993). Assessment of play and leisure: Delineation of the problem. *American Journal of Occupational Therapy, 47,* 217–222. http://dx.doi.org/10.5014/ajot.47.3.217

Eberle, S. G. (2011). Playing with the multiple intelligences: How play helps us grow. *American Journal of Play, 4,* 19–51.

Eliot, L. (1999). *What's going on in there? How the brain and mind develop in the first five years of life.* New York: Bantam Books.

Elkind, D. (2008). The power of play: Learning what comes naturally. *American Journal of Play, 1,* 1–7.

Ferland, F. (1992). Le jeu en ergothérapie: Réflexion préalable à l'élaboration d'un nouveau modèle de pratique [Play in occupational therapy: Preliminary reflection for the elaboration of a new practice model]. *Canadian Journal of Occupational Therapy, 59,* 95–101.

Folio, M. R., & Fewell, R. R. (2000). *Peabody Developmental Motor Scales* (2nd ed.). San Antonio, TX: Psychological Corporation.

Graham-Berman, S. A., Coupet, S., Egler, L., Mattis, J., & Banyard, V. (1996). Interpersonal relationships and adjustment of children in homeless and economically stressed families. *Journal of Clinical Child Psychology, 25,* 250–261.

Gray, P. (2011). The decline of play and the rise of psychopathology in children and adolescents. *American Journal of Play, 3*, 443–463.

Han, M., Moore, N., Vukelich, C., & Buell, M. (2010). Does play make a difference? How play intervention affects the vocabulary learning of at-risk preschoolers. *American Journal of Play, 3*, 82–105.

Henricks, T. (2008). The nature of play: An overview. *Journal of Play, 1*, 157–180.

Hofferth, S. L., & Sandberg, J. F. (2000). *Changes in American children's time, 1981–1997* (Report 00–456). Ann Arbor: Population Studies Center at the Institute for Social Research, University of Michigan.

Kool, R., & Lawver, T. (2010). Play therapy: Considerations and applications for the practitioner. *Psychiatry, 7*(10), 19–24.

Mayberry, W. (1990). Self-esteem in children: Considerations for measurement and intervention. *American Journal of Occupational Therapy, 44*, 729–734. http://dx.doi.org/10.5014/ajot.44.8.729

Miller, B., & Cummings, J. (Eds.). (2007). *The human frontal lobes*. New York: Guilford Press.

Miller, E., & Kuhaneck, H. (2008). Children's perceptions of play experiences and play preferences: A qualitative study. *American Journal of Occupational Therapy, 62*, 407–415. http://dx.doi.org/10.5014/ajot.62.4.407

Organization for Economic Cooperation and Development. (2004). *Five curriculum outlines*. Paris: Author.

Piaget, J. (1950). *The psychology of intelligence*. New York: Routledge & Kegan Paul.

Piaget, J. (1962). *The psychology of the child*. New York: Basic Books.

Reilly, M. (1974). *Play as exploratory learning: Studies in curiosity behavior*. Beverly Hills, CA: Sage.

Sabonis-Chafee, B., & Hussey, S. M. (1998). *Introduction to occupational therapy* (2nd ed.). St. Louis, MO: Mosby.

Soska, K. C., Adolph, K. E., & Johnson, S. P. (2010). Systems in development: Motor skill acquisition facilitates three-dimensional object completion. *Developmental Psychology, 46*, 129–138.

Spencer, J. C. (1998). Evaluation of performance contexts. In M. E. Neistadt & E. B. Crepeau (Eds.), *Willard and Spackman's occupational therapy* (9th ed., pp. 291–310). Philadelphia: Lippincott.

Tanta, K. J., Deitz, J. C., White, O., & Billingsley, F. (2005). The effects of peer-play level on initiations and responses of preschool children with delayed play skills. *American Journal of Occupational Therapy, 59*, 437–445. http://dx.doi.org/10.5014/ajot.59.4.437

Vandenberg, B., & Kielhofner, G. (1982). Play in evolution, culture, and individual adaptation: Implications for therapy. *American Journal of Occupational Therapy, 36*, 20–28. http://dx.doi.org/10.5014/ajot.36.1.20

Vygotsky, L. S. (1978). The role of play in development. In *Mind in Society* (pp. 92–104). Cambridge, MA: Harvard University Press.

Whitebread, D., Coltman, P., Jameson, H., & Lander, R. (2009). Play, cognition and self-regulation: What exactly are children learning when they learn to play? *Educational and Child Psychology, 26*, 40–52.

Willoughby, C., King, G., & Polatajko, H. J. (1996). A therapist's guide to children's self-esteem. *American Journal of Occupational Therapy, 50*, 124–132. http://dx.doi.org/10.5014/ajot.50.2.124

World Health Organization. (2001). *International classification of functioning, disability and health*. Geneva: Author.

Zemke, R., & Clark, F. (Eds.). (1996). *Occupational science: The evolving discipline*. Philadelphia: F. A. Davis.

Education as Occupation

9

It is doubtful that any child may reasonably be expected to succeed in life if he is denied the opportunity of an education. Such an opportunity, where the state has undertaken to provide it, is a right which must be made available to all on equal terms.

—Brown v. Board of Education (1954)

LEARNING OBJECTIVES

At the completion of this chapter, readers will be able to

- Describe how occupational therapy practitioners apply task analysis as an evaluation and intervention tool to develop intervention strategies that enable young clients to participate in the occupation of education;
- Define performance patterns, communication and interaction performance skills, and mental functions as these dimensions relate to the occupation of education; and
- Apply task analysis to profile the performance patterns, performance skills, and mental functions that are challenged during participation in educational activities.

KEY TERMS

Assistive technology
Cognitive skills
Collaborative consultation
Communication and social skills
Frames of reference
Habits
High technology
Individualized education program
Low technology
Mental functions
Models of practice

Occupational profile
Occupational Therapy School-Based
    Consultation model
Performance patterns
Performance skills
Roles
Routines
Sensory modulation disorder
Sensory overresponsivity
Student profile

This chapter focuses on performance skills and patterns and mental functions that may be challenged during participation in the occupation of education. Children's sense of competency in school is based on their academic achievement and their identity as a student who does schoolwork. Occupational therapy practitioners often refer to school as the "work" of the student. The task of practitioners is to examine the challenges children face and present strategies from a positive perspective.

STUDENT ROLE AND LEARNING CHALLENGES

By the time children enter school, they typically have grown accustomed to a high level of activity through the occupation of play as infants, toddlers, and preschool-age children. Once children take on the role of student, typically ages 5–6 years, they are expected to adapt to new rules of classroom and playground conduct and to quickly transition between these two environmental contexts.

As children change contexts and mature, they experience a decline in physical activity; less time is available for play, because teachers place increasing emphasis on directing children's energy and attention span toward the education occupation (Gray, 2011). Children's abilities to endure and pace academic tasks are nurtured within the school by their teachers, and children are guided in establishing more formal daily routines and habits by both parents and teachers.

Children perform many tasks each day while engaging in their student role. They also establish new performance patterns (e.g., daily routines) with a scheduled school day, week, and year (i.e., temporal contexts). Occupational therapy services for students with disabilities have been recognized as having a substantial impact on children and adolescents adapting to the student role. In addition to assisting with the accommodations a school must make to create suitable environmental conditions, occupational therapy practitioners augment educators' knowledge and skills in developing and implementing an appropriately *individualized education program* (*IEP*; Frolek Clark & Chandler, 2013; Villeneuve,

2009). The IEP is a written document that describes the special education and related services that will be provided to meet a student's educational needs (Chandler, 2013).

Villeneuve's (2009) literature review of research on occupational therapy services in schools identified two fundamental conditions for collaboration between educators and occupational therapy practitioners. First, teachers need a clear understanding of the roles and responsibilities of occupational therapy practitioners and of what practitioners can offer to the education process. Practitioners also need an understanding of school board policies, the curriculum, and classroom practices of teachers. Second, educators and occupational therapy practitioners need adequate time to collaborate and share information. The essence of the relationship is collaborative partnership.

Occupation is temporal; it structures time with purposeful activity (McColl, 2011). Although the education occupation consumes many hours in the life of a child, perceptions of the importance of the student role and academic achievement vary among children, families, and cultures. Children's interests, values, and needs, as well as their personal and environmental contexts, shape the meaning and purpose they attribute to different educational activities. In other words, the meaningfulness of an activity depends on a personal interpretation of its value or importance. Thus, the initial step of the occupational therapy process involves creating an *occupational profile* that captures the essence of the child's occupational history, interests, values, performance patterns, and personal context. Then practitioners conduct a broader analysis of the child's occupations, performance, and contexts.

Occupational therapy practitioners must be aware of whether family resources or situations support therapeutic and supportive services (e.g., whether unmet medical needs complicate performance in educational settings). Benedict (2005) conducted a study of family resources in U.S. households with children with functional limitations and found disparities in type of health insurance and household education level, reflecting inequitable access to resources among U.S. policies and programs serving children with limitations.

Increased family income and education appeared to give some families an advantage in obtaining services and in identifying unmet needs of their child (Benedict, 2005), even though Medicaid and the State Children's Health Insurance Programs were found to have improved the system. Eligibility for funding varies across programs and service settings, but criteria typically include the child's diagnosis, location, or family income. Unfortunately, some children who would benefit from cross-disciplinary services do not fit the criteria set out by the funding agency (e.g., diagnosis, age, school; Benedict, 2005). It is realistic to assume that with unmet needs, both children and families are disadvantaged in that they must cope with fewer services. Therefore, occupational therapy practitioners must examine challenges beyond those of personal factors, such as the child's diagnosis, and consider the contextual aspects beyond the family and the classroom.

SCHOOL-BASED CONSULTATION

School-based occupational therapy is directed not only to furthering general education goals but also to adding to the child's functional profile for use by the educational team. Before 1996, much of occupational therapy services in the schools consisted of direct treatment. Since then, *collaborative consultation,* which is an "interactive team process focused on student performance and influenced by critical personal and contextual variables" (Hanft & Shepherd, 2008, p. xix), and integration of intervention into the education plan have increasingly been recognized in school systems in the United States and Canada (Reid, Chiu, Sinclair, Wehrmann, & Naseer, 2006). Reid and colleagues (2006) described the *Occupational Therapy School-Based Consultation (OTSBC) model,* designed "to facilitate the developmental needs of students and enhance their occupational performance in school" (p. 216). The OTSBC model focuses on two major components—assessment and consultation—and is a functional guide to establishing the collaborative process.

Reid and colleagues (2006) noted that the primary challenge for occupational therapy practitioners is the interface between the occupational therapy assessment and consultation with other professionals. Teacher awareness of the role and purpose of occupational therapy within the classroom, in particular, was determined to be a key intermediate outcome. Reid et al. considered consultation a way to promote teachers' understanding of a student's special needs and to enhance the student's education plan by providing salient information about assistive accommodations and interventions. During this collaborative process, the teacher identifies and implements techniques and strategies to accommodate the student's needs. Long-term outcomes focus on improvement of the student's functional performance at school.

Reid et al. (2006) also found that the most frequently identified performance categories in school consultation were writing and printing (e.g., legibility), organization skills (e.g., remembering a sequence of tasks), and desk skills (e.g., using scissors). Other problems they identified included attention problems, being able to work independently, and social skills problems. Villeneuve (2009) provided important insight into the outcome of consultation:

> In stark contrast to direct intervention, the outcome of consultation is a change in the human and nonhuman environment. Providing intervention at the level of environmental change can include adapting the social environment, such as developing strategies for interpreting student behaviour to enable more effective interaction. (p. 208)

Occupational therapy practitioners may visit schools and make recommendations after assessment. The strongest approach, however, is to fully integrate occupational therapy services within the school team, enabling an interdisciplinary approach to educational planning for children with special needs. Working closely to address the challenges each child faces within the school environment allows all team members a greater understanding of the reality of school life (Hutton, 2008). The knowledge base represented on a school team, especially regarding the sensory and motor development of children with and without disability, is diverse (Hutton, 2008). Sharing knowledge is the foundation of collaborative consultation.

STUDENT PROFILE

The occupational therapy practitioner assesses a student and develops a *student profile,* which describes a child's performance and limitations within the context of the school or learning environment. The student profile includes the child's academic history, patterns of learning and strategies implemented, and assessment details (including client factors, such as body functions and structures related to diagnosed or undiagnosed limitations). Task analysis examines the action demands of school-related tasks relative to the strengths and limitations of the child. Performance expectations within the school curriculum are important factors, particularly related to a teacher's perception of a child's abilities and limitations.

Performance Skills and Patterns

Through observation of performance skills and patterns within the school context, the practitioner develops a profile of the child's challenges, skill gaps in the classroom, and family stresses related to special needs. *Performance skills* include skills "used in managing and modifying actions on route to the completion of daily life tasks" (Fisher & Kielhofner, 1995, p. 120). In the school context, performance skills related to successful learning include motor and praxis skills (e.g., printing), sensory–perceptual skills (e.g., visual scanning for reading), emotional regulation skills (e.g., accepting direction), cognitive skills (e.g., learning capacity), and communication and social skills (e.g., initiating and answering questions).

Performance patterns include a student's roles, routines, and habits (American Occupational Therapy Association [AOTA], 2014). The performance patterns expected of the student include arriving to school on time, organizing one's desk, and so forth. Case Example 9.1 describes the performance skills of a young girl struggling with fine motor delays.

Roles are "sets of behaviors expected by society and shaped by culture and context" (AOTA, 2014, p. S8). Certain behaviors or roles are expected of students, such as showing mastery of what they are learning as a measure of success. To children, achievement indicates control over their own outcomes. *Routines* are activities that have established sequences that provide structure at school (e.g., school bell to return to the classroom), whereas *habits* are automatic behaviors that are ingrained in the everyday activities within the school environment (e.g., storing outerwear and books in a locker). Habitual behavior either supports or interferes with performance.

According to McColl (2011), "Habits increase skill, decrease fatigue, free attention, and protect the individual against the stressful effects of difficult situations" (p. 95). Development of roles, routines, and habits occurs through support from parents, siblings, teachers, occupational therapy practitioners, and the community or social system. Roles, routines, and habits support engagement and participation in school and establish a sense of belonging associated with health and wellness or connectedness.

Occupational therapy practitioners must understand the purpose of school policies and routines and how these may affect a child's capacity to adapt to and engage in school and to develop realistic roles, routines, and habits. Practitioners also promote school policies (e.g., classroom inclusion) to support students who have physical, mental, and emotional challenges.

Occupational therapy practitioners observe and engage with children in schools to gather significant information about the patterns and routines of the school day, which is part of the task analysis process. Concurrently, practitioners obtain information about the specific student's family and roles in preparation for a school day, as well as the school's expectations of the parents to commit time to tutoring their child (e.g., helping with homework). Understanding the contextual framework and classroom expectations ensures that practitioners are not unrealistic in developing program aims and expectations.

Communication and social skills

Communication and social skills are the behaviors a person uses to interact with others (Fisher, 2006), such as looking where and when appropriate, gesturing to emphasize intentions, maintaining appropriate physical space, initiating and answering questions, taking turns verbally and physically, and acknowledging the other person's

CASE EXAMPLE 9.1. AVA: FINE MOTOR DELAYS

Note. Use the Client Profile and Task Analysis Form (CPTA; Appendix A) as you read this case. Complete the form with the information provided about Ava.

Client profile and referral: An occupational therapy practitioner received a referral about a **6-year-old child in first grade, Ava,** who had difficulty keeping up with classroom work and showed fine motor delays related to printing and producing numbers. The teacher indicated that Ava held her pencil with an immature grasp; took a long time to complete pencil-and-paper tasks, including craft activities; and regularly dropped items she held in her hands.

Tasks analyzed and performance skills: The practitioner conducted an assessment and noted that Ava had bilateral intrinsic and extrinsic hand muscle weakness, wrist flexor and extensor muscle weakness, and decreased fine motor coordination, and she held her pencil in her right hand in a modified thumb wrap grasp. The practitioner recognized that Ava's condition could affect a broad range of activities in and out of school. Because public resources supporting school-based occupational therapy were limited, the practitioner focused on the issues directly related to the classroom concerns, specifically, on interventions to improve Ava's performance skills pertaining to pencil-and-paper tasks and craft activities. Moreover, any homework the practitioner assigned to Ava needed to be realistic in the context of her home environment and family routine. The practitioner could not expect Ava's parents to conduct a complex home program, so the home activities needed to be purposeful and a natural extension of Ava's normal routines.

School context and analysis of performance skills: The occupational therapy practitioner initiated a meeting with Ava's teacher to share assessment findings and provide information about the underlying limitations influencing Ava's school performance. The practitioner prepared discussion points to share important information about specific difficulties Ava was having with lower-than-normal muscle tone, sensory disturbance, and difficulty with motor planning. The practitioner asked the teacher to describe specific strategies used that had worked and that had failed. Together they planned an approach for the coming term and included a way to measure outcomes.

Assignment 9.1. Ava

Review Case Example 9.1. Design a 15-minute home program that Ava's parents can help her with each evening. What specifically is your aim with this intervention, and how will it improve Ava's printing and completion of arts and crafts projects?

---

perspective during an interchange. Communication and interaction performance skills require or are dependent on mental functions such as language and emotional functions (Canadian Association of Occupational Therapists, 1997). When children enter school, they rapidly expand their circle of friends and acquaintances and the size of their social network, so the student role requires continual development and refinement of communication and social skills.

As students progress in school, measurement of academic achievement is increasingly based on written communication. Written communication in the form of paper-and-pencil or computer-generated documents is the principal way that children demonstrate their acquisition of higher-level cognitive functions, such as concept formation and problem solving. Perceptual functions required for written communication coincide with the development of visual–spatial perception and memory functions and the sensory integration of tactile, proprioceptive, and visual stimuli.

Cognitive skills

Cognitive skills include orientation, attention, perception, problem solving, memory, judgment, language, reasoning, and planning. *Mental functions* contribute to developing cognitive skills and are categorized as global (e.g., consciousness, orientation, temperament and personality, energy and drive, sleep) and specific (e.g., higher-level cognition, attention, memory, perception, thought, sequencing complex movement, emotional, experience of self and time; AOTA, 2014). Conformity to the student role is often measured in the classroom by evaluation of a child's energy level, attention span, and temperament. Academic performance is often rated primarily on the basis of success at tasks requiring cognition (e.g., reading and math acquisition, sequencing tasks needed for a school project). Teachers learn about students' mental functions and cognitive skills through the actions and words students use to communicate, and these performance skills serve as one of the primary measures of academic achievement.

Examples of abilities that teachers look for in kindergarten through Grade 3 to assess the maturity of cognitive functions include the abilities to recognize shapes, sizes, and objects; to sort and categorize information and objects; and to generalize concepts. The ability to understand language and express oneself through speech is vital to the interactive process of learning and the measurement of the outcome of knowledge acquisition. As students mature, performance skills in the area of written communication develop; cognitive and motor functions are refined to enable students to print and write in cursive. For example, a mature tripod grasp supports the acquisition of those graphic skills.

Sensory processing and sensory–perceptual skills

Sensory overresponsivity to tactile and auditory input presents as impairments within the educational context, because these sensitivities interrupt a child's participation and performance. Sensory overresponsivity was first described by Dr. A. Jean Ayres (1964), an occupational therapist and neuroscientist. Some children have significant difficulties regulating their response to sensory input manifested in atypical emotional responses observed as defensiveness and a fight-or-flight impulse (Ben-Sasson, Carter, & Briggs-Gowan, 2009; Brett-Green, Miller, Schoen, & Nielsen, 2010).

Impairments in regulating responses to sensory input are often referred to as *sensory*

modulation disorder. Decreased capacity to modulate responses to what is perceived as noxious stimulation interferes with performance, especially in activities intended to be self-initiated. Children with developmental disorders, such as autism spectrum disorder, and brain injury frequently have sensory modulation disorder. Social–emotional problems manifest, with associated problems of competence in self-care, problem solving, and social participation. Such children show high stress levels and may be easily irritated and distracted, making learning alongside their peers difficult. Behavior may include psychopathology in the form of withdrawal, defiance, resistance, and so forth; all can disrupt a classroom. The key consideration for occupational therapy practitioners and other school team members is to distinguish sensory disturbance from child behavioral problems.

Assignment 9.2. Performance Skills in Schools

1. Review and familiarize yourself with the definition of terms from the *Occupational Therapy Practice Framework: Domain and Process,* (AOTA, 2014) in the areas of performance skills.
2. From the following suggestions, select and perform 1 activity that a child might engage in at school. What process skills, communication and interaction performance skills, and mental functions are used during participation in the educational activity you selected?
   a. *Preschool level:* Place a circle, square, and triangle into a form board. Color a picture. Play "Simon Says."
   b. *Elementary level:* Use a pattern to construct a three-dimensional object. Draw a clock that tells the current time. Build a fort. Print the letters of the alphabet. Tie shoelaces.
3. Complete a CPTA form (Appendix A) profiling the activity demands of completing puzzles, using scissors, and spelling a name. You may limit your approach to subsections of the full form that reflect the focus of this chapter: performance patterns, mental functions, and performance skills.

OCCUPATIONAL THERAPY'S ROLE

Promotion of Engagement and Participation in School

Occupational therapy practitioners, who understand engagement from a holistic perspective, must address all aspects of performance when providing intervention designed to support engagement in occupations (AOTA, 2014). Student clients may be individual children, groups of children, or an entire population of students (Frolek Clark & Chandler, 2013). Practitioners work toward enabling these clients to engage in the education occupation in varied classroom contexts by developing strategies that enhance performance patterns, performance skills, and client factors and by altering activity demands and promoting enabling school contexts.

The majority of elementary school class time is spent on paper-and-pencil and manipulative tasks, a problem for the majority of children with learning difficulties who demonstrate fine motor and handwriting difficulties (McHale & Cermak, 1992). In work with preschoolers and young students with learning disabilities or motor performance delays, occupational therapy practitioners evaluate the client factors required to perform functional classroom activities and then use strategies and techniques to improve these skills (see Case Example 9.2).

Occupational therapy services can also prepare children to adjust to residual activity limitations after trauma, disorder, or disease. Practitioners direct intervention toward providing purposeful activities (i.e., remediation or restoration), altering or restructuring activity demands *(text continues on page 154)*

CASE EXAMPLE 9.2. KEISHA: SCHOOL-BASED OCCUPATIONAL THERAPY CONSULTATION

Note. Use the CPTA form (Appendix A) as you read this case example. Complete the form with the information provided about Keisha.

Keisha was about to turn age 6 years. She had attended the same day care and kindergarten center since she was 9 months old. Keisha was an only child and lived with her father, who, concerned about Keisha's development, requested an occupational therapy consultation.

According to her father, Keisha was always a very active child. Although she was uncoordinated for her age, she loved gross motor activities and was usually a daredevil on the playground. Her social skills were immature. She liked to play in the same area as the other children but did not play with them in a cooperative or collaborative fashion. She listened well but did not ask for things she needed or wanted and had to be encouraged to do so. Over the past year, Keisha's father became increasingly concerned about her short attention span and lack of interest in tabletop or quiet-time activities. She had great difficulty completing puzzles and became frustrated when trying to use scissors. She could cut a straight line, but the teacher had to explain how to turn the paper to cut around shapes. Keisha loved to color pictures but tended to color quickly and seemed unconcerned about staying within the form of the picture. Although she put great effort into printing, Keisha could not print letters in sequence to spell her name.

After spending a half-hour interviewing staff members, the occupational therapy practitioner realized that the center provided a very unstructured approach to learning. Children were encouraged to pursue whatever activities interested them. Although the teachers offered projects to facilitate learning, the students could choose not to participate.

After Keisha's evaluation was complete, the occupational therapist determined that she had poor fine motor coordination and very immature pencil grasp and had not yet established hand dominance. Her temporal and spatial organization, visual–spatial perception, and sequencing skills were also below average. Keisha appeared to be very self-conscious about her verbal skills and about her performance when completing puzzles and paper-and-pencil activities. She loved animals, the circus, and gymnastics.

Assignment 9.3. Keisha

1. Using the information in Case Example 9.2, profile Keisha's performance patterns and process skills and her communication and interaction performance skills. Also profile her mental abilities and cognitive skill deficits.
2. What cognitive skills are required for completing puzzles, using scissors, and spelling a name? List Keisha's abilities, and rate her limitations.
3. To complete the analysis of Keisha's performance skills, answer the following questions. Notice that you will be creating and, over the course of the intervention, will have the opportunity to test hypotheses regarding the performance skills, activity demands, and client factors that support or hinder Keisha's participation in play.
   a. Why do you think Keisha has difficulty completing puzzles, using scissors, and spelling her name? What cognitive and sensory–perceptual skills are required for successful participation in these activities? Does the case study indicate that Keisha has difficulty with these performance skills? Does she have impairments in mental functions (a client factor) pertinent to these performance skills?
   b. Why do you think Keisha "liked to play in the same area as the other children but did not play with them in a cooperative or collaborative fashion" and "listened well but did not ask for things she needed or wanted and had to be encouraged to do so"? What communication and social performance skills are required for more age-appropriate social skills?
   c. The father indicated that Keisha was a very active child, but he was concerned about her short attention span and lack of interest in tabletop or quiet-time activities. How do temporal contextual factors, such as chronological and developmental age, and the social and cultural contextual factors at the day care center affect Keisha and her role performance patterns?
   d. What performance skills does Keisha need to support her engagement in school activities in which she is expected to participate?
4. Use the information you have compiled to list Keisha's client goals in Table 9.1,

TABLE 9.1
Client Goals for Keisha

Long-Term Goal (Primarily client driven, measurable, global task, or activity achievements)	**Short-Term Objective** (Primarily practitioner driven, measurable, incremental, stepwise, or mini-achievements)
1. Keisha will print her name by forming letters in the correct sequence.	1.a. Keisha will trace the letters in her name to learn the required motor plan.
	1.b. Keisha will sequence the letters in her name by copying from a template on her first try, then print her name without cues immediately afterward.
2.	2.a.
	2.b.
3.	3.a.
	3.b.
4.	4.a.
	4.b.

Assignment 9.3. Keisha *(Cont.)*

which has been started for you. Ensure that the goals fit the concerns, priorities, and resources of this family and day care center. In the clinical setting, you would establish these goals on behalf of Keisha in collaboration with her father, the teacher, and any other special education professionals and staff at the day care center.

5. During the first intervention session, Keisha participated in a therapeutic activity that the occupational therapy practitioner developed for the class. The activity allowed the children a degree of movement around the classroom to seek supplies and facilitated a positive outcome on a paper-and-pencil craft activity to be a gift for the children's parents. The project required the children to find a shape or object in the room to represent the center of a sunflower and then trace it onto a piece of construction paper. Keisha found a can of the right size and successfully traced around the bottom of the can to make a circle. The next step was to go outside with a partner and find leaves or flower petals to paste around the circle as petals. Once Keisha and her partner were back at the table, the practitioner asked them to tell others about the shapes and colors they found. Keisha then glued the petals onto the paper. She shredded tissue paper and glued it to the center of the flower. The practitioner held the stems and waited for the children to ask for a stem. Keisha stood at the table to perform this craft.

   a. Why was the activity designed to include structured movement?
   b. Why was Keisha asked to trace around an object? What are the activity demands?
   c. Why did Keisha shred rather than cut the paper to decorate the center of the sunflower?
   d. How do the strategies relate to noted client factors and the challenge of the task?
   e. What are the activity demands of locating an object, tracing it, collecting leaves, shredding paper, and gluing everything together?

   f. What communication and social performance skills were required? What strategies might be used to enhance communication among the students?
   g. Assume that Keisha has mastered this activity. How could you increase the activity demands to enhance the challenge and further nurture Keisha's motor and praxis skills?

6. The purpose of therapeutic activities is to enhance participation in student activities and the education occupation by promoting the development of specific client factors and performance skills. The focus of a remediation or restoration approach to therapy is to change client factors and establish a skill or ability that has not yet been developed. Develop therapeutic activities, and identify the features of these activities that make them particularly attractive for use with children with limitations in motor and process performance skills.

   After analyzing these activities for their potential to address intervention objectives aimed at Keisha's goals, you realize that adjustments can be made to maximize therapeutic value. Explain how the activity demands of these projects can be adjusted to ensure success while challenging Keisha. Explain why purposeful activities can balance achievement with challenge. Would you recommend assistive equipment to support Keisha's efforts to improve her skills, such as pencil grips or specially designed scissors? The compensatory or adaptation approach to therapy guides occupational therapy practitioners in revising the current context or activity demands to support performance in natural settings.

7. Role-play Keisha and her occupational therapy practitioner with another person to increase the accuracy of your task analysis and enable you to practice the communication and interaction style you might use with a young child. The verbal and nonverbal interactive relationship between practitioner and client provides a source of encouragement, motivation, and feedback to reinforce and facilitate learning.

(Continued)

Assignment 9.3. Keisha *(Cont.)*

Assume that the manager of the day care center has asked for consultation regarding how the staff might provide an enriched environment and therapeutic activity experiences to enhance the performance of all children while integrating strategies for children with special needs. What therapeutic activities would you recommend that the staff at this day care center integrate into their activity planning? What recommendations do you have regarding enrichment of the social and cultural context to promote the healthy development of all children to enhance their occupational performance at school?

8. Explore the process of integrating the Person–Environment–Occupation model of practice with the frame of reference outlined in the *Framework*, which further guides evaluation and intervention. *Models of practice* give general guidance for practice, explain complex relations among concepts, and are

"a set of ideas derived from various fields of study which are organized to form a synthesis and integration of elements of theory and practice" (Hagedorn, 1997, p. 144). By comparison, *frames of reference* reflect the knowledge and theories within the basic sciences and provide a paradigm through which practitioners view the world, solve problems, and prescribe solutions (Hagedorn, 1997). Research and identify frames of reference used in occupational therapy. What frames of reference could you use to interpret Keisha's occupational performance profile in the education occupation?

9. According to the National Center for Education Statistics (2012), the number of children and youth ages 3–21 receiving special education services was 6.5 million in 2009–2010, or about 13% of all public school students. As an occupational therapy practitioner, how might you contribute to the promotion of health among this population?

(i.e., compensation or adaptation) directed at providing opportunities for students to practice new methods, training and consulting with teachers and parents to create an enriched context for all children (i.e., health promotion), and reducing the occurrence of barriers to optimal participation (i.e., disability prevention).

When selecting therapeutic activities to challenge a particular child's abilities and promote more advanced performance skills, the practitioner directs initial intervention at lower-order performance processes such as orientation and attention (Abreu & Toglia, 1987). Elements that can be graded to enhance the therapeutic value of an activity include environmental structure, activity familiarity, directions for completion, number of items, spatial arrangement of items, and response rate required (Wheatley, 1996). Purposeful and meaningful activity is the foundation for motivation (Hess & Campion, 1983; Kirscher, 1984; Trombly, 1995), personal satisfaction (Thibodeaux & Ludwig, 1988), learning and adaptation (Yuen, 1988), and motor skills development and performance (Hsieh, Nelson, Smith, & Peterson, 1996; Yuen, 1988).

To design effective and efficient evaluation and intervention, occupational therapy practitioners partner with student clients, parents, teaching and support staff, and others to identify educational goals that are important to a student and his or her family (or a group of students and their families). An individual student's educational goals are documented as part of an educational team's contribution to an IEP. Communication is vital to the process of goal setting; the process of sharing their interests, needs, values, and priorities is vital to clients' sense of autonomy in directing their own services. Parents, teachers, and other stakeholders may act as proxies for a child by providing information on the activities that have meaning and purpose to the child.

Equipment and Assistive Technology

According to the World Health Organization (WHO; 2001),

Restrictions in participation in education are brought about by the features of the physical and social environment of a person that make it difficult, or perhaps impossible, to have the opportunity to learn and to perform in the education setting. (p. 153)

The consequence of an impairment in body function or body structure may be disability; limitations and restrictions may arise as a direct consequence of impairments at the organ level or as the person's response to the impairment (WHO, 1980). Many people have disabilities, activity limitations, and participation restrictions that can be ameliorated through the application of preparatory methods or purposeful activities using a remedial or restorative approach to intervention.

Technology has provided educators with flexibility in customizing and individualizing educational strategies for all students and in restructuring the contexts of learning and classrooms. The availability and accessibility of technological devices enable teachers to formulate learning goals that maximize the potential for all learners, including those who have a disability (Center for Applied Technology [CAT], 2002). *Assistive technology (AT)* can be considered a scaffold supporting students with (or without) disabilities as they participate in education. The opportunity to engage in tasks using AT is motivating to students and provides opportunities to practice, receive immediate feedback, and demonstrate skills. Occupational therapy practitioners help clients use AT to engage in occupations (AOTA, 2014).

AT refers to a broad range of devices, services, strategies, and practices that are conceived and applied to lessen the problems faced by people who have disabilities. The Technology-Related Assistance Act of 1988 (Pub. L. 100–407) was most recently reauthorized in 2010 (Twenty-First Century Communications and Video Accessibility Act of 2010, Pub. L. 111–260). The act seeks to provide assistive technologies to enable people with disabilities to participate in education, work, and daily living at their best achievable level. The legislation covers people of all ages with all disabilities in all environments. *AT* was defined in the 1998 version (Assistive Technology Act of 1998, Pub. L. 105–394) as "any item, piece of equipment, or product system, whether acquired commercially, modified, or customized, that is used to increase, maintain, or improve functional capabilities of individuals with disabilities" (§ 3.3).

For people whose disabilities result from impairments that cannot be ameliorated through technological interventions, services are directed toward using technology to alter activity demands or environmental contexts to promote participation. For example, some children who are not able to articulate speech clearly can use AT to communicate. Similarly, some children do not have the upper-limb control and hand dexterity to operate a standard computer keyboard, and AT (e.g., switches, voice recognition software) can help them operate devices such as a computer or tablet.

AT includes both *low-technology* and *high-technology* devices. Low-technology devices are simple to program and inexpensive and include typing and writing aids. High-technology devices are more expensive, complicated, and customizable, and many include such features as switches, computers, power wheelchairs, and environmental control units (ECUs). Children and adults who have a constellation of activity limitations can maximize their participation in day-to-day occupations with the use of AT. For example, ECUs can enable children to manage their environments by remote control and to maintain an interest in interacting with their world. The use of AT may prevent learned helplessness in some children (Swinth, 1996).

AT, even high-technology devices (e.g., computers), cannot substitute for intervention to change curricular demands by creating IEPs and altering classroom environments to be more enabling for all students (CAT, 2002). Indeed, changes to activity demands and environments may result in more appropriate contexts and fewer requirements for AT. Whereas the use of AT focuses responsibility for adaptation on the child, the alteration of activity demands and environmental contexts focuses responsibility for adaptation on others. The key to services for children who have disabilities is to apply the principles of participation and engagement; best fit of strategies, techniques, and devices; and diversity in approaches.

The role of the occupational therapy practitioner is to ensure to the extent possible that impairments do not restrict participation in meaningful occupations. The practitioner may use AT to alter activity demands and restructure environmental contexts, an approach to intervention that enables clients to minimize the impact of the disability and promotes adaptation. AT may also be used as a purposeful activity to establish or restore performance skills, particularly in the motor and communication dimensions. In this context, AT is used as a preparatory method for remediation or restoration of client skills or abilities (AOTA, 2014).

Occupational therapy practitioners must be careful when recommending the use of AT devices to ensure that such devices are not seen as a substitute for other initiatives that foster greater engagement of students in the curriculum and classroom. For example, it is easy to assume that the use of a software program will enable a student with disabilities to learn concepts, but children (and adults) typically need to learn, rehearse, and generalize concepts through participation in a full range of activities. AT devices prepare clients for more purposeful and occupation-based activities. Clients will not improve the performance skills and client factors they need for engagement in the full range of education occupations exclusively through the use of AT; they improve these skills and factors through engagement in curricular and classroom activities.

SUMMARY

In education settings, occupational therapy practitioners are consultants whose purpose is to help improve students' ability to participate and learn in their school environment. Student clients may be individual children, groups of children, or an entire population of students. Practitioners collaborate with individual students or groups of students, teaching and support staff, and family members to create focused, realistic, and measureable evaluation and intervention plans. During the evaluation and intervention process, task analysis can assist practitioners in constructing an occupational profile of performance patterns and skills, environmental and personal contexts, activity demands, and client factors. Information from initial and ongoing task analyses provides a basis for intervention planning and adjustments during implementation, which includes ensuring the useful and appropriate application of technology.

The client and family guide the use of technology in intervention planning and implementation according to their values and needs, sociocultural and environmental factors, financial resources, and judgment of the cost-effectiveness of the technology (DeCoste, 2013; Shuster, 1993; Swinth, 1996). When planning an intervention, practitioners should keep in mind that learning to use AT can be a slow process for the learner, both physically and cognitively. Therefore, the intervention plan and the recommended technology should be attractive, motivating, and engaging for the client.

REFERENCES

Abreu, B. C., & Toglia, J. P. (1987). Cognitive rehabilitation: A model of occupational therapy. *American Journal of Occupational Therapy, 41,* 439–448. http://dx.doi.org/10.5014/ajot.41.7.439

American Occupational Therapy Association. (2014). Occupational therapy practice framework: Domain and process (3rd ed.). *American Journal of Occupational Therapy, 68*(Suppl. 1), S1–48. http://dx.doi.org/10.5014/ajot.2014.682006

Assistive Technology Act of 1998, Pub. L. 105–394, § 2, 29 Stat. 3628.

Ayres, A. J. (1964). Tactile functions: Their relation to hyperactive and perceptual motor behavior. *American Journal of Occupational Therapy, 18,* 6–11.

Benedict, R. E. (2005). Disparities in the use of and unmet need for therapeutic and supportive services among school-age children with functional limitations: A comparison across settings. *Health Research and Educational Trust, 41,* 103–124.

Ben-Sasson, A., Carter, A. S., & Briggs-Gowan, M. J. (2009). Sensory over-responsivity in elementary school: Prevalence and social–emotional correlates. *Journal of Abnormal Child Psychology, 37,* 705–716.

Brett-Green, B. A., Miller, L. J., Schoen, S. A., & Nielsen, D. M. (2010). An exploratory event-related potential study of multisensory integration in sensory over-responsive children. *Brain Research, 1321,* 67–77.

Brown v. Board of Education, 347 U.S. 483 (1954).

Canadian Association of Occupational Therapists. (1997). *Enabling occupation: An occupational therapy perspective.* Ottawa, ON: Author.

Center for Applied Technology. (2002). *Universal design for living.* Retrieved from www.cast.org/udl/index.cfm?i111

Chandler, B. E. (2013). Best practices in accessing and negotiating the system by understanding public education. In G. Frolek Clark & B. E. Chandler (Eds.), *Best practices for occupational therapy in schools* (pp. 55–67). Bethesda, MD: AOTA Press.

DeCoste, D. C. (2013). Best practices in the use of assistive technology to enhance participation. In G. Frolek Clark & B. E. Chandler (Eds.), *Best practices for occupational therapy in schools* (pp. 499–511). Bethesda, MD: AOTA Press.

Fisher, A. (2006). Overview of performance skills and client factors. In H. Pendleton & W. Schultz-Krohn (Eds.), *Pedretti's occupational therapy: Practice skills for physical dysfunction* (pp. 372–402). St. Louis, MO: Mosby/Elsevier.

Fisher, A., & Kielhofner, G. (1995). Skill in occupational performance. In G. Kielhofner (Ed.), *A model of human occupation: Theory and application* (2nd ed., pp. 113–128). Philadelphia: Lippincott Williams & Wilkins.

Frolek Clark, G., & Chandler, B. E. (Eds.). (2013). *Best practices for occupational therapy in schools.* Bethesda, MD: AOTA Press.

Gray, P. (2011). The decline of play and the rise of psychopathology in children and adolescents. *American Journal of Play, 3,* 443–463.

Hagedorn, R. (1997). *Foundations for practice in occupational therapy.* New York: Churchill Livingstone.

Hanft, B., & Shepherd, J. (Eds.). (2008). *Collaborating for student success: A guide for school-based occupational therapy.* Bethesda, MD: AOTA Press.

Hess, K. A., & Campion, E. W. (1983). Motivating the geriatric patient for rehabilitation. *Journal of the American Geriatric Society, 31,* 586–589.

Hsieh, C., Nelson, D. L., Smith, D. A., & Peterson, C. Q. (1996). A comparison of performance in added-purpose occupations and rote exercise for dynamic standing balance in persons with hemiplegia. *American Journal of Occupational Therapy, 50,* 10–16. http://dx.doi.org/10.5014/ajot.50.1.10

Hutton, E. (2008). "Back to school"—Piloting an occupational therapy service in mainstream schools in the UK. *Reflective Practice, 9,* 461–472.

Kirscher, M. A. (1984). Motivation as a factor of perceived exertion in purposeful versus nonpurposeful activity. *American Journal of Occupational Therapy, 38,* 165–170. http://dx.doi.org/10.5014/ajot.38.3.165

McColl, M. A. (2011). *Spirituality and occupational therapy.* Ottawa, ON: CAOT Publications.

McHale, K., & Cermak, S. A. (1992). Fine motor activities in elementary school: Preliminary findings and provisional implications for children with fine motor problems. *American Journal of Occupational Therapy, 46,* 898–903. http://dx.doi.org/10.5014/ajot.46.10.898

National Center for Education Statistics. (2012). The condition of education overview. In *Section 1—Participation in education in the United States.* Retrieved from http://nces.ed.gov/programs/coe/overview.asp

Reid, D., Chiu, T., Sinclair, G., Wehrmann, S., & Naseer, Z. (2006). Outcomes of an occupational therapy school-based consultation service for students with fine motor difficulties. *Canadian Journal of Occupational Therapy, 73,* 215–224.

Shuster, N. (1993). Addressing assistive technology needs in special education. *American Journal of Occupational Therapy, 47,* 993–997. http://dx.doi.org/10.5014/ajot.47.11.993

Swinth, Y. (1996). Evaluating toddlers for assistive technology. *OT Practice, 1*(3), 32–41.

Technology-Related Assistance Act, Pub. L. 100–407, 29 U.S.C. §§ 2201, 2202 (1988).

Thibodeaux, C. S., & Ludwig, R. F. (1988). Intrinsic motivation in product-oriented and non-product-oriented activities. *American Journal of Occupational Therapy, 42,* 169–175. http://dx.doi.org/10.5014/ajot.42.3.169

Trombly, C. A. (1995). Occupation: Purposefulness and meaningfulness as therapeutic mechanisms [Eleanor Clark Slagle Lecture]. *American Journal of Occupational Therapy, 49,* 960–972. http://dx.doi.org/10.5014/ajot.49.10.960

Twenty-First Century Communications and Video Accessibility Act of 2010, Pub. L. 111–260, 124 Stat. 2751.

Villeneuve, M. (2009). A critical examination of school-based occupational therapy collaborative consultation. *Canadian Journal of Occupational Therapy, 76,* 206–218.

Wheatley, C. (1996). Evaluation and treatment of cognitive dysfunction. In L. W. Pedretti (Ed.), *Occupational therapy: Practice skills for physical dysfunction* (pp. 241–252). St. Louis, MO: Mosby.

World Health Organization. (1980). *International classification of impairments, disabilities, and handicaps: A manual of classification relating to the consequences of disease.* Geneva: Author.

World Health Organization. (2001). *International classification of functioning, disability and health.* Geneva: Author.

Yuen, H. K. (1988). *The purposeful use of an object in the development of skill with a prosthesis.* Unpublished master's thesis, Western Michigan University, Kalamazoo.

Activities of Daily Living as Occupation

10

Occupational therapists feel that everyday activities are significant and meaningful. They have a firm belief that it is important to be able to perform everyday activities and that those activities are essential to one's sense of self-worth.

—Fleming (1994, p. 104)

LEARNING OBJECTIVES

At the completion of this chapter, readers will be able to

- Describe how occupational therapy practitioners can use task analysis as an evaluation and intervention tool when identifying intervention strategies to enable young clients to participate in activities of daily living (ADLs);
- Describe process performance skills, client factors, and contexts as dimensions of occupational therapy relevant to ADLs; and
- Apply task analysis to profile the performance patterns, process performance skills, and client factors that are challenged during participation in a basic ADL.

KEY TERMS

Activities of daily living
Activity limitations
Body functions
Body structures
Cognitive skills
Communication skills
Communicative disabilities
Disability
Frames of reference
Identity
Impairments

International Classification of Functioning, Disability and Health
Instrumental activities of daily living
Mental disabilities
Models of practice
Motor skills
Participation restrictions
Physical disabilities
Rehearsing
Sensory–perceptual skills
Severe disability

DISABILITY AND ACTIVITIES OF DAILY LIVING

In 2011, the World Health Organization (WHO) estimated that 1 billion people (15% of the world's population), including more than 100 million children ages 0 to 14 years, have a disability. The *International Classification of Functioning, Disability and Health (ICF;* WHO, 2001) advanced the understanding and measurement of disability. In the *ICF,* problems with human functioning are categorized in three interconnected areas:

1. *Impairments* are problems in body function or alterations in body structure (e.g., paralysis, blindness).
2. *Activity limitations* are difficulties in executing activities (e.g., walking, eating).
3. *Participation restrictions* are problems with involvement in any area of life (e.g., facing discrimination in employment or transportation).

Disability refers to difficulties encountered in any or all three areas of functioning (WHO, 2011, p. 5).

The *Americans With Disabilities: 2010* report for the U.S. Bureau of the Census (Brault, 2012) categorized disabilities as *communicative, mental,* and *physical.* The report estimated the total number of Americans across age groups with a disability at 56.7 million. About 38.3 million people were considered to have a *severe disability,* which means they needed extensive, ongoing support in life activities. The survey asked respondents about difficulty performing *activities of daily living (ADLs),* which are those activities done to take care of one's own body (e.g., bathing, grooming, dressing, eating, bowel and bladder management; American Occupational Therapy Association [AOTA], 2014), or *instrumental activities of daily living (IADLs),* which are those activities done to support daily life in the home and community (e.g., child care, care of pets, home management, financial management; AOTA, 2014), and whether any assistance from another person was needed, including access into and inside the home, getting into and out of bed or a chair, taking a bath or shower, dressing, eating, and toileting.

About 12.3 million people ages 6 years or older needed personal assistance with ADLs and IADLs. Employment figures estimated that 41.1% of individuals ages 21 years or older with a disability were employed compared with 79.1% of individuals ages 21 years or older without a disability (Brault, 2012). People older than age 15 years with a severe disability were nearly 3 times more likely to be in persistent poverty (i.e., continuous poverty for 24 consecutive months) than those without a disability (Brault, 2012).

The *Americans With Disabilities: 2010* report categorized disability differently for children and adults because of differences in age-related expectations in functions and activities pertaining to roles, responsibilities, and independence levels. For children younger than age 3 years, disability involves a developmental delay or difficulty with movement of the arms and legs. Disability in children ages 3–5 years includes developmental delay and difficulty walking, running, or playing. For children ages 6–14 years, *disability* is defined more broadly to include communication difficulties, mental or emotional conditions, difficulty with schoolwork, difficulty walking or running, use of assistive devices, and difficulties with ADLs. This chapter highlights child development to illustrate task analysis, but the approach is also applicable to adults.

Disability related to adults is categorized in the communicative, mental, and physical domains. *Communicative disabilities* include blindness or difficulty seeing, deafness or difficulty hearing, and speech that is difficult for others to understand. *Mental disabilities* include learning disability, intellectual disability, developmental delay, and Alzheimer's disease, senility, or dementia. *Physical disabilities* include requiring mobility aids; transfer challenges, such as getting in and out of bed; difficulty with the capacity to walk one-quarter mile, climb a flight of stairs, or lift 10 pounds; and conditions, such as arthritis, cerebral palsy, back and spine problems, cancer, diabetes, epilepsy, head and spinal cord injury, cardiac problems, and other problems with the organs (Brault, 2012).

ADLs are the area of occupation that supports effective living. Disability and its impact or severity are tied to participation in ADLs. In simple terms, the severity of the disability depends on the extent to which it affects a person's ability to perform an ADL unaided.

DIMENSIONS OF ACTIVITIES OF DAILY LIVING

Performance Skills and Patterns

To engage in ADLs, children must acquire the requisite performance skills (i.e., motor, sensory–perceptual, cognitive, communication skills) and performance patterns (i.e., roles, routines, habits). Motor skills are integral to the performance of dressing, for example, which requires a high level of mobility, coordination, strength, and energy and requires one to change position from standing to sitting and vice versa; take items to and from dresser drawers; and move, transport, lift, and grasp objects. Putting on pants, socks, or shoes requires a person to stabilize, shift weight, reach, and bend. Fastening buttons and zippers requires bilateral coordination and the ability to grasp small objects.

Sensory–perceptual skills enable a child to position the body for bathing, grooming, dressing, and eating. Vision supports learning about ADLs such as clothing set-up for dressing, use of utensils according to different foods, and so forth. Touch relates to all actions, because manipulation is restricted without tactile input.

Cognitive skills are needed to plan and manage ADLs, and skills develop through experience and maturation. A young child learns the sequence of a dressing task through participation with the parent. As the child matures, he or she uses learned skills to select clothes and objects needed for ADLs. By school age, the child recognizes the timing necessary to accomplish ADL tasks within the plans for the day (e.g., wash, dress, eat, brush teeth before school).

Communication skills are closely linked to performance. For example, the child learns through verbal and gestural communication from a parent about progressing ADL expectations. The child must listen, understand, and respond to these cues. This pattern of learning may be required of an adult with an acquired disability (e.g., stroke).

The development of proficiency in ADLs largely occurs from age 3 years to early adolescence. Children learn through participation when parents and others guide the learning process by teaching, coaching, and cuing. Toddlers practice and eventually learn how to hold a cup, finger feed and use a spoon, wipe their face and hands,

brush their teeth, and so forth. Over time, school-age children become more skilled in bathing and showering, managing personal hygiene, grooming, and other such activities. Adolescents continue to refine their performance skills through enhanced participation in personal care and IADLs. During adulthood, skills are refined that are required for IADLs such as child rearing, caring for others, and home and financial management.

ADL routines typically occur every day according to repetitive sequences. Over time, children develop their performance skills and create their own routines and habits of engagement (i.e., performance patterns). The acquisition of performance skills and patterns related to ADLs that began when children imitated their parents engaging in these occupations continues during playtime, when children rehearse these skills by putting costumes on and taking them off, grooming dolls when playing house, and so on.

Copying is a basic component of learning. Children imitate simple motor actions between ages 1 and 2 years. They can be observed copying their parents at the dinner table as they learn to use utensils and in the bathroom as they brush their teeth during morning routines. *Rehearsing* is the repetition of a sequence of events, and children can be observed rehearsing ADLs in their role-play and imaginary activities (WHO, 2001, p. 125).

Although children acquire performance patterns and skills required for ADLs as a natural part of growth and development, the complexity of the interactive learning process is often taken for granted. Occupational therapy practitioners are aware of this complexity when they observe clients as they engage in ADLs, and practitioners use task analysis during evaluation to untangle the complex interaction among performance skills and patterns, activity demands, client factors, and contexts.

To see how performance skills work together, consider the occupation of eating. The tasks of feeding and swallowing combine motor and praxis skills, sensory–perceptual skills, cognitive skills, and communication and social skills. Occupational therapy practitioners provide essential services in the comprehensive management of feeding, eating, and swallowing problems, such as difficulty bringing food to the mouth; difficulty moving food in the mouth; dysphagia; psychosocially based eating disorders (e.g., anorexia); dysfunction related to cognitive impairments, surgical intervention (e.g., oral cancers), and neurological impairments; and positioning problems that affect feeding, eating, and swallowing. Interventions focused on ADLs include facilitating a client's ability to participate in feeding and eating activities that are valued and meaningful to that person (e.g., learning to eat independently, joining friends for lunch, feeding a child; AOTA, 2007).

Client Factors

In intervention, occupational therapy practitioners focus on client factors that may influence performance. Values, beliefs, and spirituality are client factors that influence a client's motivation, even in their personal care. For example, if a family values dressing in a specific style of clothing, adaptation to intervention strategies that are not within those values may be discouraged (e.g., button-down shirts and zippered trousers ought to be worn rather than the typically recommended larger pullover T-shirt and elastic-waist pants).

Client factors also include body functions and body structures, which can significantly affect a client's ADLs. *Body functions* are the physiological functions of body systems, including psychological functions (AOTA, 2014). If a client has a urinary dysfunction, establishing a bladder routine within the context of home, community, and work may require adaptation and assistive devices. *Body structures* are "anatomical parts of the body such as organs, limbs and their components that support body function" (WHO, 2001, p. 10 as cited in AOTA, 2014). Practitioners evaluate body functions and structures because people need these client factors to engage in occupations, including ADLs. Practitioners' knowledge of such client factors enables them to identify the body functions and structures that might change as a result of participation in therapeutic activities.

Context and Environment

The importance clients place on participation in ADLs is influenced by environmental and personal contexts. Activities are culturally prescribed and laden with cultural values about the "right" way to do them.

For example, for a person with a urinary dysfunction, the time required to maintain a catheter may cause anxiety in the workplace. The cultural definitions and values involved in ADLs can be considered as "time-tested guides to occupational experience or as oppressive systems that limit freedom and creativity" (Pierce, 2001, p. 138). Cultural role expectations govern the norms of participation, and people outside the norm, such as those who have diminished self-care abilities, may be stigmatized (Christiansen, Baum, & Bass-Haugen, 2005; Mosey, 1996). Social stigma significantly influences *identity,* "the super ordinate view of ourselves that includes both self-esteem and self-concept, but also importantly reflects and is influenced by the larger social world in which we find ourselves" (Christiansen, 1999, p. 549).

Personal and environmental dimensions involve a variety of interrelated conditions within

---

Assignment 10.1. ADLs

1. Consider the developmental sequence and timing for the acquisition of ADL performance skills involved with dressing, such as buttoning a shirt and tying shoes; feeding, such as using a spoon, cutting food, and holding a cup; and printing or drawing, such as using a mature pencil grasp and recognizing colors and letters. Select 2 examples, and describe the developmental sequence and timing for each.

2. Search for additional resources, and define *feeding, eating, swallowing,* and *adaptive feeding.*

3. How do the social norms around the ADL of feeding vary among countries such as the United States, Australia, Canada, Mexico, China, India, Egypt, or any country with which you are familiar? When working with clients, it is important to be aware of and respect the fact that some behaviors you consider acceptable in your family and culture are considered inappropriate in other countries and vice versa.

and surrounding the client that influence his or her performance. These contexts affect the development and acquisition of performance skills and patterns and may influence activity demands (e.g., social demands). The cultural, physical, and social contexts form the background for ADLs because they dictate customs, norms, beliefs, role expectations, and social routines and define the terrain and structure of the environment.

EVALUATION AND INTERVENTION IN ACTIVITIES OF DAILY LIVING

Activity demands and contexts are critical considerations during evaluation and intervention. For example, activity demands (e.g., required tools and materials), environmental contexts (e.g., social supports), and personal contexts

(text continues on page 167)

CASE EXAMPLE 10.1. LERON: ADLs

Note. Readers should refer to Exhibit 10.1, which includes the "Analysis of Performance Skills" and the "Guidelines and Checklist for Task Analysis" sections of the Client Profile and Task Analysis form (CPTA; Appendix A) when reading through the case example. Based on the information in the case, readers are to complete these two sections of the form by further rating Leron's performance skills and putting a check mark next to the items on the list that appear to be impaired.

Leron was a 5-year-old boy referred for occupational therapy services by his preschool teacher. After observing Leron's preschool performance, his teacher expressed concern about general delays in his participation in ADLs, development of fine motor and gross motor skills, and acquisition of preschool concepts such as colors, numbers, and shapes. **Raya, the occupational therapy practitioner** who provided evaluation and intervention services to Leron's preschool, requested that the teacher and Leron's parents get together to share information regarding Leron's occupational history and levels of participation in preschool activities. Leron's grandparents also attended the meeting.

At the meeting, Raya learned about Leron's developmental history. He sat at 12 months, crawled at 14 months, and walked at 20 months. He was a happy toddler who was content to listen to music and play with his toys. He was difficult to toilet train and eventually accomplished the skill at age 4.

Leron's family had established daily routines and habits for his care. Both parents left home for work at 6:00 a.m. before Leron awoke. His grandparents lived with the family and cared for Leron in the morning. His grandfather woke him and ensured that Leron ate his breakfast. Leron had difficulty using a spoon and often resorted to finger feeding. He also drank out of a sippy cup to avoid spills. Leron was easily distracted from this and other tasks. Each morning, his grandfather reinforced that Leron could watch a bit of TV if he finished breakfast, groomed, and dressed for school. His grandmother dressed and groomed Leron because he needed much assistance with initiating or completing the steps of putting clothes on and brushing his teeth. Both grandparents expressed concern that Leron's ADL skills were delayed compared with the other children they had raised.

Leron attended preschool from 9:00 a.m. until 3:00 p.m., when his mother picked him up. His father returned from work in time to join the family for dinner. His parents reported that Leron had shown little developmental progress in ADLs since he was 3½ years old. Leron's teacher reported that he had difficulty feeding himself, was often distracted during lunch time, and required a change of shirt after meals. He also had trouble putting on his coat and shoes, putting his shoes on the right feet, using the hook-and-loop fasteners on his shoes, and managing his clothing during toileting. The teacher shared with the parents her observations that he was continually engaged in classroom activities and interested in playing with his peers. She reported that he loved books about animals and "building houses like my dad" with large foam blocks. She shared her concerns about his balance and coordination in gross motor activities, fine motor skill development, and knowledge of basic academic concepts.

(Continued)

CASE EXAMPLE 10.1. LERON: ADLs *(Cont.)*

Raya observed Leron in the preschool and noted that he could not orient his coat and shoes to put them on correctly and did not attempt to do the zipper. His body posture and movement suggested that he had low body tone that affected his ability to balance. For example, when he threw a ball and shifted his weight forward, he fell. Leron held a crayon with an immature palmar grasp, and his pictures looked like random squiggles. When asked to draw a picture of a boy, Leron's illustration consisted of a circle for a head, random smaller circles for facial features, and lines extending out from the head for limbs. Leron tried to cut out his drawing of a boy with scissors, but he could not cut along a thick line when Raya drew a frame around his picture. Leron recognized his favorite color, green, but was inconsistent when Raya asked him to identify the colors of his crayons. When Raya asked him to count his crayons, Leron missed numbers in an attempt to count 10 of them. When Raya drew shapes, Leron correctly identified the circle and square but could not label the triangle or rectangle. He quickly became bored with the activity.

At lunch time, Raya observed Leron while he was sitting in the middle of three long tables with all of his classmates. He spent more time watching his friends and chatting with them than he did eating. When he did feed himself, he repeatedly dropped his spoon and sippy cup and inadvertently pushed food off the plate, and at the end of the meal his shirt looked as if he had just lost a food fight.

Raya completed a formal evaluation with Leron outside the classroom to reduce environmental distractions. The formal evaluation identified fine and gross motor foundation abilities at a 3½-year-old level, low body tone, decreased balance and equilibrium, poor manual dexterity, and delays in visual–perceptual (developmental age of 3.2 years) and visual–motor (developmental age of 4.1 years) development, with the greatest weakness in spatial relations and sequencing.

**EXHIBIT 10.1. ANALYSIS OF PERFORMANCE
SKILLS AND TASK ANALYSIS CHECKLIST: LERON**

Performance Skills	Client Challenges (performance qualifier)
Rating: 0 = *no restriction*, 1 = *mild limitation*, 2 = *moderate restriction*, 3 = *severe restriction*, 4 = *complete impairment*	
Motor and praxis	**Rating**
Posture	
Mobility *decreased balance*	2
Coordination *decreased manipulation skills*	3
Strength *decreased body tone*	2
Effort	
Energy	
Execution *poor execution in feeding and paper-and-pencil tasks*	2
Process skills	**Rating**
Mental energy	
Knowledge *delayed development of ADL and preschool skills*	3

Organization	
Adaptation	
Social interaction skills	**Rating**
Communication posture	
Gestures	
Initiation *engages in play but uncertain about initiation*	query
Information exchange	
Acknowledging	
Taking turns	

GUIDELINES AND CHECKLIST FOR TASK ANALYSIS

Areas of Occupation

Activities of daily living
☐ Bathing and showering
☐ Bowel and bladder management
☐ Dressing
☐ Eating and swallowing
☐ Feeding
☐ Functional mobility
☐ Personal device care
☐ Personal hygiene and grooming
☐ Sexual activity
☐ Toileting and toilet hygiene

Instrumental activities of daily living
☐ Care of others
☐ Care of pets
☐ Child rearing
☐ Communication management
☐ Driving and community mobility
☐ Financial management
☐ Home establishment
☐ Home management and maintenance
☐ Meal preparation and cleanup
☐ Religious and spiritual observance
☐ Safety and emergency maintenance
☐ Shopping

Rest and sleep
☐ Rest and relaxation
☐ Sleep participation
☐ Sleep preparation

Play
☐ Peer interaction
☐ Play exploration
☐ Play participation

Leisure
☐ Customary activities or hobbies
☐ Leisure exploration
☐ Leisure participation

Social participation
☐ Community
☐ Family
☐ Peer or friend

Education
☐ Access issues
☐ Formal education participation
☐ Informal personal education or exploration
☐ Informal personal education participation

Work
☐ Employment interests and pursuits
☐ Employment seeking and acquisition
☐ Job performance
☐ Retirement preparation and adjustment
☐ Volunteer exploration
☐ Volunteer participation

(Continued)

EXHIBIT 10.1. ANALYSIS OF PERFORMANCE SKILLS AND TASK ANALYSIS CHECKLIST: LERON (Cont.)

Client Factors

Body functions and structures	Body functions and structures
Physical	*Sensory and pain*
☐ Cardiovascular and hematological systems	☐ Hearing functions
☐ Digestive, metabolic, and endocrine systems	☐ Pain grading and description
☐ Genitourinary and reproductive functions	☐ Seeing and related functions
☐ Movement-related functions	☐ Tactile functions
☐ Respiratory and immunological systems	☐ Taste and smell functions
☐ Skin and related structure functions	☐ Temperature and pressure reception
☐ Voice and speech functions	☐ Vestibular and proprioceptive functions
Body functions: Mental	**Body functions: Mental**
Specific mental functions	*Global mental functions*
☐ Attention	☐ Consciousness
☐ Emotional	☐ Energy and drive
☐ Experience of self and time	☐ Orientation
☐ Higher-level cognitive	☐ Sleep
☐ Motor sequencing	☐ Temperament and personality
☐ Memory	
☐ Perception	
☐ Thought	

Values, Beliefs, and Spirituality

Values	Beliefs and spirituality
☐ Meaningful qualities	☐ Cognitive content health as true
☐ Principles	☐ Guiding actions
☐ Standards	☐ Life meaning and purpose

Activity and Occupational Demands

Objects and their properties	Space demands
☐ Inherent properties (e.g., heavy, light)	☐ Size, arrangement, surface, lighting
☐ Required tools, materials, equipment	
Social demands	**Sequence and timing**
☐ Cultural context	☐ Sequence and timing
☐ Social environment	☐ Specific steps
Required actions and performance skills	**Required body functions and structures**
☐ Cognitive	☐ Anatomical parts
☐ Communication and interaction	☐ Level of consciousness
☐ Emotional and social	☐ Mobility of joints
☐ Motor and praxis	
☐ Sensory–perceptual	

Performance Skills

Motor skills	Process skills
☐ Movement actions or behaviors	☐ Judgment

☐ Skilled purposeful movements ☐ Ability to carry out learned movement	☐ Select and sequence objects or tools ☐ Organize and prioritize ☐ Create and problem solve ☐ Multitask

Social interaction skills
☐ Identify, manage, and express feelings
☐ On a one-to-one basis
☐ In groups
☐ Communication and interaction skills

Performance Patterns

Habits	**Routines**
☐ Automatic behavior ☐ Repeated activities ☐ Good, bad, or impoverished	☐ Observable patterns of behavior ☐ Time commitment ☐ Satisfying, promoting, or damaging
Roles	**Rituals**
☐ Set of expected behaviors ☐ Social or cultural ☐ Within context	☐ Symbolic actions ☐ Spiritual, cultural, or social ☐ Link to values and beliefs

Contexts and Environments

Cultural	**Personal**
☐ Customs and beliefs ☐ Activity patterns ☐ Expectations	☐ Age and gender ☐ Socioeconomic status ☐ Educational status
Temporal	**Virtual**
☐ Location of performance in time ☐ Experience shaped by engagement	☐ Communication environment
Physical	**Social and political**
☐ Natural environment (e.g., geography) ☐ Built environment (e.g., building, furniture)	☐ Relationship to individuals ☐ Relationship to organizations or systems

Note. ADLs = activities of daily living.

(e.g., expectations) support or hinder participation. In essence, people acquire performance skills through participation in ADLs, and because engagement promotes development, it can be used as a therapeutic intervention.

Practitioners use ADLs as occupation-based or purposeful activity during the intervention phase of therapy to promote engagement and participation. Using Case Example 10.1, readers can establish an occupational profile and an analysis of Leron's performance to identify the performance skills and patterns, contexts, activity demands, and client factors that affect his participation in ADLs. A priority for the family is Leron's development of independence in feeding, dressing, and toileting. All of the dimensions of occupational performance influence a person's participation in the ADL occupation: performance skills and patterns, contexts, activity demands, and client factors.

Assignment 10.2. Interventions in School and at Home

1. Read the case example of Leron, and complete the "Activity Demand" section of the CPTA form by analyzing the task of putting underwear, pants, and a T-shirt on and taking them off.
2. Table 10.1 suggests some client goals for Leron. Define 1 or more additional client goals and treatment objectives to improve his feeding both to increase his food intake and to eat with less mess while at preschool. In practice, you would establish these goals and objectives in collaboration with Leron's family, teacher, and any other caregivers.
3. Design an occupation-based therapeutic activity for Leron to do during 1 30-minute session to address 1 of the goals. This purposeful activity should address the concerns and priorities of this family and teacher, meet the developmental needs of this child, and satisfy the criteria for a purposeful activity delineated by AOTA (1993). What

approaches to occupational therapy intervention have you used to address this goal?
4. Design an occupation-based activity for Leron to do at home with his family. What approaches to occupational therapy intervention have you used?
5. Explore the process of integrating the Person–Environment–Occupation model of practice with the frame of reference outlined in the *Occupational Therapy Practice Framework* (AOTA, 2014), which further guides evaluation and intervention. *Models of practice* give general guidance for practice, explain complex relations among concepts, and are "a set of ideas derived from various fields of study which are organized to form a synthesis and integration of elements of theory and practice" (Hagedorn, 1997, p. 144). By comparison, *frames of reference* reflect the knowledge and theories within the basic sciences and provide a paradigm through which practitioners view the world, solve problems, and prescribe solutions (Hagedorn, 1997). Research and identify frames of reference used in occupational

TABLE 10.1
Client Goals for Leron

Long-Term Goals	Short-Term Objectives
1. Leron will independently put his clothes on during his morning routine by the beginning of kindergarten in 8 months.	1.a. Leron will improve his ability to put on his underwear and T-shirt from maximum to minimum assistance with cuing within 6 months. 1.b. Leron will improve his ability to put his coat on from maximum to minimum assistance with cuing within 6 months. 1.c.
2. Leron will improve his fine motor dexterity through practice while learning how to fasten large buttons and hook-and-loop fasteners on his shoes, and these improved skills will transfer to his ability to manipulate crayons and scissors.	2.a. Leron will learn to unfasten large buttons on a play button board within 2 months and will transfer the skills to unfastening his pajama top within 6 months. 2.b. Leron will pull up the zipper on his jacket once it is started (within 1 month).
3.	3.a. 3.b.
4.	4.a. 4.b.

Assignment 10.2. Interventions in School and at Home *(Cont.)*

therapy. What frames of reference could you use to interpret Leron's occupational performance profile in the occupation of ADLs?

6. Many children, adolescents, and adults have ADL limitations. How might a school group (e.g., parent–teacher association) or community group (e.g., boys and girls club) support the ADL occupation among the population? Consider how these organizations could influence activity demands and environmental contexts in support of a goal to enhance engagement of children in ADLs and IADLs. How might these groups collaborate to define goals, objectives, and an implementation plan to contribute to a reduction in limitations and participation restrictions in this area?

SUMMARY

ADLs are affected by performance skills, client factors, and context. Occupational therapy practitioners must consider all of these components when proposing intervention strategies to reflect the needs, values, and goals of the client. The CPTA form assists the practitioner as a guide to evaluation and intervention needs. When assessing children, understanding of developmental norms is critically important in developing a client profile. Practitioners must keep in mind the interaction of the person, his or her environment, and how performance limitations affect his or her capacity to engage in customary occupations, tasks, roles, and responsibilities.

REFERENCES

American Occupational Therapy Association. (1993). Position paper: Purposeful activity. *American Journal of Occupational Therapy, 47,* 1081–1082. http://dx.doi.org/10.5014/ajot.47.12.1081

American Occupational Therapy Association. (2007). Specialized knowledge and skills in feeding, eating, and swallowing for occupational therapy practice. *American Journal of Occupational Therapy, 61,* 686–700. http://dx.doi.org/10.5014/ajot.61.6.686

American Occupational Therapy Association. (2014). Occupational therapy practice framework: Domain and process (3rd ed.). *American Journal of Occupational Therapy,* 68(Suppl. 1), S1–48. http://dx.doi.org/10.5014/ajot.2014.682006

Brault, M. W. (2012). *Americans with disabilities: 2010.* Washington, DC: U.S. Bureau of the Census.

Christiansen, C. (1999). Defining lives: Occupation as an identity—An essay on competence, coherence, and creation of meaning (Eleanor Clark Slagle Lecture). *American Journal of Occupational Therapy, 53,* 547–558. http://dx.doi.org/10.5014/ajot.53.6.547

Christiansen, C., Baum, C., & Bass-Haugen, J. (Eds.). (2005). *Occupational therapy: Enabling function and well-being* (3rd ed.). Thorofare, NJ: Slack.

Fleming, M. H. (1994). A common sense practice in an uncommon world. In C. Mattingly & M. H. Fleming (Eds.), *Clinical reasoning: Forms of inquiry in a therapeutic practice* (pp. 94–116). Philadelphia: F. A. Davis.

Hagedorn, R. (1997). *Foundations for practice in occupational therapy.* New York: Churchill Livingstone.

Mosey, A. C. (1996). *Applied scientific inquiry in health professions: An epidemiological orientation* (2nd ed.). Bethesda, MD: American Occupational Therapy Association.

Pierce, D. (2001). Untangling occupation and activity. *American Journal of Occupational Therapy, 55,* 138–146. http://dx.doi.org/ 10.5014/ajot.55.2.138

World Health Organization. (2001). *International classification of functioning, disability and health.* Geneva: Author.

World Health Organization. (2011). *World report on disability.* Geneva: Author.

Adolescence and Emerging Adulthood

11

Those who believe that they master their own fate are much less likely to become anxious or depressed than those who believe that they are victims of circumstances beyond their control.

—Gray (2011, p. 449)

LEARNING OBJECTIVES

At the completion of this chapter, readers will be able to

- Describe the use of task analysis in evaluation and intervention to develop strategies that enable adolescents and emerging adults to develop performance skills, healthy patterns for social and occupational participation, and effective living skills, and
- Describe the role of occupational therapy practitioners with adolescents and young adults presenting with challenges involving sleep disorders, mental health issues, new technologies, and economic disadvantages.

KEY TERMS

Abstract thinking	Occupational enablement
Adolescence	Self-expression
Concrete thinking	Self-identity
Cyberbullying	Sexting
Effective living skills	Sleep disturbances
Emerging adulthood	Social media
Instrumental activities of daily living	Social isolation
Mental health problems	Social participation

---

*A*dolescence (ages 11–17 years) and *emerging adulthood* (ages 18–25 years) are times of rapid change and transitional steps from childhood roles to adult roles. The life tasks in adolescence are establishing self-identity, developing value systems around sexuality, and moving toward greater self-sufficiency. In emerging adulthood, life tasks include achieving economic self-sufficiency, establishing a home away from parents, attaining personal autonomy, and developing a personally satisfying lifestyle (Gorski & Miyake, 1985). This chapter describes the developmental stages of adolescence and emerging adulthood, highlights some of the challenges adolescents and young adults face, and describes principles of occupational therapy practice with this population.

ADOLESCENCE

Personal contexts shift during adolescence. Adolescents experience change in the way they view themselves (i.e., *self-identity*) in relation to their capacity to function independently. Being independent is more than feeling independent; one must be able to make one's own decisions and select a sensible course of action (Steinberg, 1998). Continued development of self-identity is linked to the sense of autonomy achieved through independence. Kenny (1996) argued,

> It is important to recognize the coherence or continuity in development across life stages, as well as the factors that contribute to discontinuity. Understanding the interplay of developmental and contextual factors is important to assessing risk and opportunity in adolescent development and in planning appropriate interventions. (p. 476)

Developmental (i.e., client) and contextual (i.e., environment) factors can provide opportunities for adolescents to expand and enhance their social participation and strengthen their self-identity, but these factors can also place adolescents at risk for ill health and dysfunctional behavior.

The interaction of persons, environments, and occupations is complex in the adolescent phase and is commonly perceived as perplexing. The dynamic interaction among adolescents, environments, and occupations promotes rapid growth and development and requires adaptation. Steinberg (1998) noted, "Generally speaking, most young people are able to negotiate the biological, cognitive, emotional, and social transitions of adolescence successfully" (p. 9). However, as Gray (2011) pointed out, "Humans are extraordinarily adaptive to changes in their living conditions, but not infinitely so" (p. 443).

Biological and Mental Changes in Adolescence

Adolescents undergo rapid changes in client factors, particularly in the areas of reproductive and mental functions. Adolescence is also marked by changes in performance patterns related to sleep, temperament, personality and emotional stability, and energy and drive. Performance skills expand in the areas of energy, knowledge, and adaptation. Biological transformations of body structures associated with puberty accompany changes in adolescents' sense of their body functions. Communication and interaction performance skills develop in response to increasingly complex occupations involving social participation and more challenging social environments.

During the first few years of adolescence, people undergo biological transformations associated with puberty and become capable of reproduction. Physical changes related to puberty, coupled with the responsibilities associated with the ability to procreate, require adolescents to adjust to new life circumstances in a short time. In adolescence, physical prowess supports the development of identity, and physical abilities lead to specialization in skill acquisition, which in turn directs potential vocational choices. Becoming comfortable with a changing experience of self in relation to body image, self-concept, and self-esteem requires the ability to adjust and adapt. Adaptation is linked to the maturation of mental functions.

Maturation of mental functions in early adolescence is associated with a cognitive transition from *concrete thinking,* which is limited to what is real in the here and now, to higher-level, *abstract thinking* that involves the ability to think hypothetically and to observe reality as a backdrop for what is possible (Watson & Wilson, 2003). As adolescents move into emerging adulthood, they use higher-level thinking in constructing prospects for their own (and society's) future. Adolescents can apply advanced reasoning to understand social situations and consider ideological concepts, alternative courses of action, and the consequences of choices and decisions. Indeed, as adolescents mature, they become better able to apply the mental functions of judgment, problem solving, reason, and logic to address challenging social circumstances and life situations.

Social Changes in Adolescence

Newly formed cognitive and psychological attributes allow adolescents to interact with others, establish and maintain friendships and kinship bonds, cope with challenging situations, and manage their own behavior (Case-Smith, 1996). *Self-expression* is the use of a variety of styles and skills to express thoughts, feelings, and needs. Formal operational thought is a highlight of adolescence, and adolescents can conceptualize complex material, use reasoning in problem solving, and evaluate relationships (Shortridge, 1989). Communication and interaction skills mature as adolescents learn new ways to communicate with others and begin to seek and establish intimate relationships. Adolescents also learn and use new ways of interacting nonverbally with others through gestures and social media.

Social participation is a central occupation of adolescence as adolescents transition to and learn how to participate in the adult world. The *Occupational Therapy Practice Framework: Domain and Process* (3rd ed., hereinafter referred to as the *Framework*; American Occupational Therapy Association [AOTA], 2014) describes *social participation* as occupations that support engagement in community, family, peer, and friend activities or "involvement in a subset of activities that involve social situations with others and that support social interdependence" (p. S21). Social

participation can occur in person or through remote technologies such as telephone, computer interaction, and video conferencing. The components of social participation for adolescents include successful interaction with family, peers, and friends and activities at the community level within neighborhoods, organizations, work, and school.

Leisure, often the setting for social participation, provides the context for much of adolescent behavior and development (Bradley & Inglis, 2012). Social participation creates avenues to form friendships, develop self-concept, and determine a sense of the meaning of life (Kang et al., 2010). Occupations provide a

> mechanism for social interaction and societal development and growth, forming the foundation of community, local, and national identity, because individuals not only engage in separate pursuits, they are able to plan and execute group activity. (Wilcock, 1998, p. 25)

Assignment 11.1. Adolescence and Emerging Adulthood

1. Review the adolescent developmental literature, and establish a checklist of occupations and related tasks and performance competencies expected of adolescents starting at age 11 years, noting progressive expectations through to age 17 years. What skills and patterns should be in place before the adolescent enters the next stage of the emerging adult?
2. Break these adolescent occupations and tasks into the performance skills and patterns required to develop your understanding of the contexts in which these occupations and tasks typically occur. Include (1) the action demands of the tasks in relation to social and cultural expectations and (2) the competencies required to be considered successful at the tasks. Consider the various social and cultural expectations embedded in specific environments, such as schools, clubs, ethnic backgrounds, and so forth.

EMERGING ADULTHOOD

Jeffrey J. Arnett (2004), a researcher on adolescence, emerging adulthood, and culture, suggested rewriting the timeline on becoming an adult, given the significant cultural changes that have evolved since the 1970s. He divided the process of becoming an adult (i.e., taking adult roles) into two periods: (1) adolescence (ages 11–17 years) and (2) early or emerging adulthood (ages 18–25 years). Arnett attributed the lengthening of the road to adulthood to the rise in age on entering marriage and parenthood, the lengthening of higher education, and prolonged job instability. His research on this evolution provides insight into the interface of culture and human performance, which is important in the occupational therapy frame of reference (Arnett, 2012).

Among the most important tasks of emerging adulthood is learning *effective living skills,* which are skills that enable self-reliance and support self-sufficiency and social responsibility. Effective living skills include the development of education and work competence as a foundation for entering the workforce as an adult, financial management, responsible sexuality, and social integration into cultural norms and role expectations. Effective living skills are closely related to *instrumental activities of daily living,* which are "activities to support daily life within the home and community that often require more complex interactions than those used in ADLs" (AOTA, 2014, p. S19).

Effective living skills refers to the capacity to implement IADLs within the context of roles, responsibilities, and the environment. IADLs include care of others, care of pets, child rearing, communication management, community mobility, financial management, health management and maintenance, home establishment and management, and so forth. Effective living skills thus involve the interaction between occupation and actions, values, and cultural roles and expectations.

Within IADLs and effective living skills are client factors that include global and specific mental functions (AOTA, 2014). For effective living, an emerging adult continues to refine abilities that began developing in adolescence (e.g., effective planning and decision making, coping strategies, conflict resolution, sense of personal responsibility, good use of time).

CHALLENGES IN ADOLESCENCE AND EMERGING ADULTHOOD

During the developmental transition from childhood to adulthood, adolescents may be vulnerable to a range of problems (Carnegie Council on Adolescent Development, 1995), such as difficulty adjusting to biological and psychological changes and increased pressures (e.g., related to education, employment, and time management), responsibilities and performance expectations, opportunities to make independent choices and mistakes, financial pressure while striving for more financial independence, and financial decision making.

Sleep Disturbances

The *Framework* includes rest and sleep as occupations addressed by occupational therapy (AOTA, 2014). This section focuses on rest and sleep because of adolescents' widespread lack of sleep, which significantly affects their physical health, cognitive function, mental health, and general well-being (Weissbluth, 2005).

Approximately 15 million American children are affected by inadequate sleep (Smaldone, Honig, & Byrne, 2007). The National Sleep Foundation (NSF; 2000) highlighted sleep as a basic drive of nature, describing how sufficient sleep "helps us think more clearly, complete complex tasks better and more consistently and enjoy everyday life more fully . . . . Scientific studies have shown that sleep contributes significantly to several important cognitive, emotional and performance-related functions" (p. 1). Insufficient sleep can be harmful, even life-threatening. According to the Centers for Disease Control and Prevention (CDC; 2002),

> While we often consider sleep to be a "passive" activity, sufficient sleep is increasingly being recognized as an essential aspect of health promotion and chronic

disease prevention in the public health community. Insufficient sleep is associated with a number of chronic diseases and conditions—such as diabetes, cardiovascular disease, obesity, and depression.

Causes and effects of inadequate sleep

According to NSF (2000), sleep research has identified several changes associated with puberty that cause irregular sleep patterns (e.g., going to bed later and rising later, keeping late nights, needing to wake up early for school). Environmental factors that also contribute to insufficient sleep include early school start times and too much time spent using technological devices (e.g., smartphones, television, computers) instead of sleeping (Bronson & Merryman, 2009; see Case Example 11.1).

Inadequate rest and sleep are associated with reduced attention, concentration, short-term memory, and learning ability, as well as negative mood, inconsistent performance, poor productivity, and loss of some forms of behavioral control (NSF, 2000). In fact, "scientists hypothesize that such sleep-related problems are due largely to conflicts between physiologically driven sleep needs and patterns, and behavioral and psychosocial factors that influence sleep habits" (NSF, 2000, p. 2).

Smaldone and colleagues (2007) reported that children affected by inadequate sleep experience associated health, school, and family factors. Parent participants in this study reported depressive symptomatology in their children and disruption in family dynamics (e.g., arguing, loss of trust). Smaldone et al. argued, "Inadequate

---

CASE EXAMPLE 11.1. RIC: POOR SLEEP

Note. Readers are to refer to the Client Profile and Task Analysis form (CPTA; Appendix A) along with this case study in preparation for Assignment 11.2, Question 2.

Hanna, an occupational therapist working in a rural region with very limited health care resources and supports, saw a vast array of clientele in divergent settings. She also had a close working relationship with some of the local doctors, who often turned to her for assistance with clients who did not require medical intervention but needed assistance from someone with a mix of clinical abilities. Hanna received a referral for **Ric, a 15-year-old boy with mild spastic cerebral palsy** living with his mother. Ric had recently undergone a tremendous growth spurt; he had fallen in the home, and in school he was sometimes unable to stay awake.

Hanna interviewed Ric and **his mother, Jen,** in their home. Because of spasticity in his left leg, Ric walked only short distances and used a cane. He walked in the house, in class, during quick stops at the store, or into the movie theater, but he did not walk between classes or during extended shopping trips. He preferred to use his manual wheelchair for distance traveling in school and in the community. He reported having grown 6 inches during the past 7 months, but the growth spurt seemed to have stopped, and his arms and legs no longer hurt. His wheelchair was too small, causing him to hunch over with his knees way up high. His bed was too small and hurt his hips when he lay on his side.

Ric had been sleeping poorly since he started the growth spurt. He thought that a combination of growing fast and sleeping poorly contributed to his falls, which mostly occurred when he went to the bathroom at night or first thing in the morning. He had fallen asleep in class, which was embarrassing because he had snored and annoyed his teachers. He admitted to sometimes lying in bed gaming on his tablet when he should have been sleeping; time slipped away, and he would later realize that he should have gone to sleep far earlier.

Jen did not want to purchase a new bed until they had seen an occupational therapist for advice. The occupational therapist who had provided the old wheelchair was no longer working in the region, so Jen wanted Hanna's advice on purchasing a wheelchair, too. Jen was hoping Hanna could assist with funding ideas for a bed and a chair because their insurance would not cover it.

Assignment 11.2. Sleep and the Transition to Adulthood

1. Read the AOTA fact sheet "Occupational Therapy's Role in Sleep" (AOTA, 2012; see Appendix C).
2. Explain the various issues facing Ric. What areas of occupation are being affected by his inadequate sleep? Using the CPTA form, do an analysis of Ric (Case Example 11.1) relative to the occupations, activities, and expectations within the contexts of home and school. The purpose is to understand the basic aspects that would guide intervention planning. Identify the interventions you would consider if you were Hanna, and arrange the interventions in terms of their priority in a therapeutic sequence.
3. What are the sleep patterns and needs of adolescents? How do they differ from those of adults? How did the start and stop times of a school day at your middle or high school meet (or not meet) your needs as a student?
4. What are some of the reasons for adolescent sleep disturbances? Think beyond the example of Ric. What are some of the psychosocial issues that lead to sleep disturbances, and how might they affect chronic sleep disturbance?
5. Explore the current federal and state or provincial legislation concerning insurance coverage for someone with a congenital health condition. How might availability of resources, specifically limited resources, affect Ric's transition to adulthood?
6. The term *effective living skills* is based on the context and role expectations for an emerging adult. Review the case example of Demi (Case Example 11.2), and develop strategies to assist a young adult with a mental health issue and impoverished living skills. Complete the following challenges:
   a. Choosing depression, posttraumatic stress disorder, or bipolar disorder as the clinical challenge, predict possible barriers to achieving effective living skills.
   b. Create a task analysis chart that identifies the roles, responsibilities, and expectations for achieving effective living skills required in college and, separately, a work environment. Keep in mind that effective living skills include basic and instrumental activities of daily living, managing a home environment, being productive in one's school or work activities, and integrating into the community.
   c. What barriers might an adolescent living with depression experience that would restrict his or her full participation in daily life? What are the social ramifications of the disorder?
   d. Identify the knowledge, skills, and strategies that an occupational therapy practitioner could use to enable a client to deal with the barriers of depression.

---

sleep during childhood is an invisible phenomenon that fails to receive attention from primary care providers until it interferes with the child's behavior, mood or performance" (p. 530). Occupational therapy practitioners can, through task analysis, address the multifaceted and complex nature of inadequate or disturbed sleep in adolescents.

Treatment of sleep disturbances

Sleep disturbances often reflect underlying physical or psychological issues. Some underlying issues are quick to resolve (e.g., sports injury, broken relationship), some take a long time to resolve, and some never resolve (e.g., chronic pain, social anxiety). Occupational therapy practitioners can use task analysis to help determine the specific causes and effects of the underlying sleep issues and to formulate effective intervention strategies. The client and practitioner may establish an immediate goal such as developing strategies that aid falling asleep and returning to sleep on awakening. Alternatively, they may choose to focus on the underlying issues to treat the root causes such as anxiety.

Mental Health Issues

Mental health problems may lead to poor school and work performance, school dropout, strained family relationships, involvement in the justice system, substance abuse, and risky sexual behaviors. In recent years, population research has suggested that the health and well-being of adolescents are increasingly challenged. For example, tobacco and substance abuse are increasing, as are rates of mental illness, antisocial behavior, and suicide (Patel, Fisher, Hetrick, & McGorry, 2007). In addition, concerns are ongoing about healthy eating and obesity in childhood and adolescence, which ultimately affect the ability to maintain a healthy body and body image into adulthood and achieve a longer lifespan (CDC, 2013; Plotnikoff et al., 2009; Raine, Lobstein, & Spence, 2013).

In 2012, the World Health Organization (WHO) reported mounting evidence that the antecedents of adult mental disorders can be detected in adolescents. WHO strongly declared that the continued neglect of the mental health needs of adolescents is unacceptable. According to the WHO, 8% of teens ages 13 to 18 years have an anxiety disorder (e.g., obsessive–compulsive disorder, posttraumatic stress disorder, social phobia, specific phobia, generalized anxiety disorder), with symptoms emerging as early as age 6 years. The National Center for Children in Poverty (2012) reported that approximately 20% of adolescents have a diagnosable mental health disorder, 20%–30% have at least one major depressive episode before reaching adulthood, and suicide is the third leading cause of death in adolescents and young adults.

Depression

Depression is complex and is generally interrelated with comorbid psychosocial problems; for example, dysfunctional or maladaptive process skills and communication and interaction skills may lower a person's capacity to cope with challenging life situations. Wilcock (1998) noted, "If individuals are under- or overstressed in the use of emotional, intellectual, or spiritual capacities because of physiological, environmental, or social factors, or

because of occupational deprivation, alienation, or imbalance, health and well-being may be undermined" (p. 102).

According to the National Institute of Mental Health (NIMH; 2013a),

> When a person has major depressive disorder, they experience a severely depressed mood and activity level that persists two weeks or more. Their symptoms interfere with their daily functioning and cause distress for both the person with the disorder and those who care about him or her.

About 11% of adolescents have experienced a dysthymic or major depressive disorder, which, notably, is the leading cause of disability among Americans ages 15 to 44 (NIMH, 2013b).

Duggal (2000) found that 97% of adolescents with a depressive disorder reported having experienced a severe negative life event either in preadolescence or during adolescence (e.g., family crisis, parental health issue, educational problems, difficulty with peer relationships). Suicidal behavior and substance dependence, two of society's most serious problems, are often comorbid with depressive disorders, psychological distress, or disruption in the family system (Cavaiola, 1999).

Gray (2011) examined the rise of psychopathology in children and adolescents relative to the historical decline in play. He referred to the work of Jean Twenge and her colleagues (2010) at San Diego State University, whose meta-analysis in a longitudinal study of adolescent mental health showed that anxiety and depression, as well as various other indexes of psychological disorder, increased between 1950 and 2007 (cited in Gray, 2011). Gray noted, "The changes seem to have much more to do with the way young people view the world than with the way the world actually is" (p. 449). Mental health practitioners have consistently observed that anxiety and depression correlate strongly with a person's sense of control or lack of control in their lives. This observation coincides with the occupational therapy understanding of the power of values, beliefs, and spirituality in people's lives (AOTA, 2014).

Social isolation

One important factor discussed by the aforementioned researchers is that social isolation and decreased sense of community appear to be significant factors in the rising mental health issues among adolescents and young adults. Within families, the sense of interconnectedness may have declined to the extent that adolescents are unclear about family and community values. In play and in school, when adults decide what children and adolescents should do, solve their problems for them, and manage their physical and social environments, a sense of loss of control on the part of the child and adolescent may in fact be realistic.

As early as the 1930s, developmental psychologist Lev Vygotsky (1933) argued that play provides an opportunity for a child to practice self-control and that the development of problem-solving skills through self-directed learning leads to the understanding of social rules and development of self-regulation (Rieber & Robinson, 2004). Gray (2011) noted that a general shift away from interdependence and toward independence, a rise in social isolation, and a shift toward extrinsic values contribute to increasing mental health issues (e.g., narcissism, antisocial behavior).

New Technologies

The transition from childhood to adulthood and the influences of expanding environments can make adolescents, young adults, and parents vulnerable to a range of challenges. Developmental literature recognizes that adolescents begin to exert their autonomy by defining areas in their lives that are outside of parental control. The Internet has emerged as a means for adolescents and young adults to meet their global developmental need to "socially interact and make social comparisons" (Israelashvili, Kim, & Bukobza, 2012, p. 418). For example, social media have emerged in everyday society as a mode of communication and can be considered an environment. Any Internet-based application that allows social interaction is included in social media (e.g., Facebook, Twitter, Instagram).

In 2011, the American Academy of Pediatrics issued a clinical report on the positive and negative impacts of social media on children, adolescents, and families (O'Keeffe, Clarke-Pearson, & Council on Communications and Media, 2011). The report indicated that using social media as a form of communication entails risk for children, adolescents, and young adults because of their limited capacity for self-regulation. Risky behaviors include cyberbullying, or "deliberately using digital media to communicate false, embarrassing, or hostile information about another person" (O'Keeffe et al., 2011, p. 801); sexting, or sending, receiving, or forwarding sexually explicit messages, photographs, or images via cell phone, computer, or other digital devices; and other types of harassment (O'Keeffe et al., 2011).

Scientists and psychologists became concerned about video game addiction in children and adolescents in the early 1990s. Fisher (1994) noted that scholars in the study of gambling saw similarities in arcade videogame playing and were concerned that these similarities suggested videogame addiction. During the following decade, researchers examined how videogames interfered with time spent on other activities while interested in videogames (Cummings & Vanderwater, 2007). School neglect and increased negative behaviors were highlighted in the research.

Studies also examined the correlation of videogame violence with increased hostility in adolescents (e.g., argumentative behavior with teachers and others, fighting with peers; Gentile, Lynch, Ruh Linder, & Walsh, 2004; Willougby, Adachi, & Good, 2012). Although some games are educational, many games emphasize negative themes such as killing people and animals, disrespect of authority, and violence). Some are concerned that children and adolescents may become immune to the horror of violence (American Academy of Child and Adolescent Psychiatry, 2012).

Barriers to Economic Independence

Financial independence and self-reliance are important criteria for adulthood, but economic downturns make financial self-sufficiency (e.g., financially establishing a household separate from one's parents) more difficult for young adults to achieve (Danziger & Rouse, 2009). A young adult may be economically forced to remain in the family home longer than would be developmentally desirable, which may result in social stigma, difficulty forging intimate adult relationships, and atypical and continued acceptance of or compulsion to accept parental authority as an adult. In turn, mental health and coping issues can arise when independence does not occur as expected or when other adolescent-to-adult transition problems arise.

OCCUPATIONAL THERAPY WITH ADOLESCENTS AND EMERGING ADULTS

Occupational therapy practitioners use task analysis as an evaluation and intervention tool to analyze the dynamic interaction among adolescents and young adults, their environments, and their occupations to identify factors that support or hinder healthy social participation. In task analysis, the practitioner considers the influence of the environment on the adolescent and young adult facing the challenges of integrating, adapting to, and functioning within the norms of society. Adolescents and young adults experiencing the consequences of maladjustment can benefit from occupational therapy when this maladjustment interferes with their social competency, quality of life, and healthy lifestyle.

Environmental factors influence social participation. During the evaluation phase, the occupational therapy practitioner interviews adolescent and young adult clients, inviting them to be reflective and articulate their interests, needs, and priorities (Watson & Wilson, 2003).

CASE EXAMPLE 11.2. DEMI: SCHOOL-BASED OCCUPATIONAL THERAPIST

Demi was an occupational therapist who worked 3 days a week at a public school for adolescents who were not thriving in their traditional high school settings. Students had experienced physical disabilities, coping and mental health issues, drug or truancy problems, or bullying or simply did not fit into the typical high school model. The purpose of the school was to reduce dropout by meeting the unique educational needs of each student. Diversity in curriculum design, class timetables, and courses of study and low student–teacher ratios were some of the offerings at the school, which was funded by federal and state funds, private donations, and research grants.

Demi's salary was funded through several joint research projects with the education, occupational therapy, and psychology departments at the local university. The focus of the research related to enhancing adolescent mental health and educational opportunities to facilitate high school graduation and advancement to tertiary education. Demi loved working at the school because she could use her skills as a school-based occupational therapist and a mental health therapist. Demi's contribution to the research involved submitting anonymized results of her assessments, reassessments, and observational notes to the researchers at the university.

One of Demi's most important contributions included developing and implementing mandatory social science and art courses for all students that included a curriculum to help the students understand and manage their emotions and behavior and improve the coping skills they needed to graduate from high school. This portion of the curriculum came about through a research project Demi had participated in that found that social sciences courses could give students the knowledge that they were not crazy, misfits, or broken and that most of their thought processes were normal and similar to those of other kids their age. The curriculum also helped students learn that it was okay to admit they sometimes felt lonely, scared, or upset and that they could manage those feelings and improve their outlook on life and self-image. The art program, also based on research evidence, allowed the students to express not only their creativity but also their emotions, thoughts, and moods in a nonthreatening and positive learning environment.

The first step in developing the course content was to understand the school context. In this case, the school was the client. To begin a task analysis, Demi interviewed key school personnel, including the school psychologist, to fully understand the values and beliefs held by each individual and collectively by the school.

(Continued)

CASE EXAMPLE 11.2. DEMI: SCHOOL-BASED OCCUPATIONAL THERAPIST *(Cont.)*

The school functioned within a community context, so the cultural and socioeconomic strengths and limitations of the community were explored. Demi identified that students had few venues in which to engage with each other in a healthy and supportive community environment. Because of the known links between mental health and how adolescents occupy their time in leisure and social participation activities, and given the limitations of the community, Demi identified the need to work with an adolescent focus group to conduct a task analysis of typical leisure and social activities.

Demi was known to the students as the occupational therapist who often shared the classroom with their teachers. The kids liked the fact that she did not grade their work and was kind. They also liked her because she talked quietly with them one-on-one and had a way, when discussing their classroom projects, of getting them to talk about the meaning of the project in their personal context. The students appreciated that Demi used a focus group of their peers to identify the activities that were affecting how the student group interacted and when negative behaviors affected individual and group mental health outcomes.

The students also appreciated Demi's ability to help them figure out for themselves how to address some of their personal concerns. Demi helped the students build their own capacity to develop an intervention plan that would help change how individuals and student groups could support each other by describing and encouraging healthy attitudes, providing mental health resource information, developing peer support groups, and designing inclusive leisure activities that could occur in the school. They liked that she did not tell them what they should do to solve their problems or try to "fix" them. They felt empowered by Demi's approach to inquiry-based learning. She simply listened and asked questions that helped them broaden their thinking about their contexts and options and heighten their understanding of the perspectives of others. Demi provided the students with a task analysis tool to help them focus on identifying the fundamental components of accomplishing a task (e.g., emotional regulation, communication and social skills, habits, routines, roles, rituals).

As the students developed course content, they learned about foundational components of developing a sustainable program (e.g., resource needs, projected impact of information, long-term outlook for change). Demi helped the students to focus on their future in a positive light and provided real examples of how what they were doing now could be useful to them after they graduated from high school at a job, in college, or at a trade school.

The practitioner both listens for information and seeks to appreciate the spirit of the communication. Establishing rapport and trust is critical to the therapeutic relationship. Open-ended questions require skillful application and therapeutic use of self, particularly with adolescents and young adults who perceive a power imbalance between the practitioner and themselves (see Case Example 11.2).

Occupational enablement is based on the premise that "creating opportunities for choice and control ensures that clients are doing the things they wish to do in the ways, time frames, and places they wish to do them" (Townsend & Polatajko, 2007, p. 72). Occupational enablement is consistent with the concept described by Gray (2011) and Twenge et al. (2010) that lack of choice and control produce negative outcomes in adolescents and young adults. Occupational therapy practitioners are charged with the task of delineating, understanding, and removing contextual barriers (e.g., personal, social, environmental) to participation in occupations. The practitioner enables adolescents and young adults facing challenges by guiding adaptation, providing coaching in effective living strategies, coordinating environmental accommodations, and engaging directly with the adolescent or young adult through the assessment and intervention process.

When working with adolescents and young adults, the occupational therapy practitioner must first recognize that the changes these clients may want or need are not necessarily related partly or fully to performance skills (i.e., sensory–perceptual skills, motor and praxis skills, emotional regulation skills, cognitive skills, communication and social skills) but may also be related to performance patterns (i.e., habits, routines, roles, rituals). Context and environment often play a substantial role in the circumstances the adolescent or young adult is experiencing; researchers believe that the increase in external locus of control is causally linked to the rise of anxiety and depression in adolescents and young adults (Newsom, Archer, Trumbetta, & Gottesman, 2003; Twenge, Zhang, & Im, 2004; Twenge et al., 2010).

SUMMARY

Adolescence can be the most turbulent time of life and is filled with tremendous cognitive, physiological, and psychological change and growth. It is a period of increasing independence and responsibility and realizing the opportunities and pitfalls that accompany it. It is also a life stage of great need for boundaries with flexibility, compassion, empathy, friendship, open communication, and stability.

Adolescence is marked by rapid physiological and emotional changes that are the cornerstone of the acquisition of effective living skills, enabling progressive independence from parental guidance toward the establishment of self-identity in emerging adulthood. Effective living skills attained in this developmental period enable self-reliance and support self-sufficiency and social responsibility.

Delays and interruptions in the developmental process can lead to severe and long-term coping issues, mental health issues, and delays in the learning and implementation of effective living skills. Interventions by occupational therapy practitioners using task analysis can help adolescents or young adults gain or regain a sense of personal control, laying the groundwork for successful adulthood.

REFERENCES

American Academy of Child and Adolescent Psychiatry. (2012). *Children and video games: Playing with violence*. Retrieved from www.aacap.org/AACAP/Families_and_Youth/Facts_for_Families/Facts_for_Families_Pages/Children_and_Video_Games_Playing_with_Violence_91.aspx

American Occupational Therapy Association. (2012). *Occupational therapy's role in sleep*. Retrieved from www.aota.org/en/About-Occupational-Therapy/Professionals/HW/Facts/Sleep.aspx

American Occupational Therapy Association. (2014). Occupational therapy practice framework: Domain and process (3rd ed.). *American Journal of Occupational Therapy, 68*(Suppl.1), S1–48. http://dx.doi.org/10.5014/ajot.2014.682006

Arnett, J. J. (2004). *Emerging adulthood: The winding road from the late teens through the twenties*. Oxford, England: Oxford University Press.

Arnett, J. J. (2012). *Adolescence and emerging adulthood: A cultural approach* (5th ed.). Boston: Prentice Hall.

Bradley, G. L., & Inglis, B. C. (2012). Adolescent leisure dimensions, psychosocial adjustment, and gender effects. *Journal of Adolescence, 35*, 1167–1176.

Bronson, P., & Merryman, A. (2009). *NurtureShock: New thinking about children*. New York: Hachette.

Carnegie Council on Adolescent Development. (1995). *Great transitions: Preparing adolescents for a new century*. New York: Carnegie Corporation.

Case-Smith, J. (1996). An overview of occupational therapy for children. In J. Case-Smith, A. S. Allen, & P. N. Pratt (Eds.), *Occupational therapy for children* (3rd ed., pp. 3–17). St. Louis, MO: Mosby.

Cavaiola, A. A. (1999). Suicidal behavior in chemically dependent adolescents. *Adolescence, 34*(136), 735–744.

Centers for Disease Control and Prevention. (2002). *Sleep and sleep disorders*. Retrieved from www.cdc.gov/sleep/

Centers for Disease Control and Prevention. (2013). *Childhood obesity facts*. Retrieved from www.cdc.gov/healthyyouth/obesity/facts.htm

Cummings, H. M., & Vanderwater, E. A. (2007). Relation of adolescent videogame play to time spent in other activities. *Archives of Pediatric Adolescent Medicine, 161*, 684–689.

Danziger, S., & Rouse, C. E. (Eds.). (2009). *The price of independence: The economics of early adulthood*. Ann Arbor, MI: National Poverty Center.

Duggal, S. (2000). Assessment of life stress in adolescents: Self-report versus interview methods. *Journal of the American Academy of Child and Adolescent Psychiatry, 39*, 455–452.

Fisher, S. (1994). Identifying video game addiction in children and adolescents. *Addictive Behaviors, 19*, 545–553.

Gentile, D. A., Lynch, P. J., Ruh Linder, J., & Walsh, D. A. (2004). The effects of violent videogame habits on adolescent hostility, aggressive behaviors, and school performance. *Journal of Adolescence, 27*, 5–22.

Gorski, G., & Miyake, S. (1985). The Adolescent Life/Work Planning Group: A prevention model. *Occupational Therapy in Health Care, 2,* 139–150.

Gray, P. (2011). The decline of play and the rise of psychopathology in children and adolescents. *American Journal of Play, 3,* 443–463.

Israelashvili, M., Kim, T., & Bukobza, G. (2012). Adolescents' overuse of the cyber world: Internet addiction or identity exploration? *Journal of Adolescence, 35,* 417–424.

Kang, L. J., Palisano, R. J., Orlin, M. N., Chiarello, L. A., King, G. A., & Polansky, M. (2010). Determinants of social participation—with friends and others who are not family members—for youths with cerebral palsy. *Physical Therapy, 90,* 1743–1757.

Kenny, M. E. (1996). Promoting optimal adolescent development from a developmental and contextual framework. *Counseling Psychologist, 24,* 475–481.

National Center for Children in Poverty. (2012). *Facts about adolescent mental health.* Retrieved from www.nccp.org/publications/pub_878.html

National Institute of Mental Health. (2013a). *Major depressive disorder in children.* Bethesda, MD: Author. Retrieved from www.nimh.nih.gov/statistics/1MDD_CHILD.shtml

National Institute of Mental Health. (2013b). *The numbers count: Mental disorders in America.* Bethesda, MD: Author. Retrieved from www.nimh.nih.gov/health/publications/the-numbers-count-mental-disorders-in-america/index.shtml#MajorDepressive

National Sleep Foundation. (2000). *Adolescent sleep needs and patterns.* Retrieved from www.sleepfoundation.org/sites/default/files/sleep_and_teens_report1.pdf

Newsom, C. R., Archer, R. P., Trumbetta, S., & Gottesman, I. I. (2003). Changes in adolescent response patterns on the MMPI/MMPI–A across four decades. *Journal of Personality Assessment, 81,* 74–84.

O'Keeffe, G. S., Clarke-Pearson, K., & Council on Communications and Media. (2011). The impact of social media on children, adolescents, and families. *Pediatrics, 127,* 800–804. http://dx.doi.org/10.1542/peds.2011-0054

Patel, V., Fisher, A. J., Hetrick, S., & McGorry, P. (2007). Mental health of young people: A global public health challenge. *Lancet, 369,* 1301–1313.

Plotnikoff, R. C., Karunamuni, N., Spence, J. C., Storey, K., Forbes, L., Raine, K., . . . McCargar, L. (2009). Chronic disease–related lifestyle risk factors in a sample of Canadian adolescents. *Journal of Adolescent Health, 44,* 606–609.

Raine, K. D., Lobstein, T., & Spence, J. C. (2013). Restricting marketing to children: Consensus on policy interventions to address obesity. *Journal of Public Health Policy, 34,* 239–253.

Rieber, R. W., & Robinson, D. K. (Eds.). (2004). *The essential Vygotsky.* New York: Kluwer Academic.

Shortridge, S. D. (1989). The developmental process: Prenatal to adolescence. In P. N. Pratt & A. S. Allen (Eds.), *Occupational therapy for children* (pp. 48–64). St. Louis, MO: Mosby.

Smaldone, A., Honig, J. C., & Byrne, M. W. (2007). Sleepless in America: Inadequate sleep and relationships to health and well-being of our nation's children. *Pediatrics, 119,* 529–537.

Steinberg, L. (1998). Adolescence. In *Gale Encyclopedia of childhood and adolescence* [Abstract]. Retrieved from www.findarticles.com/cf_dls/g2602/0000/2602000013/print.jhtml

Townsend, E. A., & Polatajko, H. J. (2007). *Enabling occupation II: Advancing an occupational therapy vision of health, well-being, and justice through occupation.* Ottawa, ON: CAOT Publications.

Twenge, J. M., Gentile, B., Dewall, C. N., Ma, D., Lacefield, K., & Schurtz, D. R. (2010). Birth cohort increases in psychopathology among young Americans, 1938–2007: A cross temporal meta-analysis of the MMPI. *Clinical Psychology Review, 30,* 145–154.

Twenge, J. M., Zhang, L., & Im, C. (2004). It's beyond my control: A cross-temporal meta-analysis of increasing externality in locus of control, 1960–2001. *Personality and Social Psychology Review, 8,* 308–319.

Vygotsky, L. (1933). *Play and its role in the mental development of the child.* Retrieved from www.marxists.org/archive/vygotsky/works/1933/play.htm

Watson, D. E., & Wilson, S. A. (2003). *Task analysis: An individual and population approach* (2nd ed.). Bethesda, MD: AOTA Press.

Weissbluth, M. (2005). *Happy sleep habits, happy child* (3rd ed.). New York: Ballantine.

Wilcock, A. A. (1998). *An occupational perspective of health.* Thorofare, NJ: Slack.

Willoughby, T., Adachi, P. J., & Good, M. (2012). A longitudinal study of the association between violent video game play and aggression among adolescents. *Developmental Psychology, 48,* 1044–1057.

World Health Organization. (2012). *Adolescent mental health: Mapping actions of nongovernmental organizations and other international development organizations.* Geneva: Author.

Adulthood: Maintaining Meaningful Lifestyles

12

Meaning is the essence of what makes an activity purposeful and critical for occupation-based intervention.

—Blount, Hinojosa, and Kramer (2014, p. 421)

LEARNING OBJECTIVES

At the completion of this chapter, readers will be able to

- Describe how occupational therapy practitioners use task analysis to match community resources and social support systems to the needs of adults and their families and
- Understand how task analysis applies to intervention strategies for adults in various settings.

KEY TERMS

Adaptation
Adaptation approach to intervention
Adulthood
Child care
Home management
Personal causation

Return-to-work rehabilitation programs
Role competence
Roles
Self-concept
Self-efficacy

---

*A*dulthood represents an achieved state of maturity. As a phase of development, adulthood typically begins with enhanced personal freedom, choice, and responsibility as people learn to care for themselves and others emotionally, spiritually, physically, and financially. Some changes through adulthood are, as Kielhofner (1995) put it, "externally recognizable as the person passes through a series of steps, crises, or transitions: marriage or divorce, starting a family, changing jobs, and bidding farewell to grown children" (p. 446).

Adulthood is a time for choosing a lifestyle and assuming new and complex roles: friend, lover, spouse, student, colleague, boss, worker, breadwinner, parent, citizen, and so on. *Roles* "are sets of behaviors expected by society, shaped by culture and context; they may be further conceptualized and defined by a client (individual, group, or population)" (American Occupational Therapy Association [AOTA], 2014, p. S8).

Roles organize behavior, communicate expectations, and evolve across the lifespan. They add pleasure and enjoyment to life, contribute to achievement, and help maintain the self and family life (Christiansen & Baum, 1991; Watson, 1997). One's identity as an adult is often shaped by the roles one assumes in society, which are influenced by environmental and personal contexts. For example, competence in the role of worker is a primary expectation of adults in many societies.

Adulthood is usually a time of personal growth. A person's identity, self-concept, and life plans evolve and are influenced by unpredictable events. When a person's ability to participate in meaningful occupations is restricted, his or her life plans must undergo a transformation (Frank, 1996; Polkinghorne, 1996). Because people are holistic entities, injury, impairment, or underdevelopment in one area may affect a person's entire identity. Likewise, changes in a person's identity can influence the degree to which impairments limit participation in occupations (Polkinghorne, 1996).

ROLE COMPETENCE AND ADAPTATION

Role competence is the "ability to effectively meet the demands of roles in which the client engages" (AOTA, 2014, p. S35). It refers to the aspects of a person that imply a level of skill, achievement, and output. Traumatic injuries such as amputation, spinal cord injury, and brain injury usually cause permanent, irreversible impairments that alter a person's ability to participate in his or her customary roles and occupations.

Impairments and activity limitations, however, need not negatively affect the client's spirit, belief in personal causation, perceived self-efficacy, self-concept, or sense of mastery over life events. *Personal causation* refers to a person's belief in his or her abilities, perception of control over behavior and outcomes, and expectation of success in future endeavors (Kielhofner, 1985). Autonomy is linked with a sense of *self-efficacy,* which is a person's judgment of his or her capacity to use existing skills to attain certain levels of performance (Kielhofner, 1995). *Self-concept* refers to the value that the person places on the physical, emotional, and sexual self (AOTA, 1994).

Familiar behaviors and customary roles give people a sense of being a part of their social community and culture. When a permanent impairment suddenly alters a client's ability to engage in

occupations and participate in customary contexts, he or she is unable to rely on familiar performance patterns to continue in customary roles.

Adaptation refers to the adjustments people make to enhance their ability to survive and thrive in the context of unforeseen circumstances. Adaptation requires and is the result of changes in people, in their desired tasks and roles, and in their personal and environmental contexts (AOTA, 1993; Mosey, 1986). Adaptation skills are required to regain a sense of competency in customary roles and participation in the contexts of community and culture. To adapt, people must take an active role in responding to specific contextual demands (King, 1978).

Role competence, adaptation, and engagement in occupations are linked. Occupational therapy practitioners combine their understanding of a client's impairments, activity limitations, participation restrictions, and preexisting lifestyle with knowledge they have gained from experience in working with other clients who have similar disabilities to construct an image of the client's future potential. Clients guide the intervention process through their participation in the construction, revision, and realization of a "possible and desirable future" (Mattingly & Fleming, 1994, p. 241).

With experience, practitioners can make increasingly accurate predictions about their clients' potential functional status. Practitioners direct intervention toward enabling clients to envision and reestablish a satisfying lifestyle by establishing, reconstructing, and controlling their patterns of occupation. In this way, occupational therapy practitioners facilitate adaptation (AOTA, 1994). Occupational therapy practitioners design intervention to promote engagement and participation in desired occupations and roles and enhance clients' participation in activities for which they have high interest but low satisfaction (Yerxa & Baum, 1986).

The compensatory or *adaptation approach to intervention* involves finding ways for the client to revise activity demands and contexts to support his or her participation in natural settings (AOTA, 2014). To successfully adapt, the client must appraise his or her values and goals and work toward attainment of personal, social, and vocational plans (Versluys, 1995). Occupational therapy practitioners working with clients with long-standing impairments collaborate to define outcome goals and objectives in all areas of occupation: basic and instrumental activities of daily living, education, work, play, leisure, and social participation.

In addition, clients' dignity and self-esteem often depend on their doing or directing their own self-care. Participation in work, leisure, and social occupations commences when the client has regained enough stamina. Activity limitations in these areas result in loss of opportunity to participate in intrinsically motivating and highly rewarding occupations. For example, loss of choice in leisure pursuits may affect volition, individuality, and interpersonal relationships and can result in social exclusion (Bundy, 1993; Howard & Young, 2002; Páez & Farber, 2012). Conversely, participation in leisure may increase sense of mastery, self-esteem, adjustment to loss, social interaction, and level of physical fitness for a person with a disability (Pasek & Schkade, 1996; Sherrill & Williams, 1996; Taylor & McGruder, 1996).

Whereas some clients are initially interested in returning to their former work, play, and leisure occupations, others may benefit from being introduced to novel activities and occupations to assist in the construction of a new identity and sense of self (Taylor & McGruder, 1996). The role of occupational therapy practitioners who work with people with long-term impairments is to restructure activity demands, alter environmental contexts, teach new methods, introduce new options, and facilitate adaptation. Using task analysis to examine these dimensions enables the practitioner to match the individual's capacities with a desired activity available in the person's environment.

Home Management and Child Care

Home management is a broad term that conjures up different meanings, depending on the individual. In everyday use, the term can refer to house cleaning tasks; meal planning and preparation; grocery shopping; light household repairs; financial management; management of recycling and garbage; lawn and garden care; and vehicle maintenance, including car washing, vacuuming,

(text continues on page 193)

CASE EXAMPLE 12.1. JASMIN AND CHRIS: HOME MANAGEMENT AND CHILD CARE AFTER A MOTORCYCLE ACCIDENT

Note. Readers should review Exhibit 12.1 after reading this case example. Pay particular attention to the challenges faced by Jasmin, who must reorganize the family around Chris's injury.

Jasmin, age 40 years, and **Chris, age 42 years,** have three daughters ages 8, 10, and 13 years. Jasmin is an executive who regularly worked 10-hour days and made frequent business trips. Chris had been a librarian, but it did not take long after having their first child for them to learn that Chris was happiest managing the home and caring for the baby. In turn, this role for Chris allowed Jasmin to pursue her growing career and still have a thriving family life. Chris loved being a full-time dad and home schooling the girls. He did not care so much for household tasks, but as the girls got older he learned to incorporate nearly all aspects of home and financial management into their school curriculum, and the previously mundane tasks became wonderful learning and life skills experiences for the kids.

Chris was recently in a serious motorcycle accident resulting in a right below-knee amputation. Jasmin arranged to take 16 weeks off work by using sick leave, family medical leave, and the few days of vacation she had left. For the first several weeks, her head was spinning. She was fearful for Chris and crushed with grief for him, the kids, and herself. Not only that, but she had not had to worry about the daily household management for years, and she felt unable to home school the kids. Now she must deal with both.

They have some money in savings, but it will not cover the monthly budget and the bills related to Chris's needs for long. Besides, in Jasmin's line of work, an extended absence will compromise her ability to perform her job, so she must get back to work as soon as she can organize the resources needed in the home and enroll her children in public school, or the family income stream will simply dry up. She tells the occupational therapist, "I don't know how Chris does it all without going insane." How can Chris's occupational therapist help this family?

EXHIBIT 12.1. CLIENT PROFILE AND TASK ANALYSIS FORM: JASMIN

CLIENT PROFILE

Name: Jasmin	Birthdate:	Age at assessment: 40
Advocates: Herself, her husband	**Education:** n/a	
	Work occupation: Business executive	
Diagnoses: None	**Current interventions:** None	
Referral source: Social worker		

PERSONAL INFORMATION

Family unit	Injured husband, Chris, and three children
Caregiver(s)	Jasmin is her husband's caregiver in his postinjury, subacute phase after traumatic amputation of his leg.
Roles and responsibilities (e.g., student, spouse, parent, friend, worker)	1. Assume her husband's roles and responsibilities as stay-at-home father who managed the home, cared for the children, and provided home schooling. 2. Reorganize the family and recruit the resources needed in the home when she returns to work and establish her children in a public school for at least 1 year.
Home environment (e.g., home design, number of people living in the home)	Two-story home with the bedrooms on the upper floor. This presents as a substantial problem for Chris, who cannot manage stairs and is currently using the main floor den as his bedroom. The full bathroom is on the upper floor, and this makes bathing and showering a great challenge.
Community context (e.g., rural, urban, metro; single-family home, residential care)	Full home care services are not available to her husband.
School or work context (e.g., public, special, or private school; stationary or travel location for work)	The children are home schooled.
Client priorities	1. Manage Chris's personal care needs. 2. Take care of housekeeping and child care tasks. 3. Reorganize household duties. 4. Locate and enroll children in the public school system.
Values/beliefs/spirituality (e.g., principles, standards, beliefs, personal quest)	To ensure a continuity of the home and education for their children while Chris is rehabilitating

SUMMARY, PLAN, AND GOALS

Assessments completed (formal and observational): Interview and review of Chris's medical documentation to determine caregiving needs and long-term prognosis

Practitioner–client plan (e.g., further formal and observational assessments, inclusion of others): To explore a home and caregiving management plan that includes acquiring needed support systems (e.g., cleaning services, public school). The practitioner needs additional information on the performance patterns of the family (to complete task analysis form).

Tasks Requiring Assessment or Intervention

Short-term goals (Primarily client driven, measurable, global task, or activity achievements)	Long-term objectives (Primarily practitioner driven, measurable, incremental, stepwise, or mini achievements)
1. Jasmin will develop a daily and weekly schedule and strategies for managing her home and caregiving responsibilities. 2. Jasmin will explore local schools for the placement of her children. 3. Jasmine will develop a return-to-work plan that identifies any outstanding needs for Chris's caregiving and for household management.	1. Establish strategies to meet Chris's residual capacity needs to resume his role in the household and family. 2. Understand the psychological needs of the children regarding a changed school environment and seek counseling services when indicated. 3. Return to work with needed strategies and resources established to ensure continuity of the family lifestyle.

TASKS ANALYZED

Occupation or Activity	Tasks (specific activity component)	Context or Environment (external and internal)
Caregiving	Personal care and psychological support for Chris	Subacute care in the home
Housekeeping	Maintenance of routine Relearn skills and timing	While providing care for Chris and managing the children's home schooling
Home schooling	Planning, organizing and executing a learning schedule	While providing care for Chris and managing housekeeping tasks

OCCUPATIONAL PROFILE AND ANALYSIS OF NEEDS

Functional ability (i.e., how strengths and deficits affect ability to perform activities and tasks)	Jasmin is well educated and has the cognitive capacity to organize her family's needs. However, she has not had primary responsibility for the home and the children's routines. She will be challenged to develop a broader understanding of home and homeschooling details. She is overwhelmed and stressed. She is the primary provider for the family and cannot return to work. She is at risk for emotional burnout.

(Continued)

EXHIBIT 12.1. CLIENT PROFILE AND TASK ANALYSIS FORM: JASMIN *(Cont.)*

Activity tolerance (e.g., physical and mental fatigue levels, energy to complete activities and tasks, temporal and environmental contexts)	Customarily, Jasmin is a high-energy person. There is little concern about physical fatigue, but the stress of the situation and the complexity of her husband's and children's needs threaten her emotional endurance.
Effect on occupational performance (e.g., reflect on client roles, responsibilities, and priorities)	Family responsibilities required Jasmin to take a leave of absence from her work as a business executive. She is expected to return to work as quickly as possible. Her leave is unpaid.
Intervention needs (e.g., physical, cognitive, emotional, social)	Occupational therapy services can assist with Chris's transition to the home and seeking home care services. Jasmin needs emotional support, and referral to psychological counseling has been discussed with her.
Resource needs (e.g., assistive devices or equipment, technology)	Assistive devices for Chris's care and to increase his independence are critical for alleviating Jasmin in his care. Home care services are also essential but may not be affordable unless a reasonable solution is found (e.g., live-in assistance).
Program needs (e.g., day programs, return-to-work programs, socialization)	None
Outlook (practitioner projection of long-term needs and life care planning)	It could take some time to put care resources in place in the home. This is a substantial threat to the family's income, as Jasmin will not be able to return to work. There is also a chance that her employer would need to release her from her duties and hire a replacement, which would put Jasmin into a position of unemployment that threatens family security.

GUIDELINES AND CHECKLIST FOR TASK ANALYSIS

Occupations

Activities of daily living	**Instrumental activities of daily living**
☐ Bathing and showering	☑ Care of others
☐ Bowel and bladder management	☐ Care of pets
☐ Dressing	☑ Child rearing
☐ Eating and swallowing	☑ Communication management
☐ Feeding	☐ Driving and community mobility
☐ Functional mobility	☐ Financial management
☐ Personal device care	☑ Home establishment
☐ Personal hygiene and grooming	☑ Home management and maintenance
☐ Sexual activity	☐ Meal preparation and cleanup
☐ Toileting and toilet hygiene	☐ Religious and spiritual observance
	☐ Safety and emergency maintenance
	☐ Shopping

Rest and sleep	**Play**
☑ Rest and relaxation	☐ Peer interaction
☐ Sleep participation	☐ Play exploration
☐ Sleep preparation	☐ Play participation

Leisure	**Social participation**
☐ Customary activities or hobbies	☑ Community
☐ Leisure exploration	☑ Family
☐ Leisure participation	☑ Peer or friend

Education	**Work**
☐ Access issues	☐ Employment interests and pursuits
☐ Formal education participation	☐ Employment seeking and acquisition
☐ Informal personal education or exploration	☐ Job performance
☐ Informal personal education participation	☐ Retirement preparation and adjustment
	☐ Volunteer exploration
	☐ Volunteer participation

Client Factors

Body functions and structures	**Body functions and structures**
Physical	*Sensory and pain*
☐ Cardiovascular and hematological systems	☐ Hearing functions
☐ Digestive, metabolic, and endocrine systems	☐ Pain grading and description
☐ Genitourinary and reproductive functions	☐ Seeing and related functions
☐ Movement-related functions	☐ Tactile functions
☐ Respiratory and immunological systems	☐ Taste and smell functions
☐ Skin and related structure functions	☐ Temperature and pressure reception
☐ Voice and speech functions	☐ Vestibular and proprioceptive functions

Body functions: Mental	**Body functions: Mental**
Specific mental functions	*Global mental functions*
☐ Attention	☐ Consciousness
☑ Emotional	☑ Energy and drive
☐ Experience of self and time	☐ Orientation
☑ Higher-level cognitive	☐ Sleep
☐ Motor sequencing	☐ Temperament and personality
☐ Memory	
☐ Perception	
☐ Thought	

Values, Beliefs, and Spirituality

Values	**Beliefs and spirituality**
☑ Meaningful qualities	☐ Cognitive content health as true
☑ Principles	☑ Guiding actions
☑ Standards	☑ Life meaning and purpose

(Continued)

EXHIBIT 12.1. CLIENT PROFILE AND TASK ANALYSIS FORM: JASMIN *(Cont.)*

Activity and Occupational Demands

Objects and their properties ☐ Inherent properties (e.g., heavy, light) ☐ Required tools, materials, equipment	**Space demands** ☐ Size, arrangement, surface, and lighting
Social demands ☑ Cultural context ☑ Social environment	**Sequence and timing** ☑ Sequence and timing ☑ Specific steps
Required actions and performance skills ☑ Cognitive ☑ Communication and interaction ☑ Emotional and social ☐ Motor and praxis ☐ Sensory–perceptual	**Required body functions and structures** ☐ Anatomical parts ☐ Level of consciousness ☐ Mobility of joints

Performance Skills

Motor skills ☐ Movement actions or behaviors ☐ Skilled purposeful movements ☐ Ability to carry out learned movement	**Process skills** ☐ Judgment ☐ Select and sequence objects or tools ☑ Organize and prioritize ☑ Create and problem solve ☑ Multitask

Social interaction skills ☐ Identify, manage, and express feelings ☐ On a one-to-one basis ☐ In groups ☐ Communication and interaction skills	

Performance Patterns

Habits ☐ Automatic behavior ☐ Repeated activities ☐ Good, bad, or impoverished	**Routines** ☐ Observable patterns of behavior ☑ Time commitment ☐ Satisfying, promoting, or damaging
Roles ☑ Set of expected behaviors ☑ Social or cultural ☑ Within context	**Rituals** ☐ Symbolic actions ☐ Spiritual, cultural, or social ☐ Link to values and beliefs

Contexts and Environments

Cultural ☐ Customs and beliefs ☑ Activity patterns ☑ Expectations	**Personal** ☑ Age and gender ☑ Socioeconomic status ☐ Educational status

Temporal ☐ Location of performance in time ☑ Experience shaped by engagement	Virtual ☑ Communication environment
Physical ☐ Natural environment (e.g., geography) ☑ Built environment (e.g., building, furniture)	**Social and political** ☑ Relationship to individuals ☑ Relationship to organizations or systems

TASK ANALYSIS TEMPLATE

An individual form is required for each task that is examined.
Task:

Task Demands	Action Demands (What is required of the person to do the task)	Client Challenges (Availability of required body functions and structures)
Objects used (e.g., equipment, technology)		
Space demands (e.g., physical context)		
Social demands (e.g., social environment and context)	Jasmin must organize her husband's care during the day and reorganize her children's school and routines.	There is no available social or insurance funding for the care of her husband.
Sequence and timing (e.g., process to carry out the task)	She needs to do this quickly in order to go back to work because this is essential for the economic stability of the family.	The process of recruiting a home care service for her husband is complex and may take a substantial amount of time. This presents an economic and personal threat.
Required actions and performance skills (e.g., basic requirements)	Finding and organizing resources.	This is overwhelming for Jasmin.

GUIDELINE AND CHECKLIST FOR TASK ANALYSIS

Areas of Occupation	
Activities of daily living: Chris ☑ Bathing and showering ☐ Bowel and bladder management ☑ Dressing ☐ Eating and swallowing ☐ Feeding ☑ Functional mobility ☑ Personal device care	**Instrumental activities of daily living: Jasmine** ☑ Care of others ☐ Care of pets ☑ Child rearing ☑ Communication management ☐ Driving and community mobility ☐ Financial management ☑ Home establishment

(Continued)

EXHIBIT 12.1. CLIENT PROFILE AND TASK ANALYSIS FORM: JASMIN *(Cont.)*

☐ Personal hygiene and grooming ☐ Sexual activity ☐ Toileting and toilet hygiene	☑ Home management and maintenance ☐ Meal preparation and cleanup ☐ Religious and spiritual observance ☐ Safety and emergency maintenance ☐ Shopping
Rest and sleep: Chris ☑ Rest and relaxation ☑ Sleep participation ☑ Sleep preparation	**Play: Children** ☑ Peer interaction ☑ Play exploration ☑ Play participation
Leisure: Family ☑ Customary activities or hobbies ☑ Leisure exploration ☑ Leisure participation	**Social participation: Family** ☑ Community ☑ Family ☑ Peer or friend
Education: Children ☐ Access issues ☑ Formal education participation ☐ Informal personal education or exploration ☐ Informal personal education participation	**Work** ☐ Employment interests or pursuits ☐ Employment seeking or acquisition ☐ Job performance ☐ Retirement preparation and adjustment ☐ Volunteer exploration ☐ Volunteer participation

Values, Beliefs, and Spirituality

Values: Family ☑ Meaningful qualities ☑ Principles ☑ Standards	**Beliefs and spirituality: Family** ☑ Cognitive content health as true ☑ Guiding actions ☑ Life meaning and purpose

Performance Patterns: Jasmin

Habits ☑ Automatic behavior ☑ Repeated activities ☑ Good, bad, or impoverished	**Routines** ☑ Observable patterns of behavior ☑ Time commitment ☐ Satisfying, promoting, or damaging
Roles ☑ Set of expected behaviors ☐ Social or cultural ☐ Within context	**Rituals** ☐ Symbolic actions ☐ Spiritual, cultural, or social ☐ Link to values and beliefs

TASK ANALYSIS TEMPLATE

An individual form is required for each task that is examined.
Task: Organization of the home and family to accommodate Chris's life change.

Task Demands	Action Demands (What is required of the person to do the task)	Client Challenges (Availability of required body functions and structures)

Objects used (e.g., equipment, technology)	Consultation on equipment needs for Chris	No incapacities
Space demands (e.g., physical context)	Jasmin must explore renovations to her home to create another bathroom on the main floor or install a lift from the main floor.	Caregiving for Chris must be in place so that Jasmin can return to work. Finances are essential for home renovations.
Social demands (e.g., social environment and context)	Setting up caregiving services for Chris is required to enable Jasmin to return to work.	Full home care services are not available to Chris in the community, and Jasmin must recruit a live-in caregiver.
Sequence and timing (e.g., process to carry out the task)	Jasmin must organize her husband's needs and enroll her children in public school within 1 month.	The children's emotional health during the transition must be attended to. Recruiting a caregiver is a big challenge.
Required actions and performance skills (e.g., basic requirements)	Jasmin must maintain her emotional stability during the reorganization of her home and family.	Jasmin should access psychological counseling for herself, her children, and Chris to ensure emotional needs are met for each of them individually and to support healthy family dynamics.

and repairs. Likewise, *child care* in general use includes the care a family member provides for a child as well as professional services conducted at a child care center or in a private home.

How an injury affects an adult varies, depending on his or her own pre- and postinjury roles and those of his or her family. Case Example 12.1 focuses on the unpaid care provided by a family member and examines home management and child care roles after a father experiences a traumatic injury and a career-oriented mother is required to take on more tasks and care for her husband while reorganizing all of their lives. In this situation, the client is the husband's caregiver.

Assignment 12.1. Chris and Jasmin

1. You are Chris's occupational therapist while he is in the hospital, but you recognize that Jasmin is emotionally overwhelmed (Case Example 12.1). Be creative with a family-centered approach to care, and focus a portion of your intervention for Chris on family education and training. Estimate how long Chris will be in the hospital, and write down some ideas for helping Chris and Jasmin problem solve how they can cope with the issues of household management, child care, and home schooling and enable Jasmin to return to work until Chris returns home. Are any community groups or services available that can help the family maintain their routines with minimal disruption?

2. Chris has been discharged, and you are a community occupational therapy practitioner providing home care to him. How will the amputation influence his ability to manage the home and home school the kids? Make a list of activities of daily living (ADLs) that have not changed since before the amputation, and then make a list of those that have changed. The injury has resulted in permanent impairment and disability for certain tasks. How will you facilitate Chris's and the family's ability to resume their previous lifestyle? Remember that funders will not pay for services for Chris on a long-term basis. Review your list of the ADLs that have changed, and provide intervention strategies that will have quick and positive outcomes for independent task completion.

Return-to-Work Rehabilitation

For full-time workers, paid employment is the occupation they spend the most time performing. In the *Occupational Therapy Practice Guidelines for Individuals With Work-Related Injuries and Illnesses,* it is noted that work is often important to one's self-identity and sense of self-worth (Kaskutas & Snodgrass, 2009). Work is also a necessary means of economic self-sufficiency.

Return-to-work rehabilitation programs are designed to return the injured worker to productive employment and may include work hardening and skill retraining. Return-to-work rehabilitation is an important specialty area of occupational therapy practice with adults who have experienced illness or injury, and the timing of interventions and description of services vary across regions and countries. This specialty area may also be referred to as *industrial rehabilitation, occupational rehabilitation, work conditioning* or *work hardening, return-to-work coordination,* or *rehabilitation consulting.* Regardless of the term used, occupational therapy practitioners and insurers share a common goal of getting injured workers back to full preinjury work duties and hours as soon as is practicable (see Case Example 12.2).

In the United States and Canada, clients may attend a work-hardening or work-conditioning program for 4 or more weeks. In such programs, the client receives a variety of interventions such as psychological counseling, pain management, body mechanics, manual handling training, general conditioning, and job simulations. Treatment continues until the client is deemed fit to return to full duties; is deemed fit to return to work within the confines of a gradual or modified return-to-work program; or is deemed unfit

---

CASE EXAMPLE 12.2. CAMILLE: RETURN-TO-WORK REHABILITATION

Note. Readers can use the Client Profile and Task Analysis form in Appendix A while considering this case example and fill in information. (*Note.* See Case Example 5.7 in Chapter 5, for initial information to be used for completing the form.)

Camille had progressed markedly since her dominant hand had been amputated at the wrist after an injury in a commercial kitchen. Because of the nature of Camille's injury and the physical demands on a chef, she was on an extended gradual return-to-work program. Over time, her **occupational therapist, Nicholas,** conducted numerous task analyses on the various commercial kitchen–related duties Camille would have to undertake on her return to work. As part of his consultative methods, Nicholas educated Camille and her **prosthetist, Kelsey,** on the methods used during a task analysis. In turn, both Camille and Kelsey provided insights into the issues and challenges Camille faced and solutions that would bring her closer to a resumption of full duties. For example, Camille obtained cooking tools such as spatulas, knives, whisks, and thermometers that fit into her prosthetic tool socket and bent at 180°, 90°, 60°, and 45° angles to match the needs of specific tasks. Specific tools remained at specific work stations so Camille could readily use them as needed.

Camille began feeling discomfort in her dominant shoulder, and Nicholas suspected she might be in the early stages of shoulder strain or tendonitis. He advised Camille to discuss her shoulder issues with her treating physician and request a physiotherapy assessment. He also advised her to address the issue sooner rather than later so her discomfort would not progress to a more serious overuse syndrome and so her return-to-work program could continue to be successful and sustainable.

Camille and Nicholas further discussed her job tasks, related modifications to the tasks, and adaptations to her prosthesis. Up to this point, Nicholas had encouraged and been supportive of Camille's desire to use her dominant arm as much as possible, as she did before her injury. He was beginning to wonder, however, whether that was the best approach or whether further modifications to task methods or to her prosthesis might reduce her use of the right shoulder. Nicholas contacted Kelsey, the prosthetist, and informed her of Camille's shoulder complaint. They discussed possible prosthetic solutions, and Kelsey agreed to research some ideas and consult her colleagues to ascertain whether any long-term solutions might allow Camille to continue to use her dominant arm primarily and at the same time avoid shoulder problems.

to return to his or her previous duties, leading to alternate interventions, such as vocational rehabilitation or a pain management program.

Australia takes a different approach to return-to-work rehabilitation interventions and the timing of returning a client to work. Work-hardening programs that take place in the clinical setting are relatively uncommon, and injured workers are encouraged to work modified hours or duties, or both, as soon as they are medically stable. Often work-hardening interventions occur during work hours at the work site or, if necessary, in the clinical setting at the beginning or end of the work day. This approach has many benefits, including keeping workers attached to their employment emotionally and financially, maintaining a line of communication between employee and employer, facilitating mental health by helping employees maintain a sense of routine and purpose vs. staying at home and potentially losing that aspect of their lives, and addressing work site and work performance issues and concerns in real time in the actual work setting versus in a clinical or simulated setting.

Loss of the ability to work can lead to a loss of self-esteem and a diminished sense of purpose (Guindon, 2009; Kaskutas & Snodgrass, 2009). Occupational therapy practitioners who specialize in return-to-work rehabilitation frequently provide services to people who have diagnosed or undiagnosed depression. Sadly, it is not uncommon for treating professionals to miss signs of depression and attribute poor attendance, participation, and performance as signs of poor motivation, poor attitude, symptom magnification, or an attempt to avoid returning to work. The following questions can aid the practitioner in exploring whether a client is experiencing depression related to work roles:

- How long has the client been off work?
- How are the client's bills, such as rent, food, car, and electricity, being paid?
- Is the client in danger of losing his or her home?
- Is he or she worried about dependents?
- What support systems does the client have, and are those systems being supportive?
- What are the client's coping mechanisms?
- Does the client talk about his or her concerns pertaining to the injury and the implications

of the injury for his or her ability to function or work?
- Is the client in pain? If so, how does he or she manage the pain?
- Has the injury had an impact on the client's ability to participate in sexual activities?
- Has the client's self-image changed since the injury? If so, how?
- Is the client eating well? Has he or she gained or lost weight since the injury?
- How are the client's hygiene and appearance now different compared with before the injury?
- Is the client's means of transport different now than before the injury?
- How has the client's ability to perform activities and participate in social events changed since the injury?
- What are the client's sleep patterns now compared with before the injury?
- Is the client fearful of certain activities?
- Is he or she fearful of returning to work?

By exploring these issues with the client and in completing a task analysis, the occupational therapy practitioner will gain insight into the client's mental and physical well-being. In turn, the practitioner's subsequent actions may enable the client to take the first step in getting better pain control, counseling, or a diagnosis of and treatment for depression.

Assignment 12.2. Camille

Camille's job demands may put her at risk of overuse syndrome, whereas someone with a similar injury in a different job may not be at risk (Case Example 12.2). Whisk eggs and milk in a bowl, and conduct a task analysis with emphasis on the movements of your hand, wrist, forearm, elbow, and shoulder. Then conduct and analyze the same task as though you were Camille using her custom prosthesis, which means you do not have the ability either to change your hand grip on the cooking utensils or to move your wrist. What differences do you find in your task analyses? How can you modify the task to decrease the use of your dominant shoulder?

SUMMARY

Adulthood is "a time for choosing a lifestyle and assuming new and complex roles" (Watson & Wilson, 2003, p. 116). This chapter provided an overview of the challenges of adulthood, including the role of caregiver for a family member. Although there is an instrumental focus on the injured individual, the practitioner also has the caregiver as a client and can consult on how to manage the many roles and responsibilities of a home lifestyle. Additionally, a major component of injury as an adult is return to work, and assisting with capacity building for return to work is within the scope of the occupational therapy practitioner. Return to work or restoration as close as possible to the client's preinjury capacity are important aims of the practitioner.

REFERENCES

American Occupational Therapy Association. (1993). Position paper: Purposeful activity. *American Journal of Occupational Therapy, 47,* 1081–1082. http://dx.doi.org/10.5014/ajot.47.12.1081

American Occupational Therapy Association. (1994). *Uniform terminology for occupational therapy* (3rd ed.). Bethesda, MD: Author.

American Occupational Therapy Association. (2014). Occupational therapy practice framework: Domain and process (3rd ed.). *American Journal of Occupational Therapy, 68*(Suppl. 1), S1–48. http://dx.doi.org/10.5014/ajot.2014.682006

Blount, M.-L., Hinojosa, J., & Kramer, P. (2014). Reflections for the future: Occupation, purposeful activities, and activities. In J. Hinojosa & M.-L. Blount (Eds.), *The texture of life: Occupations and related activities* (4th ed., pp. 417–434). Bethesda, MD: AOTA Press.

Bundy, A. (1993). Assessment of play and leisure: Delineation of the problem. *American Journal of Occupational Therapy, 47,* 217–222. http://dx.doi.org/10.5014/ajot.47.3.217

Christiansen, C., & Baum, C. (Eds.). (1991). *Occupational therapy: Overcoming human performance deficits.* Thorofare, NJ: Slack.

Frank, G. (1996). Life histories in occupational therapy clinical practice. *American Journal of Occupational Therapy, 50,* 251–264. http://dx.doi.org/10.5014/ajot.50.4.251

Guindon, M. H. (2009). *Self-esteem across the life span: Issues and interventions.* New York: Taylor & Francis.

Howard, D. K., & Young, M. E. (2002). Leisure: A pathway to love and intimacy. *Disability Studies Quarterly, 22*(4), 101–120.

Kaskutas, V., & Snodgrass, J. (2009). *Occupational therapy guidelines for individuals with work-related injuries and illnesses.* Bethesda, MD: AOTA Press.

Kielhofner, G. (1985). *A Model of Human Occupation: Theory and application.* Baltimore: Williams & Wilkins.

Kielhofner, G. (1995). *A model of human occupation: Theory and application* (2nd ed.). Baltimore: Williams & Wilkins.

King, L. J. (1978). Toward a science of adaptive responses [Eleanor Clarke Slagle Lecture]. *American Journal of Occupational Therapy, 32,* 429–437.

Mattingly, C., & Fleming, M. H. (1994). *Clinical reasoning: Forms of inquiry in therapeutic practice.* Philadelphia: F. A. Davis.

Mosey, A. C. (1986). *Psychosocial components of occupational therapy.* New York: Raven Press.

Páez, A., & Farber, S. (2012). Participation and desire: Leisure activities among Canadian adults with disabilities. *Transportation, 39,* 1055–1078.

Pasek, P. B., & Schkade, J. K. (1996). Effects of a skiing experience on adolescents with limb deficiencies: An occupational adaptation perspective. *American Journal of Occupational Therapy, 50,* 24–31. http://dx.doi.org/10.5014/ajot.50.1.24

Polkinghorne, D. E. (1996). Transformative narratives: From victimic to agentic life plots. *American Journal of Occupational Therapy, 50,* 299–305. http://dx.doi.org/10.5014/ajot.50.4.299

Sherrill, C., & Williams, T. (1996). Disability and sport: Psychosocial perspectives on inclusion, integration and participation. *Sports Science Review, 5*(1), 42–64.

Taylor, L. P. S., & McGruder, J. E. (1996). The meaning of sea kayaking for persons with spinal cord injuries. *American Journal of Occupational Therapy, 50,* 39–46. http://dx.doi.org/10.5014/ajot.50.1.39

Versluys, H. P. (1995). Facilitating psychosocial adjustment to disability. In C. A. Trombly (Ed.), *Occupational therapy for physical dysfunction* (4th ed., pp. 377–389). Baltimore: Williams & Wilkins.

Watson, D. E. (1997). *Task analysis: An occupational performance approach.* Bethesda, MD: American Occupational Therapy Association.

Watson, D. E., & Wilson, S. A. (2003). *Task Analysis: An individual and population approach.* Bethesda, MD: AOTA Press.

Yerxa, E. J., & Baum, S. (1986). Engagement in daily occupations and life satisfaction among people with spinal cord injuries. *Occupational Therapy Journal of Research, 6,* 271–283.

Older Adults: Transitions for Successful Aging

13

Some people might argue that successful aging means not aging at all; most, however, understand it to mean continued health and zest for living through one's older years.

—Cole (2008, p. 155)

LEARNING OBJECTIVES

At the completion of this chapter, readers will be able to

- Show the use of logical thinking and creative analysis in developing intervention strategies to enable older adults to engage in occupations and participate in their customary contexts and
- Describe how community resource agencies and social support systems can help older adults maintain their levels of engagement in occupation and participation in contexts.

KEY TERMS

Adaptation
Aging in community approach
Aging in place
Attendant care
Cohousing

Elders' guild
Long-term care facilities
Older adults
Successful aging

People are living longer than ever before, and changes in society and everyday life are making past ideas about the process of aging obsolete (Jackson, Mandel, Zemke, & Clark, 2001). The value people place on independence and autonomy, however, remains tenacious in older adulthood. The number of older people is growing, but extended families are frequently able to provide informal care (Jackson et al., 2001). Therefore, the challenge to society and communities is to find ways to enable older adults to age successfully. Continued engagement in daily activities provides meaning and temporal rhythm in life (Zemke & Clark, 1996).

DEMOGRAPHICS OF OLDER ADULTS

In 2010, more than 40 million Americans were *older adults* (i.e., ages 65 years or older; U.S. Department of Health and Human Services [DHHS], 2011). The number of older Americans increased by more than 15% between 2000 and 2010, compared with an increase of less than 9%

for those younger than 65 years. More important, 31% of those who were ages 45 to 64 years in 2010 will be 65 years or older within the next two decades (DHHS, 2011).

As age increases, so does the prevalence of disability. According to the *World Report on Disability* (World Health Organization [WHO], 2011), older adults constitute more than 35% of all people with disabilities in Australia, Canada, and the United States. In addition, globally there are approximately 10% more women than men with disabilities from age 45 through the "oldest old" (i.e., those older than age 85 years; WHO, 2011). In 2005, among Americans ages 65 years or older, 18.1 million (51.8%) had a disability. About 12.9 million 65 years or older (36.9%) had a severe disability. People ages 80 years or older had the highest incidence of disability, at 71.0% (U.S. Bureau of the Census, 2008).

ROLE TRANSITIONS AMONG OLDER ADULTS

The roles and routines that people assume change across their lifespan. Each person's life story is unique, but typically, children become students when they enter school, adolescents become employees when they start their first job, adults become parents when they have their first child, and older adults become retirees when they leave the workforce. In older adulthood, as in earlier stages of life, engagement in occupations, participation in life situations, and role competence provide a sense of identity, add pleasure and enjoyment to life, contribute to achievement, and help maintain the self and family life. Unfortunately, rapid changes in society have left some older adults without guidelines on the "proper way to age" (Jackson et al., 2001, p. 5).

Older adults may relinquish or experience a progressive loss of roles and occupations as they age. Many typical life changes place older adults at risk for social isolation. Retirement and loss of spouse and friends bring changes in roles and performance patterns that can affect the breadth and depth of social participation. Conversely, occupations that older adults celebrate and that produce a sense of self-worth may seem mundane to others (e.g., going to movies, reading), but

from older adults' perspective, such occupations are "salient occurrences in present life that often [embody] meaningful themes" (Zemke & Clark, 1996, p. 358). People differ in the ways they respond to growing old, in part because of variability in personal experiences, societal expectations of appropriate roles, cohort effects, and personality factors that influence attitudes toward aging.

Adaptation

Just as changes and transitions at other periods in the lifespan require people to adapt, so too do the changes and transitions experienced in older adulthood. *Adaptation* refers to adjustments people make to enhance their ability to survive and thrive in the context of changing circumstances. Adaptation enables people to master life challenges and actualize their potential. It requires, and is the result of, changes in people and their desired tasks and roles as well as in personal and environmental contexts (American Occupational Therapy Association [AOTA], 1993; Mosey, 1986). To adapt, people must take an active role in responding to specific contextual demands and advocating for social change (King, 1978; Zemke & Clarke, 1996). Adaptation is also an occupational therapy outcome (AOTA, 2014).

Although older adults typically need to adapt to changes in their role as worker, many are continuing to work well into their 70s, either for financial reasons or because they have the energy, drive, skills, and ability to work longer. Each older adult's desire, need, and ability to continue working is different.

Some people become ill and must quickly adapt to undesirable change; others have the time and circumstances to plan ahead for long-term needs, including the potential need for long-term care. In Australia, Canada, and the United States, efforts by individuals, advocacy groups, and government agencies are increasing the options consumers can choose from on the basis of their unique needs. Having an array of options gives people greater power to determine how they will use their personal, insurance, and government resources and where they will live in their later years.

Occupational Therapy Role in Aging

Occupational therapy practitioners, in collaboration with other professionals and services agencies, can address the health needs of the growing number of older adults who live in their communities through the design, implementation, and evaluation of cost-effective prevention and rehabilitation services (Anderson et al., 2000; Clark et al., 1997; Hay et al., 2002).

Occupational therapy practitioners provide services to older adults who have or are at risk of having difficulty engaging in occupations and participating in contexts. They use task analysis as an evaluation and intervention tool to identify performance patterns, performance skills, contextual variables, activity demands, and client factors that limit older clients' engagement and target intervention strategies at barriers that limit and factors that support participation. Intervention approaches include health promotion, remediation or restoration, maintenance of performance capabilities, compensation, adaptation, and disability prevention.

CASE EXAMPLE 13.1. JONO: BELOW-KNEE AMPUTATION

Note. The Client Profile and Task Analysis form (CPTA; Appendix A) is to be used for answering the assignment questions related to the case examples.

Jono was a 65-year-old man who had been a farmer until he retired at age 60 years. He lived alone in his small farmhouse about 10 miles from town. He sold most of his land 5 years previously but had enough acreage for his large vegetable patch and fruit trees, which he relied on for food. He had had diabetes for 10 years. Over the past year, Jono had chronic skin breakdown on both feet. He recently underwent a left below-knee amputation and was receiving occupational and physical therapy rehabilitation services at a skilled nursing facility. His medical history included peripheral vascular disease, hypertension, cataracts, atherosclerosis, and peripheral neuropathy. Jono's physician suggested that he be discharged home in 2 weeks.

Before his wife's death, Jono spent much of his day working on the farm and maintaining the yard while his wife managed the household and cooked all their meals. Since her death, he had assumed responsibility for all of these activities, but he was having increasing difficulty because of his inability to stand for long periods of time. During his leisure time, he enjoyed woodworking and riding his horse.

Although Jono was walking with his temporary prosthesis in physical therapy, he moved around the facility in a wheelchair that belonged to the facility. He was able to walk 5 to 10 feet but relied very heavily on a standard walker because of poor standing balance. Both the physical and the occupational therapy practitioners felt that Jono's problem with postural control was secondary to peripheral neuropathy in his right leg. His left leg was swollen, and his skin was slightly red after using the prosthesis for short periods. He had only limited interest in the rehabilitation program and spoke to staff during therapy sessions only after he was asked questions. During a conference in which Jono's case was discussed, the dietician indicated that Jono appeared to have a very poor understanding of an appropriate diet. Although he stated that he cooked his meals, his answers to questions regarding his diet were vague. When Jono was not in therapy, he spent most of his time sleeping or sitting alone in his room. He rarely conversed with other residents at the facility and had few visitors.

The occupational therapy practitioner had been involved with Jono since his admission, and services were directed primarily toward achieving functional goals in basic activities of daily living (ADLs). Jono was now independent in these areas using some equipment (e.g., bath chair). He performed his ADLs from a wheelchair. The entrance to Jono's home was not wheelchair accessible, nor was he interested in purchasing or renting "one of those clunkers."

Over the past week, Jono commented that he had achieved all of his occupational goals. When instrumental activities of daily living (IADLs), work, and leisure interests were discussed, Jono indicated that he planned to get to and from town by driving his truck, which had a standard transmission. In addition, he claimed, "Once I am able to push the clutch down on my lawn mower and ride it, I can do the chores at home." He indicated several projects he would like to do after leaving the skilled nursing facility, including painting the garage, tuning up the lawnmower, replacing the rain gutters, fixing the snow blower, and chopping wood for the winter.

Assignment 13.1. Jono

1. Read the case example of Jono, and complete the CPTA form (Appendix A). Occupational therapy practitioners are responsible for determining how impairment and activity limitation affect engagement in occupations and participation in contexts. These determinations or judgments are often based on limited information about clients. To develop knowledge and skills in this area, use the information provided in the case example and supplementary research evidence to predict the impact of Jono's impairment and activity limitations on his engagement in occupations and participation in contexts.

2. Document specific, measurable, outcome-oriented client goals and objectives for Jono. In practice, you would establish these goals and objectives in collaborative consultation with Jono. He has defined some priority occupations—painting the garage, tuning up the lawnmower, replacing the rain gutters, fixing the snow blower, and chopping wood for the winter. Predict whether they are achievable, and document your rationale. In what other meaningful occupations and roles might he have participation restrictions? Are these areas in which occupational therapy services might be appropriate to offer?

3. Using the CPTA form, identify a task from the list of "Client Priorities" and complete the "Task Analyzed" section. Use the "Task Analysis Template" to specify "Action Demands" and "Client Challenges" in achieving the identified client priorities. Next, consider Jono's customary environmental contexts. Then complete the CPTA form section "Analysis (of Performance Skills)." Is there a match or fit among Jon's performance capabilities, the activity demands of this task, and contextual factors? Explain and justify your impressions.

4. Using the CPTA form's "Occupational Profile and Analysis of Needs" section, develop an initial intervention plan to address the area of occupation you chose for Question 3. Select and design a purposeful activity or occupation-based activity for use with Jono during a 30-minute session. Consider designing an intervention plan for the 2-week period before Jono's discharge to prepare him for the demands that await him at home. Consider designing an intervention plan as though you were providing home health services after discharge.

5. Describe the role of occupational therapy practitioners in promoting physical activity among older adults. Does Jono exhibit risk factors for reduced levels of physical activity? What health promotion intervention initiatives might you use with Jono to address this area of health? What role might an occupational therapy practitioner take in designing intervention for a population of older adults to promote physical activity?

6. Describe the role of occupational therapy practitioners in the prevention of suicide among older adults, keeping in mind that depression is a risk factor for suicide. What health promotion and disease and disability prevention interventions might you use with Jono to address his risk of suicide?

7. Opportunities for social participation may diminish with increasing age. Explore the social opportunities available and accessible to older adults in your community. What events and activities are offered? Are these events and activities accessible to people using wheelchairs for mobility? What health promotion and disease and disability prevention programs for older adults exist in your community? How might these options promote health and fitness?

8. Jono lives alone and is responsible for all of his ADLs and IADLs, including house and property maintenance. Do you think he has the physical and mental health to manage all of those responsibilities? With his reduced mobility and the increased time he requires to complete most of his ADLs, do you think he has the time to manage his home? If not, as an occupational therapy practitioner working for ABC Seniors Advisory Council, what services would you likely recommend to help keep Jono living independently in his home?

That older adults should be able to take part in the naturally occurring activities of society is a fundamental belief of the occupational therapy profession (AOTA, 1996). After all, people of all ages place a priority on retaining independence and autonomy and having others witness and share their lives.

Occupational therapy services directed at enhancing older adults' access to and engagement in occupations and participation in community contexts are consistent with this understanding of human motivation and behavior (see Case Example 13.1).

PLACEMENT NEEDS AND CARE CONSIDERATIONS

Older adults now have fewer health problems and disabilities, live more independently, and live healthier lives than their predecessors (Centers for Disease Control and Prevention, 2011; Chen & Millar, 2000; Menec, MacWilliam, Soodeen, & Mitchell, 2002; Sifferlin, 2013). As life expectancy increases, health promotion and prevention initiatives focus on the need for older adults to maintain healthy levels of engagement in occupations.

People remain healthier for a larger portion of their life than previously, but because they will live longer, they are more likely to experience chronic disease or disability at some point during their lives (Jackson et al., 2001; see Case Examples 13.2 and 13.3).

Demographic trends have given rise to the concept of successful aging as a key public health and policy concern (Fisher, 1995; Jackson et al., 2001). The characteristics of *successful aging* include low levels of disease and disability, high mental and physical functioning, and active engagement with life (Rowe & Kahn, 1998). Currently, three primary models of care are occurring in the United States, Canada, and Australia: (1) nursing home or long-term care, (2) attendant care, and (3) aging in place.

Long-term care facilities are health care facilities for permanent residents who have chronic or progressive illnesses or diagnoses (e.g., dementia; AOTA, n.d.). No one longs for the day they can live in a long-term-care facility, but sometimes it is the best place for a person to be, because of their level of nursing and ADL support needs. These facilities are expensive for individuals, insurers, and governments, and not everyone requires the level of care available at these facilities.

Attendant care provides a secure environment where staff are available as needed and where residents can have graded independence ranging from entirely independent with all ADLs to requiring regular facility-provided or community care assistance. Attendant care is provided in a variety of settings such as a retirement village or facility. Some couples move to attendant care facilities when one spouse requires more assistance than the other spouse can provide. Typically, when an attendant care facility is attached to a long-term-care facility, the spouse with greater needs can move into the facility if needed while the other spouse lives nearby in an attendant care facility.

Another option that is increasing in popularity is *aging in place,* which is "being able to continue living in one's own home or neighborhood and to adapt to changing needs and conditions. It is of high concern due to the increasing number of old and very old people in all societies" (Malmegren Fänge, Oswald, & Clemson, 2012, p. 1). Aging in place occurs when an individual requires home or community care assistance but is still capable of safely living in his or her own home. Aging in place is possible to the extent that community care assistance is available. This model is the least expensive option, so more insurers and governments are encouraging it because of the cost savings. In addition, the aging-in-place model has emotional benefits for the client.

A growing aspect of support for aging in place is when a person receives a fiscal allotment based on his or her needs and is responsible for allocating the funds toward needs. This funding model would enable individual autonomy because the individual consumer is the primary decision maker. Such autonomy and control allow older adults to actively participate in the effort to age in their own home, thereby enabling them to stay in their community.

Beacon Hill Village in Boston and the Canada Mortgage Housing Corporation are examples of organizations enabling aging in place. Beacon Hill Village is credited as being the United States' first Aging in Community. The *Aging in Community*

(text continues on page 206)

CASE EXAMPLE 13.2. MAX AND CELINA: A CAREGIVER'S INJURY

Max and Celina were both in their mid-70s and had been married for 48 years. They had 4 children and 8 grandchildren. Max had had Parkinson's disease for almost 20 years. Celina fell while gardening and fractured her humerus; her right arm was in a cast and would be in a sling for approximately 6–8 weeks. Celina had great difficulty caring for her husband in this condition, and her family physician arranged for home health services.

When the occupational therapy practitioner arrived to begin services, Celina answered the door and introduced herself and her husband. Max lifted his tremulous hand as if to wave hello from his seat at the dining room table. He was sitting in front of playing cards that were arranged in a row, face up and on the tabletop. The couple appeared to have been playing a game. As the interview proceeded, Celina contributed most to the conversation while her husband watched. Celina had a list of services and equipment that she wanted, including an assistant to bathe Max twice a week, someone to assist with housework, and a grab bar next to the toilet. Once provided with this assistance and equipment, Celina expected that she would once again be able to take care of her husband.

When asked about her concerns regarding bathing and access to the toilet, Celina indicated that she was unable to get her husband into the bathtub without the use of both arms. Although she assisted him on and off the toilet, this task had been very difficult for both Celina and Max, and since Celina injured herself, the task had become close to impossible. Max had begun to wear incontinence pads, which was upsetting for him. The couple did not have any assistive devices for the toilet or the bathtub. Celina indicated that Max was given a walker 5 years previously, but in her opinion he walked better and was safer with her assistance because he was unstable with the walker.

Max relied very heavily on his wife's assistance and support to stand up and sit down and to walk. The most difficult activity was getting up from the dining room chair. When the couple walked together from the dining room to the living room, Celina indicated, "Getting up is always the hardest. After he gets going, we are pretty good together." Max walked into the living room with a stooped posture and slow, shuffling gait, and his wife held him close to her using her left arm. Once in the living room, the couple slowed their pace before turning toward the piano. Max sat on the piano bench and said in a quiet monotone, "It's easier to get up from here."

Celina indicated that she was the "planner, organizer, and motivator of the family":

My husband and I spend every second Monday afternoon at the library. Max does not read very much because he has trouble with the pages, but I love to read. On the way home, we stop for dinner at a restaurant. On Tuesday or Wednesday, we go out to the bank and the grocery store. My husband stays in the car while I do the running around. Friday is our day for swimming, and my husband takes me out for an afternoon dinner date every Saturday. We often go to our favorite garden terrace restaurant. Sunday is our day of rest, although I am usually busy in the yard. By the end of the day, we are usually ready to go out for a light dinner.

Max watched his wife as she described their week together. Although he did not smile, he seemed to be very interested in the conversation.

The couple lived in a small, two-bedroom bungalow that had two sets of stairs at the entrance of the home. The property had a very large lawn and a small garage. Before her fall, Celina drove the couple around in their small two-door car. Recently they had gone out less because they now needed to use a taxi to get around in their community.

Assignment 13.2. Max and Celina

1. Read the case example of Max and Celina, and complete the CPTA form (Appendix A) with information that includes "Client Profile", "Personal Information," and "Analysis (of Performance Skills)," and "Analysis (of Performance Patterns)."

2. Occupational therapy practitioners are responsible for determining how impairment and activity limitations affect engagement in occupations and participation in contexts. These determinations or judgments are often based on limited information about clients. To develop knowledge and skills in this area, use the information provided in the case example and supplementary research evidence to predict the impact of Celina's impairment and activity limitations on her engagement in customary and desired occupations and participation in life situations.

3. Document specific, measurable, outcome-oriented client goals and objectives for both Max and Celina. In practice, you would establish these goals and objectives in consultation with the couple. Celina has described some areas of need in relation to caring for Max; how does her impairment affect her engagement in occupations, participation in contexts, and role competence? How might occupational therapy services address the needs of Max and Celina as individuals versus as a couple?

4. Using the CPTA form's "Summary, Plan, and Goals" section, document specific, measurable, outcome-oriented client goals and objectives for both Max and Celina. In practice, you would establish these goals and objectives in consultation with the couple. Celina has described some areas of need in relation to caring for Max; how does her impairment affect her engagement in her care of Max? Using the "Task Analysis Template," identify a task Celina must perform to care for Max, and analyze the action demands and her challenges in meeting these demands. To determine this, complete the "Analysis (of Performance Skills)" section to identify Celina's challenges. Ensure that you are conversant with Max and Celina's customary environmental contexts. Is there a match or fit among Celina's performance capabilities, the action demands in caring for Max, and contextual factors? Explain and justify your impressions. Finally, identify potential activity demands, performance limitations, and contextual factors that might limit or support Max in his engagement in occupations and activities that Celina no longer can support.

5. Develop an initial intervention plan to address participation restrictions in the task you have just analyzed. Consider different approaches and types of interventions, as well as outcomes applicable to occupational therapy practice.

6. Develop an initial intervention plan to address the couple's performance limitations. How might your strategies incorporate their individual and interdependent needs and priorities?

7. Explore transportation options for older adults in your community. Are they affordable to older adults? Do any agencies provide social participation opportunities to older adults who are mobile in the community? How about those who are confined to their homes? Are these activities affordable to older adults? Locate and consider the median income for older adults from published national and local statistical reports.

8. As an occupational therapy practitioner working for ABC Seniors Advisory Council, what services would you recommend to help Celina manage her home and care for Max? How long do you think these services will be needed?

CASE EXAMPLE 13.3. MARIA AND EDUARDO: A CAREGIVER'S DECLINING HEALTH

Eduardo was a 68-year-old man who had recently been hospitalized after having a mild heart attack. For many years he had been the primary caregiver for **his wife, Maria,** who was severely disabled with rheumatoid arthritis. The family requested assistance from a community health services agency because Eduardo was experiencing difficulties caring for Maria. Their only daughter, who lived 3 hours away, was concerned that Maria might need to be placed in a continuing care center.

Maria and Eduardo's home was a split-level with the kitchen, dining room, den, and half-bathroom on the main level and the bedrooms and a full bathroom on the upper level. There were 2 exterior stairs and 6 steps between the main and upper level. As the occupational therapy practitioner entered the home to begin the evaluation session, Eduardo asked his wife what he should make for lunch. Maria sat in an overstuffed antique chair that was positioned next to a window. From that position, she could see the front entrance to the house, the garden, and the kitchen. Magazines, 2 candy dishes, a radio, and a television surrounded the chair. The practitioner observed Eduardo walk over to the candy dish and put 2 small peppermints in his wife's mouth. He then left the room to prepare lunch as directed.

Maria had limited extension in all metacarpophalangeal (MP) joints and ulnar drift bilaterally. Although she held her left MP and proximal interphalangeal joints in flexion, she had enough active extension in these fingers to hold an object 1 inch in diameter with a cylindrical grip. She did not wear resting splints at night because "they are too clumsy and look awful." Although she had a walker and reacher, they were of minimal use to her because of her inability to hold on to the walker and the amount of finger flexion and extension and strength required to grasp and squeeze the trigger of the reacher. Maria walked very slowly around the home. She ascended and descended stairs with moderate assistance from Eduardo (Maria could perform between 50% and 75% of the task). She tended, however, to spend the vast majority of her day sitting in the chair by the window. Although she had a wheelchair, it was used exclusively for community outings. The only other assistive device in use was a raised toilet seat.

Since his heart attack, Eduardo tired more easily and found that he had to rest after making meals or doing housework. Vacuuming was particularly tiring. He seemed to have energy only for Maria's personal care and meal preparation and cleanup. He had difficulty helping Maria in and out of the tub, a daily occurrence because Maria truly enjoyed bathing: "I don't know what I would do without my daily bath. It eases the morning aches and pains." Eduardo knew that Maria loved her morning bath, but he needed to sit down for a few minutes after helping her, and he felt he couldn't continue. Eduardo no longer had the time or energy to work in the garden, an activity he enjoyed in the past. Community outings were particularly tiring for him, and lifting the wheelchair in and out of the car trunk left him exhausted and weak. They had always been able to accommodate Maria's disability to ensure that they continued to have a sex life, but nobody had talked to them about sexual health since his heart attack. Both were concerned about the effect the heart attack was having on their intimacy.

In the past, Eduardo and Maria had led an active life of gardening, walking, traveling, and socializing with friends. More recently, Eduardo continued to work in the garden for very short periods while Maria sat and watched. They liked to plan the annual garden during the winter months. Until the heart attack, they socialized on a regular basis and hosted a bridge tournament at their home once a month; Maria watched while Eduardo and their guests played the game. They were aware of their daughter's concerns about their ability to continue living at home and her opinion that her mother should be placed in a home. They were adamantly opposed to any move, although they understood their daughter's concerns and recognized that changes might be necessary.

Assignment 13.3. Maria and Eduardo

1. Read the case example of Maria and Eduardo, and complete the CPTA form's (Appendix A) "Task Analyzed", "Analysis (of Performance Skills)," "Analysis (of Performance Patterns)," "Occupational Profile and Analysis of Needs," and "Task Analysis Template" sections (to the extent possible with the information provided and for each individual).

2. Occupational therapy practitioners are responsible for determining how impairment and activity limitation affect engagement in occupations and participation in contexts. These determinations or judgments are often based on limited information about clients. To develop knowledge and skills in this area, use the information provided in the case study and supplementary research evidence to predict the impact of Eduardo's newly diagnosed impairment and activity limitations on his engagement in customary and desired occupations and participation in contexts.

3. Using the completed CPTA forms for Maria and Eduardo, determine the areas of need that should be addressed to ensure that both have their needs met. What is Maria's potential to modify her occupational engagement and participation in contexts? What is Eduardo's potential?

4. Occupational therapy practitioners working in home health services enter private homes and have the opportunity to observe family relationship patterns firsthand. Given that Maria expected to answer the practitioner's interview questions while Eduardo made lunch, role-play how you might engage both partners in the interview and goal-setting process.

5. Complete the CPTA form's "Summary, Plan, and Goals" section by documenting specific, measurable, outcome-oriented client goals and objectives for both Maria and Eduardo. In practice, you would establish these goals and objectives in consultation with each individual and with the couple. How might the occupational practitioner address this couple's needs?

6. Identify a task from the list of goals and objectives that is a priority for both Maria and Eduardo, and analyze the activity and occupational demands using the checklist in the CPTA form. Using the information you collected for Question 1, and considering the couple's environmental and personal contexts, determine if there is a match or fit among the couple's performance capabilities, the occupation or activity demands, and the contextual factors? Explain and justify your impressions. Finally, identify potential occupation or activity demands, performance limitations or restrictions, and contextual factors that might limit or support their engagement as a couple.

7. Develop an initial intervention plan to address this area of occupation. Consider the different approaches and types of interventions as well as outcomes applicable to occupational therapy practice.

8. What type of intervention could or should be provided through a home health service agency? If you receive a referral to see Eduardo, can you provide services directed toward Maria? Review research evidence on the effectiveness and cost-effectiveness of home health services (also called *home care services*) for older adults. What are the characteristics of effective and efficient services?

9. Determine current and temporal trends in levels of home health services nationally and in your community. Become familiar with the availability and accessibility of home health and institutional care options in your community. How affordable are these housing options to older adults?

10. Imagine that Maria and Eduardo live in your community. Identify available community resources that serve the needs of older adults like Maria and Eduardo (e.g., volunteer, advocacy). Given the information provided in the case study and your understanding of the role of ABC Seniors Advisory Council and DEF Home Health and resources available in your community, do you agree with the daughter that Maria should be placed in a continuing care center? What is your rationale?

11. Western countries such as the United States, Canada, and Australia are building the capacity to enable older adults to age in place. Explore these developments, and determine the common aspects across countries.

approach was designed to help older adults thrive through retirement. This approach to community planning is multifaceted and encompasses environments, such as cohousing, senior cohousing, and elder's guilds and facilitates networks of similar communities. *Cohousing* may include shared common areas either indoors or outdoors and voluntary shared duties (e.g., cooking). An *elders' guild* uses the wisdom and power of groups of older adults to promote positive change in the lives of aging adults and in all of society. By linking to other like-minded community planners, Aging in Community networks support these groups with idea sharing and with legal advice and facilitate further growth of these communities to provide a more enriching life for others across the country (Aging in Community, 2012).

Canada Mortgage Housing Corporation (2008) released *Community Indicators for an Aging Population* in which researchers identified six indicators that support or hinder the ability of older adults to age in their own home:

1. Neighborhood walkability
2. Transportation options
3. Access to services
4. Housing choice
5. Safety
6. Community engagement in civic activities.

This report demonstrates the Canadian government's awareness that aging in place requires more than funding for in-home service; it also requires local governments and city planners to anticipate the needs of the aging population and make amenities available to meet those needs and keep people in their homes.

SUMMARY

The number of older adults in all societies are increasing and will continue to do so for some time. The challenge to society and communities is to find ways to enable older adults to age successfully and in place for as long as possible. Older adults are challenged to adapt to transitions, including changing roles and diminishing functional capacity, to manage their customary and desired tasks. Task analysis is a tool for the occupational therapy practitioner to assess the needs of the older adult and to assist with seeking resources, making home alterations, and providing rehabilitation services.

Assignment 13.4. Resources for Older Adults

You are an occupational therapy practitioner working for ABC Seniors Advisory Council, a nonprofit organization in the community where Jono, Max, Celina, Maria, and Eduardo live. The council's mandate is to offer community education to older adults on how to maintain their health and independent lifestyle. Assume that this community has the same supports for older adults as your own local community.

1. How might you work for the council to enhance or enrich services and resources in your community that support achievement of the council's mandate? How could you work to ensure that older adults are linked with these resources? How would you design an injury prevention program to support the council's goal to prevent falls among older adults in the community? If you would like some assistance with this challenge, review the literature to identify the components of cost-effective injury prevention programs.

2. How might you work with DEF Home Health, a nonprofit organization with a mandate similar to the council's? DEF Home Health has a tradition of directing services toward individual clients, whereas ABC Seniors Advisory Council has a tradition of designing and implementing initiatives that enable older adults as a population to understand and participate in occupations that contribute to health.

3. Health promotion and disability prevention can be used with individuals, organizations, and populations. Imagine that you work for DEF Home Health. What health promotion and disability prevention initiatives might you implement with Jono, Max and Celina, or Maria and Eduardo?

REFERENCES

Aging in Community. (2012). Aging in community: *New models for retirement.* Retrieved from www. agingincommunity.com

American Occupational Therapy Association. (1993). Position paper: Purposeful activity. *American Journal of Occupational Therapy, 47,* 1081–1082. http://dx.doi.org/10.5014/ajot.47.12.1081

American Occupational Therapy Association. (1996). OT practitioners work more with elderly patients. *OT Practice, 1*(3), 17.

American Occupational Therapy Association. (2014). Occupational therapy practice framework: Domain and process (3rd ed.). *American Journal of Occupational Therapy, 68*(Suppl. 1), S1–48. http://dx.doi.org/10.5014/ajot.2014.682006

American Occupational Therapy Association. (n.d). *Occupational therapy's role in skilled nursing facilities.* Retrieved from www.aota.org/-/media/Corporate/ Files/AboutOT/Professionals/WhatIsOT/RDP/ Facts/FactSheet_SkilledNursing Facilities.ashx

Anderson, C., Mhurchu, C. N., Rubenach, S., Clark, M., Spencer, C., & Winsor, A. (2000). Home or hospital for stroke rehabilitation? Results of a randomized controlled trial: II. Cost minimization analysis at 6 months. *Stroke, 31,* 1032.

Canada Mortgage Housing Corporation. (2008). *Research highlight: Community indicators for an aging population.* Retrieved from www.cmhc-schl. gc.ca/odpub/pdf/66099.pdf?lang=en

Centers for Disease Control and Prevention. (2011). *Deaths and mortality: 2010.* Retrieved from www.cdc.gov/nchs/fastats/deaths.htm

Chen, J., & Millar, W. J. (2000). Are recent cohorts healthier than their predecessors? *Health Reports, 11,* 9–23.

Clark, F., Azen, S. P., Zemke, R., Jackson, J., Carlson, M., Mandel, D., . . . Lipson, L. (1997). Occupational therapy for independent living older adults. *JAMA, 278,* 1321–1326.

Cole, M. B. (2008). Theories of aging. In S. Coppola, S. J. Elliot, & P. Toto (Eds.), *Strategies to advance gerontology excellence: Promoting best practice in occupational therapy* (pp. 135–161). Bethesda, MD: AOTA Press.

Fisher, A. (1995). Successful aging, life satisfaction, and generativity in later life. *International Journal of Aging and Human Development, 41,* 239–250.

Hay, J., Labree, L., Luo, R., Clark, F., Carlson, M., Mandel, D., . . . Azen, S. P. (2002). Cost-effectiveness of preventive occupational therapy for independent living older adults. *Journal of the American Geriatrics Society, 50,* 1381–1387.

Jackson, J., Mandel, D. R., Zemke, R., & Clark, F. A. (2001). Promoting quality of life in elders: An occupation-based occupational therapy program. *World Federation of Occupational Therapists Bulletin, 43,* 5–12.

King, L. J. (1978). Toward a science of adaptive responses [Eleanor Clarke Slagle Lecture]. *American Journal of Occupational Therapy, 32,* 429–437.

Malmegren Fänge, A., Oswald, F., & Clemson, L. (2012). Aging in place in late life: Theory, methodology, and intervention. *Journal of Aging Research, 2012,* 1–2. http://dx.doi. org/10.1155/2012/547562

Menec, V., MacWilliam, L., Soodeen, R., & Mitchell, L. (2002). *The health and health care use of Manitoba's seniors: Have they changed over time?* Winnipeg: Manitoba Centre for Health Policy.

Mosey, A. C. (1986). *Psychosocial components of occupational therapy.* New York: Raven Press.

Rowe, J. W., & Kahn, R. L. (1998). *Successful aging.* New York: Pantheon Books.

Sifferlin, A. (2013). *We're living longer—and healthier.* Retrieved from http://healthland.time.com/2013/07/ 29/were-living-longer-and-healthier/

U.S. Bureau of the Census. (2008). *Americans with disabilities: 2005.* Washington, DC: U.S. Department of Commerce. Retrieved from www.census. gov/prod/2008pubs/p70-117.pdf

U.S. Department of Health and Human Services. (2011). *A profile of older Americans 2011.* Washington, DC: Administration on Aging. Retrieved from www.aoa.gov/aoaroot/aging_statistics/Profile/ 2011/3.aspx

World Health Organization. (2011). *World report on disability.* Geneva: Author.

Zemke, R., & Clark, F. (Eds.). (1996). *Occupational science: The evolving discipline.* Philadelphia: F. A. Davis.

Healthy Communities

14

By locating our programs in the community defined by locale or spirit, we are accepting the challenge of responding to that community's need with what must be new and innovative ways of being.

—Fazio (2001, p. 5)

LEARNING OBJECTIVES

At the completion of this chapter, readers will be able to

- Define the similarities and differences among the medical, behavioral, and socioenvironmental models of health intervention;
- Describe how health promotion initiatives can be advanced through a community development process;
- Describe how occupational therapy practitioners use task analysis in the context of health promotion and community development; and
- Describe how occupational therapy practitioners use research and relevant evidence in planning health interventions.

KEY TERMS

Asset mapping
Behavioral model
Communities
Community action
Disability
Epidemiological reasearch
Evidence-based practice
Health
Health education
Health promotion
Healthy Cities and Healthy Communities movement

Healthy People 2010
Healthy People 2020
Incidence
MAP–IT
Medical model
Ottawa Charter for Health Promotion
Population-based research
Population health research
Prevalence
Program evaluation research
Socioenvironmental model
Workplace health

Occupational therapy practitioners have been increasingly involved with local, national, and international projects and decision making about facilitating health and wellness initiatives across communities and populations. "Chunking" processes down to doable components is achieved through task analysis. The process enables a group to set priorities and to assign components of the work to be accomplished to participants on a task force. The Client Profile and Task Analysis Form (CPTA; Appendix A) demonstrates how practitioners might develop a task analysis model that can be adapted for use when working with communities and groups.

HEALTHY PEOPLE, COMMUNITIES, AND POPULATIONS

Health promotion is a "prevention strategy that allows people to manage and improve their overall health status" (American Occupational Therapy Association [AOTA], 2013b). It includes both health education and the provision of supports for environmental contexts that enable healthy behavior (Green & Kreuter, 1999). It "goes beyond health care" (para. 1), because

> Our societies are complex and interrelated. Health cannot be separated from other goals. The inextricable links between people and their environment constitutes the basis for a socioeconological approach to health. . . . Changing patterns of life, work and leisure have a significant impact on health. Work and leisure should be a source of health for people. (World Health Organization [WHO], 1986, para. 4)

Health professionals use several approaches to guide the development of strategies and interventions to improve the health status of communities. These approaches have evolved over time to include medical, behavioral, and socioenvironmental models of practice. Practitioners across disciplines who use these approaches have made and continue to make an impact on the health of individuals and populations. When considering health interventions targeted toward populations, these approaches are indivisible, and all come into play.

Medical Model

Proponents of the *medical model* view *health* as the absence of disease, trauma, or other health condition and *disability* as an activity limitation or participation restriction resulting from a health condition or impairment. Health professionals who use this approach focus on individual clients and the management of physiological risk factors, disease, or impairment. Examples of interventions using the medical model approach to health maintenance would be to reduce activity levels to manage the risk of cardiac disease and to exercise to improve fitness and reduce physiological risk.

Behavioral Model

Proponents of the *behavioral model* view health as being controlled by individuals; therefore, intervention focuses on promoting healthy lifestyles and addressing behavioral risk factors. Examples of this approach to intervention include health education programs that teach clients about risk factors for back injuries and ways to reshape their task methods to reduce their risk or lifestyle counseling programs that inform adolescents how to prevent violence and avoid drug addiction. Public policies that require people to use seat belts and bike helmets and public health monitoring to prevent falls are other examples of a behavioral approach to intervention.

Socioenvironmental Model

Proponents of the *socioenvironmental model* view health as a function of social and environmental determinants. The premise is that changes at the community level, rather than the individual level, will have the most significant influence on the health of the population (McBeth & Schweer, 2000). Health professionals who use this approach point to research and practice indicating that differences among populations in health status are attributable to variability in their exposure to ecological contexts that create and sustain inequities in health. Therefore, these practitioners direct health intervention toward altering socioenvironmental conditions to create healthy environments and improve health status.

Socioenvironmental models acknowledge that the health and well-being of a population go beyond traditional biomedical determinants of health to include broader conditions and resources for health in the social, political, cultural, and physical environments. Such conditions as peace, shelter, education, food, income, employment, literacy, a stable ecosystem, social justice, and equity are seen as key determinants of the health of populations (U.S. Department of Health and Human Services [DHHS], 1979, 2000; Wallerstein, 1992; WHO, 1984, 1986, 2000). These determinants of health and wellness require health promotion strategies and a community development process. In comparison to biomedical and behavioral models, ecological models that rely on community-focused approaches to improving health change the focus from "us and them" to "us being them" (McKenzie & Smeltzer, 2001).

Community groups, associations, coalitions, and organizations are central to socioenvironmental health intervention models; communities implement their own health promotion and disability and disease prevention strategies. The socioenvironmental model views each community as a geopolitical entity with its own unique environment, personality, characteristics, power structure, health status, and resources for sustainable change (Kaufman, 1990; McKenzie & Smeltzer, 2001).

An example of a socioenvironmental intervention is a welfare-to-work initiative that covers an array of needs of dislocated workers through stress and financial management workshops, lessons on writing résumé and preparing for employment interviews, and employee assistance programs. Significant and necessary relations exist among medical, behavioral, and socioenvironmental models, which are all necessary to address the complex phenomenon of health. After all, the goal of all three models of health intervention is to serve and fulfill society's interest in ensuring conditions to support healthy people, communities, and populations (DHHS, 1998; Kaufman, 1990; WHO, 1980, 2001).

Assignment 14.1. Understanding Population Health and Healthy Communities

1. Familiarize yourself with Healthy People 2020 (DHHS, 2010a).
2. Explain the similarities and differences among the medical, behavioral, and socioenvironmental models and their approaches to health intervention.

A SYSTEMATIC APPROACH TO IMPROVING THE HEALTH OF POPULATIONS

In response to international recognition that the health of North Americans and Europeans was not improving despite large and increasing investments in health care focused on biomedical and behavioral interventions, the *Healthy Communities and Healthy Cities movement* emerged. Similarly, the Healthy Cities movement emerged after the WHO's (1986) publication of the *Ottawa Charter for Health Promotion*. The Healthy Communities and Healthy Cities movement built its interventions on a merging of the medical, behavioral, and socioenvironmental models of health intervention, and the movement's philosophies have coalesced to become what is now the strategy for health promotion espoused by most health leaders, including DHHS.

The Healthy Communities movement seeks to build and strengthen multisectoral partnerships to improve the social and health conditions in the spaces where people live, advocate for the formulation of health-related public policy, maintain healthy environments, and promote healthy lifestyles.

In 2000, DHHS presented *Healthy People 2010*, which set forth 10-year goals and objectives that address the health of the nation. This document included a conceptual framework titled Healthy People in Healthy Communities (HPHC) that identified the DHHS's view of the determinants of health. Ten years later, *Healthy People 2020* advanced the initiative (DHHS, 2010a). The determinants of the health of populations defined in the 2020 HPHC framework are strikingly similar to the dimensions of concern to occupational therapy practitioners as defined by AOTA (2014; DHHS, 2010a). The determinants of health are identified as physical and social environments, individual behavior, biology and genetics, and health services.

Occupational therapy practitioners strive to establish and optimize the fit among persons, environments, and occupations, and the HPHC framework identifies factors related to the individual (biology, behavior) and to the social, physical, and cultural contexts that must be optimized to promote and maintain health. Occupational therapy practitioners who seek to influence the health and behaviors of populations can incorporate the goals, objectives, and intervention processes recommended by DHHS to help guide and focus their services on improving the health of local communities to contribute to the improved health of the nation.

The primary focus of Healthy People 2020 is on wellness (DHHS, 2010a). It articulates four overarching goals:

1. Attain high-quality, longer lives free of preventable disease, disability, injury, and premature death.
2. Achieve health equity, eliminate disparities, and improve the health of all groups.
3. Create social and physical environments that promote good health for all.
4. Promote quality of life, healthy development, and healthy behaviors across all life stages.

The mission of the initiative is to

- Identify nationwide health improvement priorities.
- Increase public awareness and understanding of the determinants of health, disease, and disability and the opportunities for progress.
- Provide measurable objectives and goals that are applicable at the national, state, and local levels.
- Engage multiple sectors to take actions to strengthen policies and improve practices that are driven by the best available evidence and knowledge.
- Identify critical research, evaluation, and data collection needs. (DHHS, 2010a, para. 4)

The focus, goals, and objectives of this national strategy for health parallel the vision and mission of occupational therapy. The primary focus of occupational therapy is enabling clients to enhance functional status, engage in occupations, participate in life situations, prevent disability, and promote health. The DHHS goal of reducing inequities in health parallels occupational therapy's consistent focus on providing services to vulnerable populations and people most in need of amelioration of activity limitations and participation restrictions.

In addition to defining goals and accompanying objectives, Healthy People 2020 includes indicators to help health professionals and communities target actions to improve health and to focus state governments, local communities, health care organizations, professional organizations, and others in targeting health care services, risk prevention programs, and health promotion initiatives (DHHS, 2010a). The Healthy People 2010 and Healthy People 2020 initiatives have generated much interest in health promotion and disease and disability prevention and in activities and interventions that support attainment of its goals and objectives: "Imagine an integrated, holistic health system that serves people throughout their lifespan. Imagine achieving not just the vision but the reality of healthy people living in healthy communities" (McBeth & Schweer, 2000, p. ix).

Health services professions and organizations in the United States and worldwide are increasingly shifting from a focus on illness and disability to one of keeping communities and populations healthy (WHO, 2009). Consequently, many professionals and organizations are designing and evaluating health interventions, and the materials they generate can be used in designing programs to achieve the vision of Healthy People 2020. For example, the Healthy People 2020 MAP–IT tool kit is available to provide guidance in the creation of public health initiatives (DHHS, 2010b). This task-based tool kit walks the public health promoter through the entire process, from considering stakeholders for engagement to prioritizing issues and objectives, implementing the initiative, and measuring progress.

HEALTH PROMOTION AND INJURY PREVENTION

In initiatives with a capacity-building health promotion and injury prevention orientation, certain community processes are considered necessary to enhance personal health, and environments can be created that simultaneously protect health and support healthy personal behaviors. Green and Kreuter (1999) suggested that *health promotion* is "the combination of education and ecological supports for actions and conditions of living conducive to health" (p. 27).

Health education is aimed at closing the gap between what clients know promotes health (e.g., physical activity is good for one's health) and what they practice in terms of health behaviors (e.g., their fitness habits and routines). Intervention is targeted toward promoting knowledge of healthy behaviors and contexts among people, organizational leaders, and policymakers. The intent is to facilitate healthy attitudes, behaviors, social structures, and contexts for living. Health education and awareness initiatives seek to "promote healthy behavior and lifestyle by increasing understanding of how engagement in occupation can prevent illness and promote health and well-being" (Wilcock, 1998, p. 227).

Occupational Therapy Approach

Occupational therapy areas of practice include health promotion and disability prevention. AOTA "supports and promotes involvement of occupational therapists and occupational therapy assistants in the development and provision of health promotion and disease or disability prevention programs and services" (AOTA, 2013a, p. S47; see also Appendix D). Such programs and services are directed toward individuals, organizations, communities, populations, and policymakers, and their focus is to prevent or reduce illness or disease; reduce health disparities; enhance mental health; prevent secondary conditions; and promote healthy living practices, social participation, and healthy communities.

The role of occupational therapy in offering prevention services to individuals and populations is linked to the profession's focus on the impact of the interaction among persons, environments, and occupations on engagement in occupations and participation in contexts. AOTA (2008; see also AOTA, 2013a) articulated the following roles for occupational therapy practitioners offering primary prevention services:

- Evaluate occupational capabilities, values, and performance;
- Provide education regarding occupational role performance and balance;
- Reduce risk factors and symptoms through engagement in occupation;
- Provide skill development training in the context of everyday occupations;
- Provide self-management training to prevent illness and manage health;
- Modify environments for healthy and safe occupational performance;
- Consult and collaborate with health care professionals, organizations, communities, and policymakers regarding the occupational perspective of health promotion and disease or disability prevention;
- Promote the development and maintenance of mental functioning abilities through engagement in productive and meaningful activities and relationships…; and
- Provide training in adaption to change and in coping with adversity to promote mental health. (p. 698)

A task analysis approach is fundamental for analyzing the developmental needs to advance health and health promotion strategies and establishing the steps to achieve desired outcomes. For example, system strengths and weaknesses must be identified (i.e., organization factors); environments understood (e.g., institutional, political); and past, current, and future activities analyzed relative to the desired outcome (e.g., what strategies worked, are working, and are needed for change).

Workplace Health

Adults spend a large percentage of their day at work, and workplaces are a prime location in which to influence health, including personal health. Health promotion programs have been demonstrated to reduce employee-related health care expenditures and absenteeism (Aldana, Merrill, Price, Hardy, & Hager, 2005). Many programs that encourage healthy behaviors are being designed and implemented at work sites, and the most effective *workplace health* programs are those that provide comprehensive programming and counseling (Pelletier, 2001): "A comprehensive approach to workplace health . . . . [addresses] issues related to the physical environment, the psychosocial environment, and individual health practices" (Bachmann, 2000, p. i).

To implement a successful workplace intervention, organizations need to ensure that senior management supports and provides leadership on workplace health issues; designate various people throughout the organization to be responsible for portions of the program; develop policies and programs that address the full array of issues, including physical and psychosocial well-being, work–life balance, and

---

CASE EXAMPLE 14.1. ADRIANO: PREVENTING INJURY IN A COMMUNITY WORKPLACE

GHI Wood Fabrications contracted **Adriano, an occupational therapist,** to complete a risk analysis of the plant environment and to develop injury prevention and health promotion programs to promote safety among employees. The management team was motivated to act because of rising injury claims, which consisted primarily of back, shoulder, and wrist injuries.

GHI Wood Fabrications manufactured large, heavy-duty wooden items such as doors, workbenches, desks, and boardroom tables. Adriano first interviewed the managers of the firm to determine the nature of current efforts to avoid injuries. The health promotion manager described, among other initiatives, a program that ensured that all employees engaged in a health awareness "toolbox talk" for 5 minutes at the beginning of each day. The health promotion manager developed short fact sheets to promote discussion of health-related topics, and at the end of the discussion employees completed a form that asked how the presentation had affected them and what they could do to improve their health or increase their safety awareness. One company goal was to eventually have employees, rather than management, select the health promotion activities.

Adriano learned that the most prevalent claim was back injury due to repetitive lifting of weights over 50 pounds. Adriano then observed workers throughout the plant at different workstations to assess activity demands. At the first station, a conveyor belt moved large units of lumber to tables for cutting. Two men were required to guide 8-foot by 16-foot, 60-pound units of lumber as they were conveyed, then to lift them off the conveyor onto the 36-inch-high table. At the table, one man sanded the lumber on one side using a power sander, then turned the board over to sand the other side. The same worker slid the lumber horizontally along the table to the next area, where the lumber was cut in two. Two workers were stationed to cut, one to guide the lumber into the saw and switch the saw on, and the other to guide the piece on the other side as it came through the saw. The next step was a fine sanding of each board, a one-man operation using power tools. Each board weighed approximately 30 pounds, and one man carried each board to the staining booth.

Adriano interviewed workers to identify their perceptions of risk. He noted as he talked to the workers that loud music interfered with his ability to hear their responses. Workers indicated that they were happy with their jobs, in part because they were encouraged to rotate through the stations to decrease repetitive action and mental and physical fatigue. They felt that their employer was generous in providing membership to the local fitness club to promote good physical health. They were given sufficient breaks throughout the day that allowed them to rest. A major concern they voiced was the combined weight and awkward postures involved with the repetitive lifting of the boards. In addition, several workers had been in the job for more than 15 years and were experiencing chronic back, shoulder, and wrist pain. The employer was eager for a prevention plan and was not hesitant about exploring options and costs.

Assignment 14.2. Workplace Injury Prevention

1. Read Case Example 14.1. How can an occupational therapy practitioner's knowledge and task analysis skills be used to profile the unique characteristics of individuals among a population of workers at risk for injury, the activity demands of the job tasks, and the performance context of this industry? What dimensions of workers, their job tasks, and the performance contexts are of concern?

2. Determine the incidence of workplace injuries and prevalence of work-related lower back disorders. Use information from the literature to identify factors that contribute to risk of injury. Consider starting your search at the Centers for Disease Control and Prevention's National Institute for Occupational Safety and Health Web site (www.cdc.gov/niosh).

3. Review *Occupational Therapy in the Promotion of Health and Well–Being* (AOTA, 2013a; Appendix D). Identify how this statement applies to occupational therapy practice in the workplace. How might you use this information in describing the role of occupational therapy to the workplace client or employer?

4. The client in the case example of GHI Wood Fabrications is the population of factory workers employed there. To begin the evaluation, design an interview and develop an occupational profile to better understand the occupational history of the work site and the industry. What performance skills and patterns are required of the workers? Identify body structures and functions that are at risk for injury. Then analyze the activity demands of the job tasks and features of the performance contexts that promote or hinder engagement in occupations and participation in contexts at this work site. To complete your analysis, answer the following questions:

   a. What are the physical demands of the job? What body structures and functions are required of workers while on the job? How might the physical environment (i.e., work site space) and objects affect performance?

   b. What process and motor performance skills are required for the job? Consider the concepts and objects used on the job, required actions, and sequencing and timing of the work.

   c. What are the communication and interaction performance skills required for the job? What are the social interaction demands of the job?

   d. What are the required performance patterns of the job? How might you determine whether there is a match between a person and an activity?

   e. Identify the risk factors for injury within the context of the factory environment.

5. Define the long-term goal and measurable short-term objectives of an injury prevention and health promotion program. Consider that intervention can be targeted to workers, performance contexts, and job demands. In practice, you would establish the goals and objectives of a prevention program and develop the intervention plan in collaboration with stakeholders, especially those directly affected by proposed changes, who would both define priorities and identify opportunities for targeted intervention.

6. Consider the features of an injury prevention program to ameliorate the risks you identified in your analysis. What might be the features of a comprehensive workplace injury prevention program for this workplace? Bear in mind the following five-step hierarchy to control risk: (1) Eliminate the hazardous task, (2) substitute the task with a less hazardous task, (3) engineer to isolate the task (e.g., safety guards on equipment), (4) train staff on safe work procedures, and (5) provide personal protective equipment such as gloves.

7. If health education is a component of your plan, what educational modalities might work with this population in the context of the work environment?

8. What resources are needed to support implementation of the intervention plan and evaluation of its effectiveness? Identify policies that may support or hinder implementation of the program.

individual health practices; and recognize and influence external forces in the larger community that influence health (Bachmann, 2000).

It appears that low-intensity, short-duration educational programs aimed at increasing awareness of health and safety issues among employees may not be sufficient to provide desired change in improved health and reduced workplace injury. Yet there is strong evidence that individualized risk reduction for high-risk employees within the context of comprehensive programming and counseling is effective (Pelletier, 2001).

Occupational therapy practitioners can use task analysis to compare the factors that influence the health of workers by evaluating sample cases in the group, comparing them with a sample group of high-risk employees, and then using these findings to provide information to the employer about the person–environment–occupation interactions that affect workplace performance (see Case Example 14.1).

HEALTHY COMMUNITIES THROUGH COMMUNITY DEVELOPMENT

Communities are not just geographic entities; any social aggregation constitutes a community, whether of students, people with disabilities, older adults, or other people with common interests. According to the DHHS (2000), outcomes and research evidence support the idea that "individual health is closely linked to community health—the health of the community and environment in which individuals live, work, and play" (p. 3).

Health promotion initiatives increasingly focus on communitywide efforts to promote healthy behaviors, create healthy environments, and enhance access to high-quality health care. Raeburn and Rootman (1998) indicated that to build healthy communities, "the control of and resources for this enterprise need to be primarily in the hands of the people themselves" (p. 11).

One example of a successful community development process that is recognized internationally is the North Karelia Project in Finland.

Puska et al. (1995) summarized the process required to ensure positive outcomes related to lifestyle change in this and other communities:

> The gaping contrast between existing medical knowledge and the situation in everyday society stems from a host of formidable obstacles to healthy change—cultural, political, economic, psychological, and so on. The aim of a community program is to build a bridge for people and communities to overcome these obstacles, or at least to minimize them. (p. 32)

Developing good public policy and health promotion initiatives requires the combination of health professionals and coalitions working with communities to identify needs and priorities, establish a political voice, and work toward sustainable change with policymakers and organizational leaders incorporating the will of the community and research evidence into their decision making. The challenge is to link actions and create synergies among these stakeholders with the aim of building their capacity to empower the community to identify, lead, and manage strategies in support of health using available professional, institutional, and government resources. Head Start, Smart Start, and California's Children and Families Commission are U.S. initiatives designed to promote health and healthy life trajectories of young children through partnerships and joint initiatives among governments, organizations, businesses, community leaders, child care workers, teachers, and parents.

Establishing a participatory culture among communities, health professionals, and policymakers requires a paradigm shift from a top-down consultation approach to a community-centered and community-driven approach. Occupational therapy practitioners who use health promotion approaches to improve the health of populations consider the community to be the client and use intervention strategies informed by the Healthy Communities movement. The underlying philosophy of the Healthy Communities movement, and the approach to health promotion and community development recommended by both DHHS and WHO, emphasizes starting where people live and creating healthy places to live, work, and play. Indeed, these health intervention strategies are appropriate to use whether services are targeted toward disabled populations (i.e., a community of similar people) or to all people who reside in a specific location (i.e., a geographically defined community).

Occupational therapy practitioners "develop a collaborative relationship with clients to understand their experiences and desires for intervention" (AOTA, 2014, p. S12). Clients define the goals and objectives of intervention and provide the primary resources and structures for sustainable change: "Community partnerships, particularly when they reach out to non-traditional partners, can be among the most effective tools for improving health in communities" (DHHS, 2000, p. 4). Earls (2001) observed,

> There is a broad recognition within most sectors of society that the quality of civic engagement is of critical importance to community effort to improve the health and well-being of children. This is true for all communities and families, regardless of their levels of material wealth and educational achievement. (p. 693)

MOBILIZING COMMUNITY ACTION

Occupational therapy practitioners offer a unique approach to assessing community needs, assets, and resources by conducting task analysis of population characteristics (i.e., people), environments (i.e., performance contexts), and *community actions* (i.e., tasks and activities) that support or hinder health. Just as the concept of person–environment–occupation (PEO) fit guides the establishment of a client profile and analysis of occupational performance for individual clients, this construct guides work with community clients. The creation of a client profile for communities is referred to as *asset mapping.*

At the community level, the PEO model (Law et al., 1996) translates to a community–context–action model. The community is a collective of people with performance skills and patterns, and body structures and functions are analogous to the community's assets. The context includes cultural, physical, social, temporal, and virtual environments, as well as personal factors such as values, beliefs, and goals. The targeted action or occupation of a community is its members' level of participation in healthy lifestyles and behaviors. The occupational therapy process with individual clients involves assessing and optimizing the interaction and fit among person, environment, and occupation, and this procedure is equally applicable with community clients (see Case Example 14.2).

CASE EXAMPLE 14.2. RONNI: COMMUNITY DEVELOPMENT FOR HEALTH PROMOTION

A **rural First Nations community** faced the closure of a public health unit that had historically offered services. **Ronni, an occupational therapy practitioner,** became the project manager responsible for reestablishing rehabilitation services for community members and ensuring their consistency with community values, one of which was the integration of health promotion initiatives for this population. Ronni worked with the community and federal funders to collaborate and develop consensus on a service delivery model. She understood that the critical components in service planning were communication strategies and cultural sensitivity. It was essential to bring together the perspectives of the community and the funder through collaboration, demonstration, and discussion.

Ronni served as facilitator in the collaborative development of an interdisciplinary service model through a community development process that ensured communication among the stakeholders. She interviewed key spokespeople to get a sense of the community's needs and objectives for services. The funder expected to provide conventional individual and small group rehabilitation services, but community members requested that the funder respect their interest in being responsible for their own health care issues

(Continued)

CASE EXAMPLE 14.2. RONNI: COMMUNITY DEVELOPMENT FOR HEALTH PROMOTION (Cont.)

and allow them to design rehabilitation services that would meet the distinct health and cultural needs of their community. Clearly, there was a desire among the community members that all initiatives have a health promotion focus and all services be based on a holistic concept of *health* that included mental, physical, and spiritual well-being, in addition to education, economic opportunity, and social participation.

Mental health services and parenting initiatives to promote performance patterns and skills in parents and communication and interaction skills between parents and children were priority community concerns. In fact, the community described mental health intervention as specifically encompassing health promotion and community development issues. Ronni remained flexible and responsive to the changing and conflicting demands by designing services that would evolve through phases and demonstrating how integrated services would work. She identified a natural starting point that would lead to a model that complied with the funders' mandate and that answered one of the health promotion issues of the community.

As a result of historical decisions to separate Native Canadian youth from their communities for the purposes of education and cultural assimilation, a generation of the community's members grew up in boarding schools away from their parents. This generation had now become parents, and many had not had the opportunity to develop parenting skills through role modeling. An interdisciplinary team worked with the community to integrate a parenting program into all intervention sessions with children; children received the mandated services, and their parents received services to enhance their success in child rearing. Many of the mental health issues appeared to be related, at least in part, to the impact of the parents' early childhood experiences and the stresses of raising their own children without a foundation of exposure to parenting performance patterns.

The service outcome demonstrated that through innovative approaches, the fixed amount of funding available for individuals could be spread across families. Community leaders had the evidence to support parenting programs, which were sanctioned and funded as a result of the evidence-based outcomes. The idea of parent education sessions so inspired two community spokespeople who worked in the education system that they designed and funded program opportunities and educational materials. Another community representative who was a member of the First Nation's Band Council and an employer of many parenting-age adults encouraged the community to establish a day care center to support working parents and to provide respite options for other parents.

The program was so successful that the First Nation's Band Council sanctioned other initiatives that various members of the community took the lead in developing. The day care coordinator developed nutrition educational materials for the children and their parents in collaboration with a local nutritionist to respond to the growing prevalence of diabetes and obesity among all community members. She also initiated family picnic days and included the parents and children in the menu planning. One by one, community members began to identify and act on opportunities to contribute to the development of parenting skills among parents in the community and to nurture healthy families. By meeting regularly, the spokespeople began to identify the initiatives that were most effective in achieving the goals they had for improving the health of the community. Over time, the policymakers began to identify and support the mechanisms the community identified as effective interventions to improve health.

Mobilizing key individuals to assess the community's needs, strengths, and resources is a necessary requisite to the establishment of intervention goals, objectives, and priorities, which in turn become the vision, goals, and guiding principles embedded in service delivery. The challenge of sustaining community involvement in the process of change is best met by agreeing as early as possible on a vision for the community. This vision should emerge from the most important needs, values, and goals identified by the community. The evaluation and intervention process is always client directed in that services focus on the priorities identified by key stakeholders in the community: "When community coalitions work together to set priorities and to allocate resources

---

Assignment 14.3. Community Development and Citizen Action

1. Using the *Occupational Therapy Practice Framework* (AOTA, 2014) and the Healthy People 2020 framework (DHHS, 2010a), develop a graphic illustration that superimposes the dimensions presented in each framework to demonstrate how these dimensions parallel each other.
2. Read Case Example 14.3 and describe how task analysis was used to focus the analysis of issues facing the community, to explore research into factors that contribute to this problem, and to identify intervention options for addressing the goal of reducing the prevalence of obesity.
3. Research the prevalence of obesity in the United States, and identify factors that are known to influence its prevalence. Describe the characteristics of intervention approaches that appear to show results with this growing public health epidemic.

4. Describe how you might use task analysis to enable an individual client or a group of clients who are obese to reflect on the determinants of their own health state. How might you use task analysis as a tool to guide intervention with these clients?
5. How might you use task analysis to promote the collective sharing of critical self-reflections among a group of people who are obese? Because people are often unaware of the characteristics of their customary environments that adversely influence their health, how might you use task analysis in a group context as an educational tool? How might this participation model facilitate social action by a group or community?
6. Describe how you might use task analysis to enable a group of clients who are not obese to reflect on the determinants of obesity and opportunities they can seize to contribute to national efforts to address this public health problem.

---

to these priorities, they are far more likely to continue to participate in the process and to achieve measurable results" (DHHS, 2001, p. 12).

A five-step process of community development called *MAP–IT* (DHHS, 2010b) recommends the following:

1. *Mobilize* key people who care about the health of the community.
2. *Assess* areas of greatest need in the community and strengths and resources that can be tapped to address these areas (i.e., asset mapping).
3. *Plan* your approach by starting with a vision and adding strategies and action steps.
4. *Implement* the action plan using concrete steps that can be monitored and will make a difference.
5. *Track* progress and outcomes over time.

GROUNDING COMMUNITY HEALTH INTERVENTIONS IN EVIDENCE

Intervention plans that are designed by occupational therapy practitioners to improve the health of individuals or populations must be built in collaboration with clients, designed to address targeted outcomes, and grounded in science. The challenge and rewards of evidence-based practice are in the process of obtaining, evaluating, and using evidence to inform intervention plans and demonstrate positive outcomes for clients. To ground health interventions in science, practitioners must search out evidence relative to their practice and incorporate research findings using their own judgment and in consultation with clients (Lin, Murphy, & Robinson, 2010).

In addition, practitioners can contribute to or conduct research to generate new practice knowledge. For instance, occupational therapy practitioners can use research-generated information to profile levels of engagement in occupations, identify risk factors for poor health, determine key factors to improve health, provoke action to address key health issues, establish baseline measures against which to track progress, and assess the effectiveness of alternative intervention strategies.

Evidence-based practice involves merging information, evidence, and judgment. It contributes to informed decision making and accountable intervention planning and implementation.

Accessing Evidence

Whereas information on individuals is obtained through interviews and assessments, information on communities comes through *population-based research* methods. Population-level information can be used to profile levels of health and wellness, performance skills, performance patterns, morbidity and mortality, performance contexts, and so forth.

Research evidence can be used to identify factors that contribute to health, such as engagement in occupation, or conditions that put people at risk for ill health, such as reduced levels of physical activity.

For example, population-based information can be used to determine the proportion of people who are independent in activities of daily living, who have work-related disabilities, who participate in sports, who participate in social events, and who are literate, as well as the *prevalence* (i.e., proportion of a group who experience a disease, condition, or injury at a specific time) and *incidence* (i.e., proportion of a group initially free of disease, condition, or injury who develop the disease, condition, or injury during a specific period) of health determinants such as disease, disability, obesity, substance abuse, unsafe sexual practices, smoking, and so forth.

Population-level statistics regarding health, performance skills, performance patterns, morbidity, and environmental contexts are typically reported for geographic jurisdictions or special populations (e.g., children, students, older adults). For example, the WHO publishes population-level statistics for countries, whereas U.S. federal departments such as the U.S. Bureau of the Census and the U.S. Department of Education, National Institute on Disability and Rehabilitation Research, provide population-level information for geographically defined or special populations.

Population health research explores the origins and determinants of health, whereas *epidemiological research* seeks to identify the origins and determinants of disease, impairments, and disability. Both forms of scientific inquiry profile the prevalence, incidence, and temporal trends in health, illness, and other factors that contribute to different states of health, and findings can be used to focus interventions on key issues and factors deemed to be significant determinants of activity limitations and participation restrictions. *Program evaluation research* can be used to track performance and achievement relative to the goals and objectives of services, as well as to identify effective intervention strategies.

Using Evidence

Practitioners must combine the insights they derive from research with information on the performance patterns, activity demands, and unique contexts of a community gained through observation, focus groups, and conversations with community advocates. This combined evidence can then help the practitioner establish community needs, focus attention on the most significant issues, set priorities, target outcomes, and monitor progress. Just as DHHS (2000) set health goals and objectives for the nation on the basis of population health statistics, occupational therapy practitioners and their community partners should focus health intervention goals, objectives, and activities on the basis of the research evidence they gather.

Interesting research findings can be used to prompt a community into action. For example, health education strategies that focus on communicating the prevalence of substance abuse among pregnant women, the link between parental substance abuse and infant health, and the incidence of fetal alcohol syndrome can stimulate a community to action.

Generating Evidence

Occupational therapy practitioners have a role in contributing to population health research by encouraging and supporting critical appraisal of their own hypotheses about the value of engagement in occupations and participation in contexts. To conduct research to test hypotheses regarding linkages among people and their occupations and contexts or to evaluate occupational therapy interventions directed at individuals or populations, occupational therapy practitioners require information regarding their clients (i.e., the domains and dimensions of practice) and outcomes, as well as the type, frequency, duration, and timing of interventions. If practitioners routinely collect and record this information, they can use it not only to guide intervention but also to conduct research on practice. In fact, the professions that have most consistently used information gleaned in the course of providing routine care (e.g., medicine) have the largest body of evidence regarding the use, quality, and effectiveness of their services.

Occupational therapy practitioners should seize every opportunity to collect information routinely during practice and use it to test hypotheses about the importance of occupation, the contribution of engagement in occupations and participation in contexts to health and wellness, and the effectiveness of occupational therapy services directed toward individuals and populations.

Because the dimensions of the occupational therapy profession's domain of practice align with the determinants of health of individuals and populations, practitioners routinely collect information on and monitor changes in factors that contribute to health and health outcomes such as engagement in occupations that can serve as proxy measures of well-being. Therefore, client profiles should include all the data that are needed to test hypotheses regarding the factors that contribute to the health of individuals and populations and to measure the impact of occupational therapy interventions in altering health status (see Case Example 14.3).

CASE EXAMPLE 14.3. KARLEE: CITIZEN ACTION AGAINST OBESITY

An occupational therapy practitioner, Karlee, was keenly aware of her unique role in the community as a mother and as a participant in a community development project. Project partners and stakeholders who participated in the asset mapping process identified health determinants that paralleled her understanding of key contributors to the health of children and their levels of wellness as they matured.

Many of the participants had concerns about the increasing number of children with obesity, and they wondered about changes in nutrition and physical activity. They had heard about the impact of obesity on general health and wellness across the lifespan, but they could not recall the specifics of information they had received about these effects. They asked Karlee to guide them through a focus group session to further explore the epidemiology of obesity and research on the impact of obesity on health across the lifespan. Karlee suggested that once they completed their analysis of the obesity problem in their community, she could facilitate the development of a proposal to seek funds for a research initiative. The community participants were motivated to learn more and to identify opportunities to work together with children and their families to nurture and support lifestyles and environments in support of healthy bodyweight.

The community members learned that obesity was a more complex health condition than they had anticipated and that the issue epitomized the importance of considering social, behavioral, cultural, environmental, physiological, and genetic factors as determinants of health. Because being overweight and obesity are major contributors to many preventable causes of poor health and death, nutrition, physical activity, and obesity are among the leading health indicators in the Healthy People 2020 initiative.

Karlee took community leaders through a process of examining the parameters of the problem as reflected in population health data. She focused on describing the characteristics of people that predispose them to obesity, the profiles of their typical engagement in occupations and participation in contexts, and descriptions of customary environmental contexts that contribute to or work against healthy bodyweight. It became apparent to the community members that prevention should target people who are at risk for obesity and focus on personal characteristics that are amenable to change and the environmental contexts that most influence children. One of the more immediate objectives was to conduct a survey of the physical, social, and cultural environments to learn more about how to halt the obesity epidemic in their community. Karlee would coauthor the funding proposal and be the coinvestigator on the project.

SUMMARY

Task analysis is an approach that occupational therapy practitioners can use as a unique contribution in project management, setting goals, and identifying priority steps for implementation of a task force on local, national, and international projects. The primary aim of such projects is to guide the development of strategies and interventions to improve the health status of communities and populations. Task analysis is a useful tool for comparison of medical, behavioral, and socioenvironmental factors that support or limit health promotion, injury prevention, and the development of healthy community strategies.

REFERENCES

Aldana, S., Merrill, R. M., Price, K., Hardy, A., & Hager, R. (2005). Financial impact of a comprehensive multisite workplace health promotion program. *Preventive Medicine, 40*, 131–13.

American Occupational Therapy Association. (2008). Occupational therapy in the promotion of health and the prevention of disease and disability statement. *American Journal of Occupational Therapy, 62*, 694–703. http://dx.doi.org/10.5014/ajot.62.6.694

American Occupational Therapy Association. (2013a). Occupational therapy in the promotion of health and Well-being. *American Journal of Occupational Therapy, 67*, S47–S59. http://dx.doi.org/10.5014.ajot.2013.67S47

American Occupational Therapy Association. (2013b). *Occupational therapy's role in health promotion.* Retrieved from www.aota.org/-/media/Corporate/Files/AboutOT/Professionals/WhatIsOT/MH/Facts/FactSheet_HealthPromotion.pdf

American Occupational Therapy Association. (2014). Occupational therapy practice framework: Domain and process (3rd ed.). *American Journal of Occupational Therapy, 68*(Suppl.1), S1–48. http://dx.doi.org/10.5014/ajot.2014.682006

Bachmann, K. (2000). *More than just hard hats and safety boots: Creating healthier work environments.* Ottawa, ON: Conference Board of Canada.

Earls, F. (2001). Community factors supporting child mental health. *Child and Adolescent Psychiatry Clinics of North America, 10*, 693–709.

Fazio, L. S. (2001). *Developing occupation-centered programs for the community: A workbook for students and professionals.* Upper Saddle River, NJ: Prentice Hall.

Green, L. W., & Kreuter, M. W. (1999). *Health promotion planning: An educational and ecological approach* (3rd ed.). Mountain View, CA: Mayfield.

Kaufman, M. (1990). *Nutrition in public health: A handbook for developing programs and services.* Gaithersburg, MD: Aspen.

Law, M., Cooper, B., Strong, S., Stewart, D., Rigby, & Letts, L. (1996). The Person–Environment–Occupation model: A transactive approach to occupational performance. *Canadian Journal of Occupational Therapy, 63*, 9–23.

Lin, S. H., Murphy, S. L., & Robinson, J. C. (2010). The issue is—Facilitating evidence-based practice: Process, strategies, and resources. *American Journal of Occupational Therapy, 64*, 164–171. http://dx.doi.org/10.5014./ajot.64.1.164

McBeth, A. J., & Schweer, K. D. (Eds.). (2000). *Building healthy communities.* Boston: Allyn & Bacon.

McKenzie, J. F., & Smeltzer, J. L. (2001). *Planning, implementing, and evaluating health promotion programs: A primer* (3rd ed.). Boston: Allyn & Bacon.

Pelletier, K. R. (2001). A review and analysis of the clinical- and cost-effectiveness studies of comprehensive health promotion and disease management programs at the worksite: 1998–2000 update. *American Journal of Health Promotion, 16*, 107–116.

Puska, P., Tuomilehto, J., Nissinen, A., & Vartiainen, E. (1995). *The North Karelia Project: 20-year results and experiences.* Helsinki, Finland: National Public Health Institute.

Raeburn, J., & Rootman, I. (1998). *People-centred health promotion.* Toronto, ON: Wiley.

U.S. Department of Health and Human Services. (1979). *Healthy People: The Surgeon General's report on health promotion and disease prevention.* Washington, DC: U.S. Government Printing Office.

U.S. Department of Health and Human Services. (1998). *Healthy People 2010 objectives: Draft for public comment.* Washington, DC: Author.

U.S. Department of Health and Human Services. (2000). *Healthy People 2010: Understanding and improving health.* Washington, DC: Author. Available from www.health.gov/healthypeople

U.S. Department of Health and Human Services. (2001). *Healthy people in healthy communities: A community planning guide using Healthy People 2010.* Rockville, MD: Author. Retrieved from www.health.gov/healthypeople/Publications/HealthyCommunities2001/default.htm

U.S. Department of Health and Human Services. (2010a). *Healthy People 2020.* Washington, DC:

Author. Retrieved from www.healthypeople.gov/2020/about/default.aspx

U.S. Department of Health and Human Services. (2010b). *Implementing Healthy People 2020, MAP–IT: A guide to using Healthy People 2020 in your community*. Washington, DC: Author. Retrieved from www.healthypeople.gov/2020/implement/MapIt.aspx

Wallerstein, N. (1992). Powerlessness, empowerment, and health: Implications for health promotion programs. *American Journal of Health Promotion, 6,* 197–205.

Wilcock, A. A. (1998). *An occupational perspective of health*. Thorofare, NJ: Slack.

World Health Organization. (1980). *International classification of impairments, disabilities, and handicaps: A manual of classification relating to the consequences of disease*. Geneva: Author.

World Health Organization. (1984). *The health burden of social inequities*. Copenhagen: WHO Regional Office for Europe.

World Health Organization. (1986). *The Ottawa Charter for Health Promotion*. Ottawa: Health and Welfare Canada and Author. Retrieved from www.who.int/healthpromotion/conferences/previous/ottawa/en/

World Health Organization. (2000). *Obesity: Preventing and managing the global epidemic* (Report of a WHO Consultation, WHO Tech. Rep. Series 894). Geneva: Author.

World Health Organization. (2001). *International classification of functioning, disability and health*. Geneva: Author.

World Health Organization. (2009). *Milestones in health promotion: Statements from global conferences*. Geneva: Author.

Appendix A.
Client Profile and
Task Analysis Form

CLIENT PROFILE

Name:	Birthdate:	Age at assessment:
Advocates:	Education:	
	Work occupation:	
Diagnoses:	Current interventions: 1. 2. 3. 4.	
Referral source:		

PERSONAL INFORMATION

Family unit	
Caregiver(s)	
Roles and responsibilities (e.g., student, spouse, parent, friend, worker)	1. 2. 3. 4.

Home environment (e.g., home design, number of people living in the home)	
Community context (e.g., rural, urban, metro; single-family home, residential care)	
School or work context (e.g., public, special, or private school; stationary or travel location for work)	
Client priorities	1. 2. 3. 4. 5. 6.
Values/beliefs/spirituality (e.g., principles, standards, beliefs, personal quest)	

SUMMARY, PLAN, AND GOALS

Assessments completed (formal and observational):	
Practitioner–client plan (e.g., further formal and observational assessments, inclusion of others):	
Tasks Requiring Assessment or Intervention	
Short-term goals (Primarily client driven, measurable, global task, or activity achievements)	**Long-term objectives** (Primarily practitioner driven, measurable, incremental, stepwise, or mini achievements)
1.	1.a. 1.b.
2.	2.a. 2.b.
3.	3.a. 3.b.
4.	4.a. 4.b.

TASKS ANALYZED

Occupation or Activity	Tasks (specific activity component)	Context or Environment (external and internal)

ANALYSIS (OF PERFORMANCE SKILLS)

Performance Skills	Client Challenges (Performance qualifier)
Rating: 0 = *no restriction*, 1 = *mild limitation*, 2 = *moderate restriction*, 3 = *severe restriction*, 4 = *complete impairment*	
Motor and praxis	**Rating**
Posture	
Mobility	
Coordination	
Strength	
Effort	
Energy	
Execution	
Process skills	**Rating**
Mental energy	
Knowledge	
Organization	
Adaptation	
Social interaction skills	**Rating**
Communication posture	
Gestures	
Initiation	
Information exchange	
Acknowledging	
Taking turns	

ANALYSIS (OF PERFORMANCE PATTERNS)

Performance Patterns	Daily Life Activities	Client Challenges (skill deficits and context restrictions)
Habits (Automatic and integrated behaviors)		
Routines (Regular activities that provide daily structure)		

Roles (Expected behaviors and responsibilities)		
Rituals (Customary cultural and social activities)		

Synopsis of performance skills and performance patterns (strengths, deficits, and challenges):

_____
_____
_____
_____
_____
_____
_____

OCCUPATIONAL PROFILE AND ANALYSIS OF NEEDS

Functional ability (i.e., how strengths and deficits affect ability to perform activities and tasks)	
Activity tolerance (e.g., physical and mental fatigue levels, energy to complete activities and tasks, temporal and environmental contexts)	
Effect on occupational performance (reflect on client roles, responsibilities, and priorities)	
Intervention needs (e.g., physical, cognitive, emotional, social)	
Resource needs (e.g., assistive devices or equipment, technology)	
Program needs (e.g., day programs, return-to-work programs, socialization)	
Outlook (practitioner projection of long-term needs and life care planning)	

GUIDELINES AND CHECKLIST FOR TASK ANALYSIS

Occupation

Activities of daily living
- ☐ Bathing and showering
- ☐ Bowel and bladder management
- ☐ Dressing
- ☐ Eating and swallowing
- ☐ Feeding
- ☐ Functional mobility
- ☐ Personal device care
- ☐ Personal hygiene and grooming
- ☐ Sexual activity
- ☐ Toileting and toilet hygiene

Instrumental activities of daily living
- ☐ Care of others
- ☐ Care of pets
- ☐ Child rearing
- ☐ Communication management
- ☐ Driving and community mobility
- ☐ Financial management
- ☐ Home establishment
- ☐ Home management and maintenance
- ☐ Meal preparation and cleanup
- ☐ Religious and spiritual observance
- ☐ Safety and emergency maintenance
- ☐ Shopping

Rest and sleep
- ☐ Rest and relaxation
- ☐ Sleep participation
- ☐ Sleep preparation

Play
- ☐ Peer interaction
- ☐ Play exploration
- ☐ Play participation

Leisure
- ☐ Customary activities or hobbies
- ☐ Leisure exploration
- ☐ Leisure participation

Social participation
- ☐ Community
- ☐ Family
- ☐ Peer or friend

Education
- ☐ Access issues
- ☐ Formal education participation
- ☐ Informal personal education or exploration
- ☐ Informal personal education participation

Work
- ☐ Employment interests and pursuits
- ☐ Employment seeking and acquisition
- ☐ Job performance
- ☐ Retirement preparation and adjustment
- ☐ Volunteer exploration
- ☐ Volunteer participation

Client Factors

Body functions and structures
Physical
- ☐ Cardiovascular and hematological systems
- ☐ Digestive, metabolic, and endocrine systems
- ☐ Genitourinary and reproductive functions
- ☐ Movement-related functions
- ☐ Respiratory and immunological systems
- ☐ Skin and related structure functions
- ☐ Voice and speech functions

Body functions and structures
Sensory and pain
- ☐ Hearing functions
- ☐ Pain grading and description
- ☐ Seeing and related functions
- ☐ Tactile functions
- ☐ Taste and smell functions
- ☐ Temperature and pressure reception
- ☐ Vestibular and proprioceptive functions

Body functions: Mental
Specific mental functions
- ☐ Attention
- ☐ Emotional

Body functions: Mental
Global mental functions
- ☐ Consciousness
- ☐ Energy and drive

☐ Experience of self and time ☐ Higher-level cognitive ☐ Motor sequencing ☐ Memory ☐ Perception ☐ Thought	☐ Orientation ☐ Sleep ☐ Temperament and personality

Values, Beliefs, and Spirituality

Values ☐ Meaningful qualities ☐ Principles ☐ Standards	**Beliefs and spirituality** ☐ Cognitive content health as true ☐ Guiding actions ☐ Life meaning and purpose

Activity and Occupational Demands

Objects and their properties ☐ Inherent properties (e.g., heavy, light) ☐ Required tools, materials, equipment	**Space demands** ☐ Size, arrangement, surface, lighting
Social demands ☐ Cultural context ☐ Social environment	**Sequence and timing** ☐ Sequence and timing ☐ Specific steps
Required actions and performance skills ☐ Cognitive ☐ Communication and interaction ☐ Emotional and social ☐ Motor and praxis ☐ Sensory–perceptual	**Required body functions and structures** ☐ Anatomical parts ☐ Level of consciousness ☐ Mobility of joints

Performance Skills

Motor skills ☐ Movement actions or behaviors ☐ Skilled purposeful movements ☐ Ability to carry out learned movement	**Process skills** ☐ Judgment ☐ Select and sequence objects or tools ☐ Organize and prioritize ☐ Create and problem solve ☐ Multitask

Social interaction skills
☐ Identify, manage, and express feelings
☐ On a one-to-one basis
☐ In groups
☐ Communication and interaction skills

Performance Patterns

Habits ☐ Automatic behavior ☐ Repeated activities ☐ Good, bad, or impoverished	**Routines** ☐ Observable patterns of behavior ☐ Time commitment ☐ Satisfying, promoting, or damaging

Roles	Rituals
☐ Set of expected behaviors ☐ Social or cultural ☐ Within context	☐ Symbolic actions ☐ Spiritual, cultural, or social ☐ Link to values and beliefs

Contexts and Environments

Cultural	Personal
☐ Customs and beliefs ☐ Activity patterns ☐ Expectations	☐ Age and gender ☐ Socioeconomic status ☐ Educational status
Temporal ☐ Location of performance in time ☐ Experience shaped by engagement	**Virtual** ☐ Communication environment
Physical ☐ Natural environment (e.g., geography) ☐ Built environment (e.g., building, furniture)	**Social and political** ☐ Relationship to individuals ☐ Relationship to organizations or systems

TASK ANALYSIS TEMPLATE

An individual form is required for each task that is examined.

Task:		
Task Demands	**Action Demands** (What is required of the person to do the task)	**Client Challenges** (Availability of required body functions and structures)
Objects used (e.g., equipment, technology)		
Space demands (e.g., physical context)		
Social demands (e.g., social environment and context)		
Sequence and timing (e.g., process to carry out the task)		
Required actions and performance skills (e.g., basic requirements)		

Appendix B.
Position Paper:
Purposeful Activity

The American Occupational Therapy Association (AOTA) submits this paper to clarify the use of the term purposeful activity, a central focus of occupational therapy throughout its history. People engage in *purposeful activity* as part of their daily life routines, in the context of occupational performance (AOTA, 1979). *Occupation* refers to active participation in self-maintenance, work, leisure, and play. *Purposeful activity* refers to goal-directed behaviors or tasks that comprise occupations. An activity is purposeful if the individual is an active, voluntary participant and if the activity is directed toward a goal that the individual considers meaningful (Evans, 1987; Gilfoyle, 1984; Mosey, 1986; Nelson, 1988). The purposefulness of an activity lies with the individual performing the activity and with the context in which it is done (Henderson et al., 1991). The meaning of an activity is unique to each person, influenced by his or her life experiences (Mosey, 1986; Pedretti, 1982), life roles, interests, age, and cultural background, as well as the situational context in which the activity occurs. Occupational therapy practitioners (i.e., registered occupational therapists and certified occupational therapy assistants) are committed to the use of purposeful activity to evaluate, facilitate, restore, or maintain individuals' abilities to function in their daily occupations.

Occupational therapists use activities to evaluate an individual's capacities to meet the functional demands of his or her environment and daily life. On the basis of an evaluation, the occupational therapy practitioner, in collaboration with the individual, designs activity experiences that offer the individual opportunities for effective action. Purposeful activities assist and build upon the individual's abilities and lead to achievement of personal functional goals.

Purposeful activity provides opportunities for persons to achieve mastery of their environment, and successful performance promotes feelings of personal competence (Fidler & Fidler, 1978). A person who is involved in purposeful activity directs attention to the goal rather than to the processes required for achievement of the goal. Engagement in purposeful activity within the context of interpersonal, cultural, physical, and other environmental conditions requires and elicits coordination among the individual's sensory motor, cognitive, and psychosocial systems. Purposeful activity may involve the independent use of complex cognitive processes, such as premeditation, reflection, planning, and use of symbolic cues. Conversely, it may involve less complex processes and take place in an environment of external structure, support, and supervision (Allen, 1987; Henderson et al., 1991). Engagement in purposeful activity provides direct and objective feedback of performance both to the occupational therapy practitioner and the individual.

The therapeutic purposes for which purposeful activity is used include mastery of a new skill, restoration of a deficient ability, compensation for functional disability, health maintenance, or prevention of dysfunction. To use purposeful activity therapeutically, an occupational therapy practitioner analyzes the activity from several perspectives. First, the activity is examined to identify its component parts to determine which skills and abilities are necessary to complete the task. Second, it is examined in terms of the context in which it will be performed. Third, the practitioner considers the person's age, occupational roles, cultural background, gender, interests, and preferences that may influence the meaningfulness of the activity for the individual. All this information is considered together to assist the occupational therapy practitioner in synthesizing (i.e., adapting, grading, and combining) activities for therapeutic purposes for a particular individual.

Purposeful activities cannot be prescribed on the basis of analysis of their inherent characteristics alone; rather, by definition, prescription of purposeful activity is individual-specific. An occupational therapy practitioner grades or adapts a chosen activity for an individual to promote successful performance or elicit a particular response. Grading activities challenges the patient's abilities by progressively changing the process, tools, materials, or environment of a given activity to gradually increase or decrease performance demands. These incremental modifications are made in response to the individual's dynamic changes and provide opportunities for gradual development of skill and related therapeutic benefits. The grading of activities is accomplished by modifying the sequence, duration, or procedures of the task; the individual's position; the position of the tools and materials; the size, shape, weight, or texture of the materials; the nature and degree of interpersonal contact; the extent of physical handling by the occupational therapy practitioner during performance; or the environment in which the activity is attempted. Supportive or assistive devices or techniques may be used to enhance the effectiveness of an activity or to facilitate performance (Henderson et al., 1991; Pedretti & Pasquinelli, 1990). Such techniques or devices are considered facilitative or preparatory to performance of purposeful activity and engagement in occupations.

If the therapy goal is to enhance a performance component so that an individual can engage in an occupational performance area, the selected activity and environmental conditions are manipulated to present graded challenges to the specific skills required. When an individual's successful completion of a task is a priority, occupational therapy practitioners adapt the task and the environment to facilitate performance. Adaptation is a process that changes an aspect of the activity or the environment to enable successful performance and accomplish a particular therapeutic goal. Adaptation of a task may require the use of assistive devices and techniques or grading strategies.

Occupational therapy education provides the necessary background for using activities as therapeutic modalities by instructing the student about behavioral and biological sciences related to the use and meaning of activity, about the nature of purposeful activity, about the process of activity analysis and synthesis, and about the application of activity to therapeutic problems within occupational therapy frames of reference.

In summary, purposeful activity occurs within the context of work, self-care, play, and leisure activities and is used therapeutically to evaluate, facilitate, restore, or maintain individuals' abilities to function competently within their daily occupations. The occupational therapy practitioner's commitment to those whom he or she serves is to guide them in the use of purposeful activities so as to empower them to enhance the quality of their being in the daily reality where they live as parents, children, students, homemakers, workers, or retirees (Reilly, 1966).

REFERENCES

Allen, C. K. (1987). 1987 Eleanor Clarke Slagle Lecture—Activity: Occupational therapy's treatment method. *American Journal of Occupational Therapy, 41*, 563–575.

American Occupational Therapy Association. (1979). Resolution C, 531–79: The philosophical base of occupational therapy. *American Journal of Occupational Therapy, 33*, 785.

Evans, K. A. (1987). Nationally Speaking—Definition of occupation as the core concept of occupational therapy. *American Journal of Occupational Therapy, 41,* 627–628.

Fidler, G. S., & Fidler, J. W. (1978). Doing and becoming: Purposeful action and self-actualization. *American Journal of Occupational Therapy, 32,* 305–310.

Gilfoyle, E. M. (1984). Eleanor Clarke Slagle Lectureship 1984—Transformation of a profession. *American Journal of Occupational Therapy, 38, 575–584.*

Henderson, A., Cermak, S., Coster, W., Murray, E., Trombly, C., & Tickle-Degnen, L. (1991). The Issue Is—Occupational science is multidimensional. *American Journal of Occupational Therapy, 45,* 370–372.

Mosey, A. C. (1986). *Psychosocial components of occupational therapy.* New York: Raven.

Nelson, D. L. (1988). Occupation: Form and performance. *American Journal of Occupational Therapy, 42,* 633–641.

Pedretti, L. W. (1982, May). *The compatibility of current treatment methods in physical disabilities with the philosophical base of occupational therapy.* Paper presented at the 62nd Annual Conference of the American Occupational Therapy Association, Philadelphia.

Pedretti, L. W., & Pasquinelli, S. (1990). A frame of reference for occupational therapy in physical dysfunction. In L. W. Pedretti & B. Zoltan (Eds.), *Occupational therapy practice skills for physical dysfunction* (pp. 1–17). St. Louis: Mosby.

Reilly, M. (1966). The challenge of the future to an occupational therapist. *American Journal of Occupational Therapy, 20,* 221–225.

Prepared by Jim Hinojosa, PhD, OTR, FAOTA; Joyce Sabari, PhD, OTR; and Lorraine Pedretti, MS, OTR, with contributions from Mark S. Rosenfeld, PhD, OTR, and Catherine Trombly, ScD, OTR/L, FAOTA, for The Commission on Practice (Jim Hinojosa, PhD, OTR, FAOTA, Chairperson).

Approved by the Representative Assembly April 1983. Revised and approved by the Representative Assembly June 1993.

Originally published in *American Journal of Occupational Therapy, 47,* 1081–1082. http://dx.doi.org/10.5014/ajot.47.12.1081

Appendix C.
Occupational Therapy's Role in Sleep

Sleep is essential for well-being and critical for maintaining homeostasis and participating in activities of daily living. Occupational therapists have long acknowledged the influence of sleep on occupational performance. The *Occupational Therapy Practice Framework: Domain & Process* (2nd ed.; American Occupational Therapy Association, 2008) includes rest and sleep as an area of occupation addressed by occupational therapy.

Sleep insufficiency, defined as not obtaining restorative sleep, is a public health crisis in the United States (Centers for Disease Control & Prevention, 2008) with resulting negative economic consequences due to lower productivity, increased absenteeism, decreased job performance, increased health care utilization, and potential injury. There are more than 80 defined sleep disorders, each of which results in distress or daytime difficulties in daily life tasks, or home, employment, or community life—problems that occupational therapy practitioners uniquely address. Referral to a physician for further evaluation or medical intervention is indicated for clients reporting unresolved, chronic, or potentially serious sleep problems. Persistent sleep disturbances that disrupt the daily functioning of other members of the household (e.g., sundowning in adults with Alzheimer's disease) should also be referred to the medical team. Occupational therapists work with individuals following diagnosis to create behavioral or environmental changes that facilitate daytime performance and participation.

ROLE OF OCCUPATIONAL THERAPY

Occupational therapists use knowledge of sleep physiology, sleep disorders, and evidence-based sleep promotion practices to evaluate and address the functional ramifications of sleep insufficiency or sleep disorders on occupational performance and participation. Sleep problems are framed from the perspective of health maintenance and health promotion and are addressed with all clients.

Therapists working with families of children with an autism spectrum disorder or another developmental disorder explore the impact of sleep deprivation on the family unit and the child's and caregivers' ability to function effectively during the day. They aid families to systematically trial changes in bedtime routines, habits, and patterns. Cognitive or behavioral therapy interventions, or sensory integration strategies to address sensory avoiding or sensory seeking behaviors (e.g., a picture poster for bedtime routines, stickers or consistent praise for sleeping through the night, loose or tight pajamas, lightweight or weighted blankets) are addressed. Managing the physical environment and enhancing observation skills help parents anticipate reactions to changes in clothing, toys, or family schedules. Calming activities and routines that do not burden the family and can be consistently carried out may facilitate sleep.

Therapists working in long-term-care settings for older adults develop individual sleep routines, adjust lighting in residential settings to clearly demarcate day and night, reduce staff noise, train staff to use recommended equipment for bed positioning, maintain turning schedules for individuals who are immobile, and advocate for clients' needs for privacy. Daytime activity programs, including exercise, foster socialization and facilitate arousal, engagement, and decreased involuntary daytime napping, thus improving sleep latency and maintenance. Occupational therapy practitioners address nocturnal toileting safety, bedding management, and clothing preferences for sleep. Environmental elements, such as sufficient blankets for warmth, sound machines to add white noise, and blackout curtains or eye masks may enhance quality of sleep.

Therapists working in wellness and prevention practices can facilitate sleep health by increasing physical activity in clients and well populations across the lifespan, and addressing smoking cessation, substance use, and obesity management, which have been linked to sleep disturbances (Strine & Chapman, 2005).

ASSESSMENT

Occupational therapists evaluate clients in areas that contribute to sleep dysfunction, including difficulties in sleep preparation and sleep participation; sleep latency (how long it takes to fall asleep, typically less than 30 minutes for someone without a sleep disorder), sleep duration (the number of hours of sleep, which varies by age), sleep maintenance (the ability to stay asleep), or daytime sleepiness; the impact of work, school, and life events, such as shift work or caregiving responsibilities; the influence of pain and fatigue; disturbances in balance, vision, strength, skin integrity, and sensory systems; psycho-emotional status, including depression, anxiety, and stress; the impact of caffeine, nicotine, drugs or alcohol, smoking, or medication (e.g., prescriptions or over-the-counter sleep aids); and the impact of the environment (e.g., those in acute care hospitals and long-term-care facilities report higher rates of sleep disturbance).

INTERVENTION

Occupational therapy interventions focus on promoting optimal sleep performance. These interventions include

- Educating clients and caregivers on sleep terminology, misconceptions, and expectations
- Preventing secondary conditions that may precipitate diminished sleep quality (e.g., decreased range of motion, depression, or anxiety)
- Encouraging smoking cessation, reduced caffeine intake, a balanced diet, adequate exercise, etc.
- Establishing predictable routines, including regular times for waking and sleeping
- Managing pain and fatigue
- Addressing activities of daily living, particularly for bed mobility and toileting
- Establishing individualized sleep hygiene routines (e.g., habits and patterns to facilitate restorative sleep)
- Teaching cognitive–behavioral and cognitive restructuring techniques, such as leaving the bedroom if awake and returning only when sleepy, or exploring self-talk statements regarding sleep patterns
- Increasing coping skills, stress management, and time management
- Addressing sensory processing disorders and teaching self-management or caregiver management
- Modifying the environment, including noise, light, temperature, bedding, and technology use while in bed
- Introducing complementary mind–body techniques, including progressive muscle relaxation, guided imagery, autogenic training, tai chi, yoga, meditation, and biofeedback
- Advocating on a state or national level for laws that protect workers from excessive work schedules that threaten their health or public safety.

CONCLUSION

Restful and adequate sleep provides the foundation for optimal occupational performance, participation, and engagement in daily life, a concept that is historically consistent with the development of occupational therapy. Attention to the impact of sleep is incorporated into the repertoire of occupational therapists and addressed across the lifespan. Prevention and intervention strategies to address individual, family, and population-based sleep needs lie within the scope of practice for occupational therapy and represent another way in which the profession approaches clients from a holistic perspective to help them live life to its fullest.

REFERENCES

American Occupational Therapy Association. (2008). Occupational therapy practice framework: Domain and process (2nd ed.). *American Journal of Occupational Therapy, 62,* 625–683. doi: 10.5014/ajot.62.6.625

Centers for Disease Control and Prevention. (2008). Perceived insufficient rest or sleep—Four states, 2006. *Mortality and Morbidity Weekly Report, 57,* 200–203. Retrieved February 8, 2012, from http://www.cdc.gov/mmwr/PDF/wk/mm5708.pdf

Strine, T. W., & Chapman, D. P. (2005). Associations of frequent sleep insufficiency with health-related quality of life and health behaviors. *Sleep Medicine, 6,* 23–27. doi: 10.1016/j.sleep.2004.06.003

Note. Developed by Meryl Marger Picard, MSW, OTR, for the American Occupational Therapy Association.

Appendix D.
Occupational Therapy in the Promotion of Health and Well-Being

The purpose of this statement is to describe occupational therapy's contribution in the areas of health promotion and prevention. It is intended for internal and external audiences. The American Occupational Therapy Association (AOTA) supports and promotes involvement of occupational therapists and occupational therapy assistants in the development and provision of programs and services that promote health, well-being, and social participation of all people.

HEALTH PROMOTION

It is important to frame the discussion of occupational therapy's role in health promotion by first defining the term. The World Health Organization (WHO) provides the following definition in the *Ottawa Charter for Health Promotion:*

> *Health promotion* is the process of enabling people to increase control over, and to improve, their health. To reach a state of complete physical, mental, and social well-being, an individual or group must be able to identify and realize aspirations, to satisfy needs, and to change or cope with the environment. Health is, therefore, seen as a resource for everyday life, not the objective of living. Health is a positive concept emphasizing social and personal resources,

as well as physical capacities. Therefore, health promotion is not just the responsibility of the health sector, but goes beyond healthy lifestyles to well-being. (WHO, 1986, para. 2, italics added)

Trentham and Cockburn (2005) expand on this definition by stating that

> *health promotion* is equally and essentially concerned with creating the conditions necessary for health at individual, structural, social, and environmental levels through an understanding of the determinants of health: peace, shelter, education, food, income, a stable ecosystem, sustainable resources, *social justice,*[1] and equity. (p. 441, italics added)

Since 1980, the U.S. Department of Health and Human Services (HHS) has established health promotion and disease prevention objectives to facilitate and measure improvement in health (HHS, 1980, 1990, 2000, 2010). The vision of Healthy People 2020 is the realization of "a society in which all people live long, healthy lives" (HHS, 2010, p. 2). Healthy People 2020 has four major goals:

---

[1]Some italicized terms in this statement are defined in the glossary.

1. "Attain high-quality, longer lives free of preventable disease, disability, injury, and premature death."
2. "Achieve health equity, eliminate disparities, and improve health of all groups."
3. "Create social and physical environments that promote good health for all."
4. "Promote quality of life, healthy development, and healthy behaviors across all life stages." (p. 5)

Active engagement in life and overall health status and not just longevity is emphasized. From an individual perspective, a healthy life means the use of capacities and adaptations across the life span, allowing people to enter into satisfying relationships with others, to work, and to play. From a national perspective, a healthy life means vital, creative, and productive citizens and residents contributing to flourishing communities and a thriving nation.

HEALTH DISPARITIES

It is important from a health promotion perspective to differentiate between the constructs of health and functional status. Many assessments of health status include items that measure function. As a result, these tools are negatively biased against persons with disabilities. It is possible to be physically and mentally healthy and have a high quality of life in spite of disability and functional limitations (Krahn, Fujiura, Drum, Cardinal, & Nosek, 2009). As noted earlier, one goal of Healthy People 2020 is to eliminate health disparities (HHS, 2010).

The term *health disparities* refers to population-specific differences in disease rates, health outcomes, and access to health care services. Addressing health disparities is consistent with the occupational therapy profession's official document on nondiscrimination and inclusion, which states, "Inclusion requires that we ensure not only that everyone is treated fairly and equitably but also that all individuals have the same opportunities to participate in the naturally occurring activities of society" (AOTA, 2009b, p. 819).

Persons with disabilities may be the largest population experiencing health disparities. "The differences in health status between people with disabilities and without disabilities are increasingly recognized as preventable and therefore unacceptable" (Krahn, Putnam, Drum, & Powers, 2006, p. 18). Persons with disabilities are at risk for developing secondary conditions that are physical and mental as well as social health problems that are the direct or indirect consequence of the disability. The five most frequent secondary conditions identified in a study by Kinne, Patrick, and Doyle (2004) are (1) chronic muscle and joint pain, (2) sleep disturbances, (3) extreme fatigue, (4) weight or eating problems, and (5) depression.

The prevalence of these conditions was 2 to 3 times higher among adults with disabilities than among adults without disabilities. In addition, persons with disabilities often have higher rates of diabetes, obesity, anxiety, social isolation, and unemployment (Drum, Krahn, Culley, & Hammond, 2005) and less satisfaction with care within the health system (Krahn et al., 2006) than their able-bodied counterparts. Secondary conditions, many of which are preventable, are often considered the primary cause of health disparities for this population.

Health promotion programs and services may target individuals, communities, and populations as well as policymakers. The focus of these programs is to

- Prevent or reduce the incidence of illness or disease, accidents, and injuries in the population;
- Reduce health disparities among racial and ethnic minorities and other underserved populations;
- Enhance mental health, resiliency, and quality of life;
- Prevent secondary conditions and improve the overall health and well-being of people with chronic conditions or disabilities and their caregivers; and
- Promote healthy living practices, social participation, *occupational justice,* and healthy communities, with respect for cross-cultural issues and concerns.

PREVENTION STRATEGIES

A key purpose of health promotion is improved well-being, quality of life, and social participation for individuals and populations. Health management and maintenance for persons with or without disabilities requires the implementation of prevention strategies. Prevention is generally categorized into three levels: (1) primary, (2) secondary, and (3) tertiary.

Primary prevention is defined as education or health promotion efforts designed to prevent the onset and reduce the incidence of unhealthy conditions, diseases, or injuries. Primary prevention attempts to identify, reduce, or eliminate risk factors for disease and injury. For persons with disabilities, primary prevention may include modifying the physical and social environment to address the special needs resulting from the disability. Strategies for improving nutrition; increasing physical activities; smoking cessation; weight management; and screening for heart disease, diabetes, and cancer are important for persons with disabilities as well as the general population.

Secondary prevention typically includes screening, early detection, and intervention after disease has occurred; it is designed to prevent or disrupt the disabling process. For persons with disabilities, secondary prevention involves limiting the development of secondary conditions and their subsequent impact on function and quality of life.

Tertiary prevention refers to services designed to prevent the progression of a condition. Tertiary prevention for persons with disabilities should also include strategies to promote equal opportunity, full participation, independent living, and economic self-sufficiency (Patrick, Richardson, Starks, Rose, & Kinne, 1997).

POPULATION HEALTH APPROACH

Population health focuses on *aggregates*, or communities of people, and the many factors that influence their health. A population health approach strives to identify and reduce health disparities as well as enhance the overall health and well-being of a population (Finlayson & Edwards, 1997). In addition to providing occupational therapy interventions for individuals, occupational therapy practitioners[2] can develop

and implement occupation-based population health approaches to enhance occupational performance and participation, quality of life, and occupational justice.

HEALTH PROMOTION AND OCCUPATION

Healthy People 2020 and the Ottawa Chapter of Health Promotion parallel occupational therapy's belief that engagement in meaningful occupations supports health and leads to a productive and satisfying life. Wilcock (2006) stated that

> Following an occupation-focused health promotion approach to well-being embraces a belief that the potential range of what people can do, be, and strive to become is the primary concern and that health is a by-product. A varied and full occupational lifestyle will coincidentally maintain and improve health and well-being if it enables people to be creative and adventurous physically, mentally, and socially. (p. 315)

According to Christiansen (1999), "Health enables people to pursue the tasks of everyday living that provide them with the life meaning necessary for their well-being" (p. 547). *Well-being* is a state of flourishing that consists of the following elements: positive emotion, engagement or flow, *meaning* (i.e., a sense of belonging to or serving something larger than oneself), positive relationships, and accomplishment or achievement (Seligman, 2011).

Occupational therapy services are provided to clients of all age groups, infants through older adults, from a variety of socioeconomic, cultural, and ethnic backgrounds, who possess or who are at risk for impairments, activity limitations, or participation restrictions. According to AOTA (2008), occupational therapy practitioners recognize that health is supported when individuals are able to engage in occupations and activities that allow them to achieve the desired outcome of participation in their chosen environments. The essence of occupational therapy is "supporting health and participation in life through engagement in occupation" (p. 626). This focus on

---

[2]When the term *occupational therapy practitioner* is used in this document, it refers to both occupational therapists and occupational therapy assistants (AOTA, 2006).

engagement in occupation is interwoven through the delivery of service, beginning with evaluation and continuing through the intervention phase. Health management and maintenance are included within the domain of occupational therapy as an instrumental activity of daily living; health promotion and prevention are identified as occupational therapy intervention approaches; and health and wellness, quality of life, and occupational justice are potential outcomes of occupational therapy services (AOTA, 2008).

Occupations are purposeful and meaningful daily activities that fill a person's time and are typically categorized as self-care, work, play or leisure, and rest (AOTA, 1995; Meyer, 1922). A natural, balanced pattern of occupations is believed to be health enhancing and fulfills both the needs of the individual and the demands of the environment (Kielhofner, 2004; Meyer, 1922). This belief has been supported in studies with well elderly individuals in urban communities (Clark et al., 1997, 2001, 2012).

By engaging clients in everyday occupations, occupational therapy practitioners promote physical and mental health and facilitate well-being for persons with and without disabilities. Occupational therapy practitioners promote positive mental health through competency enhancement strategies, such as skill development, environmental supports, and task adaptations, and they prevent mental illness through risk reduction strategies, such as establishing healthy habits and routines and providing training in relaxation and coping techniques (AOTA, 2010).

Occupational imbalance, deprivation, and *alienation* are risk factors for health problems in and of themselves. They may also result from or lead to the development of other risk factors, which can in turn result in larger health and social problems. Causes are varied (e.g., unanticipated caregiving responsibilities, losses in employment or housing) and can lead to occupational imbalance, deprivation, and alienation, which can then lead to individual health problems such as stress, sleep disturbance, and depression (Wilcock, 2006).

Belle et al. (2006) demonstrated that caregivers of people with dementia experienced significant improvement in quality of life and a decrease in depression after intervention that included stress management; strategies for engaging in pleasant events; and teaching of healthy behaviors, communication skills, and problem-solving skills regarding behavior management of care recipients' difficult behaviors. Elliott, Burgio, and DeCoster (2010) similarly found that a caregiver intervention enhances health and decreases depression, resulting in a decrease in perceived burden. Occupational therapy practitioners are in a prime position to recognize the occupation and health problems inherent with caregiving and offer interventions such as those described in the cited research as well as additional interventions from an occupation lens, such as task analysis and modification to minimize the physical and emotional stresses of caregiving.

ROLE OF OCCUPATIONAL THERAPY IN HEALTH PROMOTION

Occupational therapy practitioners have three critical roles in health promotion and prevention:

1. To promote healthy lifestyles;
2. To emphasize occupation as an essential element of health promotion strategies; and
3. To provide interventions, not only with individuals but also with populations.

It is important that occupational therapy practitioners promote a healthy lifestyle for all individuals and their families, including people with physical, mental, or cognitive impairments. An occupation-focused approach to prevention of illness and disability has been defined by Wilcock (2006) as

> the application of medical, behavioral, social, and *occupational science* to prevent physiological, psychological, social, and occupational illness; accidents; and disability; and to prolong quality of life for all people through advocacy and mediation and through occupation-focused programs aimed at enabling people to do, be, and become according to their natural health needs. (p. 282, italics added)

The roles of occupational therapy practitioners in evaluation and intervention in health promotion practice are based on the *Guidelines for*

Supervision, Roles, and Responsibilities During the Delivery of Occupational Therapy Services (AOTA, 2009a). Occupational therapy practitioners possess the basic knowledge and skills to carry out health promotion interventions to prevent injury and maximize well-being. However, this area of practice is very broad, and practitioners need to continually expand their knowledge in health promotion to be effective and competent members of the team.

While recognizing the unique role of occupational therapy in health promotion and prevention, it is also important to acknowledge and respect the contributions of other health care professions in this arena. Occupational therapy practitioners should operate within their scope of practice and training and partner with other health promotion disciplines with specialized expertise such as in the areas of public health, health education, nutrition, and exercise science.

As in all other areas of practice, health promotion services should be based on the best available evidence. Law, Steinwender, and LeClair (1998) conducted an extensive review of the literature on the relationship between occupation and health. The longitudinal studies that were reviewed found that activity participation had a significant effect on perceived health. Maintenance of everyday activities, social interactions, and community mobility influenced self-reported quality of life.

A long-term benefit attributable to preventive occupational therapy was shown by Clark et al. (2001) when they reevaluated participants from the Well Elderly Study and found that 90% of therapeutic gain observed after intervention was retained at the 6-month follow-up. The Well Elderly Study was replicated through the Well Elderly Trial 2 with participants from a wider array of economic and ethnic backgrounds. Occupational therapy health promotion was once again found to be a cost-effective method to enhance health and well-being among older adults in an urban context (Clark et al., 2012).

Interventions With Individuals

The following are examples of occupation-based primary prevention intervention that target individuals:

- Musculoskeletal injury prevention and management programs;
- Anger management and conflict resolution training for parents, teachers, and school-aged youth to reduce the incidence of bullying and other violence;
- Parenting skills training to enhance family health and decrease potential for abuse;
- Fall prevention programs for community-dwelling seniors; and
- Ensuring health literacy for non-English-speaking populations.

Examples of secondary prevention carried out by occupational therapy practitioners may include

- Education and training regarding eating habits, activity levels, and prevention of secondary disability subsequent to obesity;
- Education and training on stress management and adaptive coping strategies to enhance resilience for persons with mood disorders and posttraumatic stress disorder; and
- Osteoporosis prevention and management classes for individuals recently diagnosed with or at high risk for this condition.

Examples of occupation-based tertiary prevention intervention may include

- Transitional or independent-living skills training for people who have mental illness and those with cognitive impairments;
- Leisure participation groups for older adults with dementia to prevent depression, enhance socialization, and improve quality of life;
- Social participation activities at a drop-in center for adults with severe mental illness; and
- Stroke support groups for survivors and caregivers.

Occupational therapy practitioners have an opportunity to complement existing health promotion efforts by adding the contribution of occupation to programs developed by experts in health education, nutrition, exercise, and so forth. For example, when working with a person with a lower extremity amputation due to diabetes, the occupational therapy practitioner may focus on the occupation of meal preparation using foods and preparation methods recommended in the nutritionist's health promotion program. This focus enables achievement of the occupational therapy goal of functional independence in the kitchen and reinforces the importance of proper nutrition for the prevention of further disability (Scaffa, 2001).

Interventions With Populations

To be effective, health promotion efforts cannot focus only on intervention at the individual level. Because of the inextricable and reciprocal links between people and their environments, larger groups, organizations, communities, and populations may also benefit from occupational therapy intervention (AOTA, 2008; Law, 1991; Wilcock, 2006).

Examples of interventions through the intermediary of organizations include

- Consultation to businesses to promote well-being of workers through identification of problems and solutions for balance among work, leisure, and family life;
- Consultation to schools regarding implementation of Americans With Disabilities Act of 1990 (ADA; Pub. L. 101-336) requirements;
- Education for day care staff regarding normal growth and development, handling behavior problems, and identifying children at risk for developmental delays; and
- Promotion of ergonomically correct workstations in schools and offices.

Community or population-level interventions may include

- Consulting with the local transportation authority regarding accessible public transportation;
- Consulting with contractors, architects, and city planners regarding accessibility and universal design;
- Implementing a community-wide screening program for depression at nursing homes, assisted living facilities, and senior centers for the purpose of developing group and individual prevention and intervention programs;
- Conducting needs assessments and implementing intervention strategies to reduce health disparities in communities with high rates of disease or injury, such as lifestyle management programs addressing hypertension, diabetes, and obesity;
- Addressing the health and occupation needs of the homeless population by eliminating barriers and enhancing opportunities for occupational engagement; and
- Training volunteers to function effectively in special needs shelters during disasters.

Governmental or policy-level interventions may include

- Promoting policies that offer affordable, accessible health care to everyone, including people with disabilities;
- Promoting barrier-free environments for all ages, including aging in place and universal design;
- Supporting full inclusion of children with disabilities in schools and day care programs;
- Lobbying for public funds to support research and program development in areas related to improvement in quality of life for people at risk and those with disabilities; and
- Promoting policies that establish opportunities for rehabilitation in the community for people discharged from inpatient psychiatric programs.

OPPORTUNITIES FOR OCCUPATIONAL THERAPY IN HEALTH PROMOTION

Funding for health promotion programs can come from governmental agencies, foundations, nonprofit organizations, insurance companies, and large corporations, among others. In addition, fee for service is an option. Typically, health promotion and prevention programs do not rely on a single source of funding (Brownson, 1998; Scaffa, 2001).

Changes in health care brought about by the 2010 Patient Protection and Affordable Care Act (ACA; Pub. L. 111-148) have already and will continue to have an impact on health promotion, prevention, and public health service provision. Although the ACA is designed to improve individual health by increasing access to health insurance and health care, several provisions relate directly to health promotion. Specifically, Title IV calls for

- Increasing funding for prevention and public health programs;
- Providing education and outreach related to health promotion and disease prevention;
- Reviewing evidence related to preventive services and the development of recommendations;
- Providing Medicare coverage of annual well care visits and the development of personalized prevention plans;
- Improving access to preventive services for eligible adults in Medicaid;
- Eliminating patient copays for prevention services;
- Dispersing incentives for prevention of chronic diseases in Medicaid;
- Evaluating outcomes of community-based prevention and wellness programs for Medicare beneficiaries;
- Removing barriers and improving access to health promotion services for individuals with disabilities;
- Providing grants for employer-based wellness programs; and
- Funding for childhood obesity demonstration project (Kaiser Family Foundation, 2011; Network for Public Health Law, 2011).

Occupational therapy practitioners can seize opportunities to participate in the provision of health promotion and prevention services under the ACA by becoming a member of the primary care team and the patient's medical home. Failure to integrate occupational therapy into these arenas could severely limit the profession's future growth.

CASE STUDIES

The following case studies provide examples of the role of occupational therapy in health promotion and prevention of disease and injuries.

Primary Prevention—Working With a Family

A retired couple consult an occupational therapist about a home safety assessment for the purpose of remaining in their home as they age.

Assessment

The occupational therapist develops an occupational profile (AOTA, 2008) using a semistructured interview format. She gathers information about the couple's goals, occupational history, health, occupational performance, and satisfaction level within the various performance areas, as well as social connectedness and overall life satisfaction.

Both spouses are healthy and able to perform daily tasks with a high level of satisfaction. They have a strong social support network and report being very satisfied with their lives. The occupational therapist also explores the health history of their parents and learns of a history of Alzheimer's disease and diabetes. She assesses the environment (i.e., home, yard, neighborhood) for accessibility and safety using the Safety Assessment of Function and the Environment for Rehabilitation (SAFER) tool (Oliver, Blathwayt, Brackley, & Tamaki, 1993).

The occupational therapist notes that the living area is on three levels (several steps have no railings); rooms and hallways are generally poorly lit; and the rooms have too much furniture, leaving narrow or obstructed passageways. The yard has uneven and poorly defined walkways. The couple lives in a residential neighborhood with a distance of 3 miles to shopping. No public transportation is available, even for people with mobility impairments.

Intervention

For immediate consideration, the occupational therapist recommends that the couple install railings near all stairs, increase the level of lighting, and decrease the amount of furniture. She works with them to find the best configuration of furniture placement to maximize safety when walking in a room. She recommends that they consider changing the landscape to include clearly defined and level walkways that will also accommodate wheeled mobility, should that ever be needed.

A second set of recommendations includes how to retrofit the house if mobility impairments preclude climbing stairs in the future. The therapist describes optimal placement of an elevator from the first to the second floor. There is not an easy placement of an elevator from the basement to the first floor, so the therapist describes how the occupations now performed in the basement (e.g., exercise, laundry, computer use) may be transferred to the other two floors. The therapist works with the couple on problem solving around transportation, should driving become difficult.

Primary Prevention—Working With a Business

A commercial bakery contacts an occupational therapist to assess the various workstations in the bakery and make recommendations for improvements. Management goals include increasing productivity and decreasing sick days and worker compensation claims.

Assessment

The occupational therapist observes the work performed at the various workstations and interviews the workers. He notes body mechanics, repetitive motions, machine design, layout of workstations with travel distances, weights lifted and number of lifts per time unit, work speed and load, noise, temperature, air quality, clothing comfort, and length and frequency of rest breaks. He also notes worker-to-worker interaction and interaction among workers, supervisors,

and management. In general, the supervisors and management seem approachable and open to suggestions from the workers.

The occupational therapist identifies a high frequency of lifting and repetitive motion done by the workers. Workstations require a significant amount of static standing, which can contribute to many musculoskeletal problems. Travel distances are long, work speed is rapid, noise level is high in certain parts of the factory, and the temperature is uncomfortably warm.

Intervention

The occupational therapist recommends ergonomically designed workstations that can decrease the amount of static work, time standing, travel, or lifting and that can improve working positions. Because some jobs involve repetitive motions that may not be avoided, the therapist instructs the managers in the benefits of rest breaks and instructs the workers in stretching exercises. Each worker is also instructed in proper body mechanics at his or her workstation. The therapist works with the management to design a daily schedule that allows for an even workflow to decrease times of high stress. The therapist is asked to return every 6 months to reassess and instruct new employees.

Primary Prevention—Working With a School

An elementary school is planning a new playground, which must be accessible to every child in the school. An occupational therapist is consulted for input on design features that will make the playground aesthetically pleasing, fun, and challenging to use for children of all abilities.

Assessment

The occupational therapist surveys the area where the school is planning to locate the playground. He uses the guidelines for play areas developed by the U.S. Access Board (2007) to ensure minimum requirements are met. He then researches commercially available playground equipment to find equipment that will be fun and challenging to use for all populations in the school as well as encourage interaction among the children.

Intervention

The occupational therapist provides the school with a report detailing his recommendations for important features in the playground equipment and the layout of the playground. He is careful to identify all safety issues and suggests ways to make the playground as safe as possible. The report also includes recommendations for landscaping so that children using wheeled mobility can easily navigate around the playground. The therapist remains on the design team for consultation until the playground is completed.

Secondary Prevention—Working With a Local Governmental Agency

An occupational therapist working in home health has noticed that her elderly clients who no longer drive because of a variety of functional limitations have no other means of transportation to go grocery shopping, run errands, and visit friends. The therapist reviews the literature for evidence and locates the special issue of the *American Journal of Occupational Therapy* that includes several systematic reviews on the relationship between occupation and productive aging (Leland & Elliott, 2012), and she commits to taking action.

Assessment

To determine the need for alternative means of transportation, the occupational therapist conducts a needs assessment, gathering existing data from several sources, including state and local census data and information from community organizations that provide services to older adults.

Intervention

The occupational therapist contacts the county office on aging to discuss her findings and concerns. She conducts a brief presentation, including data she collected about the local community and evidence from the systematic reviews. A joint task force is formed with local senior centers to further study the transportation experience of elderly county residents and make recommendations. Cognizant of the need to balance the fiscal resources of the county with the needs of aging county residents, the task force develops a proposal for extending one bus route and including three additional stops on two other bus routes during the weekday non–rush hour time period. The proposal emphasizes the importance of transportation and social participation to the health and well-being of elders.

Tertiary Prevention—Working With a Group

A rehabilitation unit in a hospital decides to offer health promotion classes to former patients with chronic conditions. An occupational therapy assistant is chosen to lead a class for patients with chronic obstructive pulmonary disease.

Assessment

The occupational therapy assistant researches information on the disease, existing programs, and their content and outcomes. He researches optimal group size, length of each session, session frequency, and number of sessions.

Intervention

Using the assessment information, the supervising occupational therapist works with the occupational therapy assistant and a respiratory therapist to develop the health promotion class, including number of participants, length of session, and topics offered. It is decided that a maximum of 15 participants will meet monthly for 1 1/2 hours for a total of 12 sessions. Topics include self-management, assertive communication, information-seeking, and problem-solving skills. The group will also function as a support group. The occupational therapist collects data to determine the effectiveness of the program in preventing secondary conditions associated with chronic obstructive pulmonary disease and promoting independent living and quality of life.

SUMMARY

Through this statement, the AOTA described the role of occupational therapy in the promotion of health and well-being among individuals, families, communities, and populations. Three levels of prevention services were defined, and potential contributions by occupational therapy practitioners were detailed at each level.

The examples provided are just a few of the extensive, rich, and varied occupation-based approaches that can facilitate the achievement of the national goals outlined in Healthy People 2020. These approaches include, but are not limited to, the creation of health-promoting social and physical environments, improved quality of life, healthy development, and health equity for all.

REFERENCES

American Occupational Therapy Association. (1995). Occupation: A position paper. *American Journal of Occupational Therapy, 49,* 1015–1018. http://dx.doi.org/10.5014/ajot.49.10.1015

American Occupational Therapy Association. (2006). Association policies: Policy 1.44: Categories of occupational therapy personnel. *American Journal of Occupational Therapy, 60,* 683–684. http://dx.doi.org/10.5014/ajot.60.6.681

American Occupational Therapy Association. (2008). Occupational therapy practice framework: Domain and process (2nd ed.). *American Journal of Occupational Therapy, 62,* 625–683. http://dx.doi.org/10.5014/ajot.62.6.625

American Occupational Therapy Association. (2009a). Guidelines for supervision, roles, and responsibilities during the delivery of occupational therapy services. *American Journal of Occupational Therapy, 63,* 797–803. http://dx.doi.org/10.5014/ajot.63.6.797

American Occupational Therapy Association. (2009b). Occupational therapy's commitment to non-discrimination and inclusion. *American Journal of Occupational Therapy, 63,* 819–820. http://dx.doi.org/10.5014/ajot.63.6.819

American Occupational Therapy Association. (2010). Specialized knowledge and skills in mental health promotion, prevention, and intervention in occupational therapy practice. *American Journal of Occupational Therapy, 64*(Suppl.), S30–S43. http://dx.doi.org/10.5014/ajot.2010.64S30

Americans With Disabilities Act of 1990, Pub. L. 101–336, 42 U.S.C. § 12101.

Belle, S. H., Burgio, L., Burns, R., Coon, D., Czaja, S. J., Gallagher-Thompson, D., ... Zhang, S. (2006). Enhancing the quality of life of dementia caregivers from different ethnic or racial groups. *Annals of Internal Medicine, 145,* 727–738. http://dx.doi.org/10.7326/0003-4819-145-10-200611210-00005

Brownson, C. A. (1998). Funding community practice: Stage 1. *American Journal of Occupational Therapy, 52,* 60–64. http://dx.doi.org/10.5014/ajot.52.1.60

Christiansen, C. H. (1999). Defining lives: Occupation as identity: An essay on competence, coherence, and the creation of meaning. *American Journal of Occupational Therapy, 53,* 547–558. http://dx.doi.org/10.5014/ajot.53.6.547

Clark, F., Azen, S. P., Carlson, M., Mandel, D., LaBree, L., Hay, J., ... Lipson, L. (2001). Embedding health-promoting changes into the daily lives of independent-living older adults: Long-term follow-up of occupational therapy intervention. *Journals of Gerontology, Series B: Psychological Sciences and Social Sciences, 56,* 60–63. http://dx.doi.org/10.1093/geronb/56.1.P60

Clark, F., Azen, S. P., Zemke, R., Jackson, J., Carlson, M., Mandel, D., ... Lipson, L. (1997). Occupational therapy for independent-living older adults: A randomized controlled trial. *JAMA, 278,* 1321–1326.

Clark, F., Jackson, J., Carlson, M., Chou, C, Cherry, B. J., Jordan-Marsh, M., ... Azen, S. P. (2012). Effectiveness of a lifestyle intervention in promoting the well-being of independently living older people: Results of the Well Elderly 2 randomised controlled trial. *Journal of Epidemiology and Community Health, 66,* 782–790. http://dx.doi.org/10.1136/jech.2009.099754

Drum, C. E., Krahn, G., Culley, C., & Hammond, L. (2005). Recognizing and responding to the health disparities of people with disabilities. *Californian Journal of Health Promotion, 3,* 29–42.

Elliott, A. F., Burgio, L. D., & DeCoster, J. (2010). Enhancing caregiver health: Findings from the Resources for Enhancing Alzheimer's Caregiver Health II Intervention. *Journal of the American Geriatrics Society, 58,* 30–37. http://dx.doi.org/10.1111/j.1532-5415.2009.02631.x

Finlayson, M., & Edwards, J. (1997). Evolving health environments and occupational therapy: Definitions, descriptions, and opportunities. *British Journal of Occupational Therapy, 60,* 456–460.

Kaiser Family Foundation. (2011). *Summary of new health reform law.* Retrieved from www.kff.org/healthreform/8061.cfm

Kielhofner, G. (2004). *Conceptual foundation of occupational therapy* (3rd ed.). Philadelphia: F. A. Davis.

Kinne, S., Patrick, D. L., & Doyle, D.L. (2004). Prevalence of secondary conditions among people with disabilities. *American Journal of Public Health, 94,* 443–445. http://dx.doi.org/10.2105/AJPH.94.3.443

Krahn, G. L., Fujiura, G. T., Drum, C. E., Cardinal, B. J., & Nosek, M. A.; RRTC Expert Panel on Health Measurement. (2009). The dilemma of measuring perceived health status in the context of disability. *Disability and Health Journal, 2,* 49–56. http://dx.doi.org/10.1016/j.dhjo.2008.12.003

Krahn, G. L., Putnam, M., Drum, C. E., & Powers, L. (2006). Disabilities and health. *Journal of Disability Policy Studies, 17,* 18-27. http://dx.doi.org/10.1177/10442073060170010201

Law, M. (1991). The environment: A focus for occupational therapy [Muriel Driver Memorial Lecture]. *Canadian Journal of Occupational Therapy, 58,* 171–179. http://dx.doi.org/10.1177/000841749105800404

Law, M., Steinwender, S., & LeClair, L. (1998). Occupation, health, and well-being. *Canadian Journal of Occupational Therapy, 65,* 81–91. http://dx.doi.org/10.1177/000841749806500204

Leland, N. E., & Elliott, S. J. (2012). Special issue on productive aging: Evidence and opportunities for occupational therapy practitioners. *American Journal of Occupational Therapy, 66,* 263–265. http://dx.doi.org/10.5014/ajot.2010.005165

Meyer, A. (1922). The philosophy of occupation therapy. *Archives of Occupational Therapy, 1,* 1–10.

Network for Public Health Law. (2011). *Public health provisions of the Patient Protection and Affordable Care Act: Issue brief.* Retrieved from www.networkforphl.org/_asset/x4mc6h/ACA-chart-formatted-FINAL.pdf

Oliver, R., Blathwayt, J., Brackley, C., & Tamaki, T. (1993). Development of the Safety Assessment of Function and the Environment for Rehabilitation (SAFER) tool. *Canadian Journal of Occupational Therapy, 60,* 78-82. http://dx.doi.org/10.1177/000841749306000204

Patient Protection and Affordable Care Act, Pub. L. 111–148, § 3502, 124 Stat. 119, 124 (2010).

Patrick, D. L., Richardson, M., Starks, H. E., Rose, M. A., & Kinne, S. (1997). Rethinking prevention for people with disabilities, Part II: A framework for designing interventions. *American Journal of Health Promotion, 11,* 261–263. http://dx.doi.org/http://dx.doi.org/10.4278/0890-1171-11.4.261

Scaffa, M. E. (2001). *Occupational therapy in community-based practice settings.* Philadelphia: F. A. Davis.

Seligman, M. (2011). *Flourish: A visionary new understanding of happiness and well-being.* New York: Free Press.

Trentham, B., & Cockburn, L. (2005). Participatory action research: Creating new knowledge and opportunities for occupational engagement. In F. Kronenberg, S. Simó Algado, & N. Pollard (Eds.), *Occupational therapy without borders: Learning from the spirit of survivors* (pp. 440–453). Philadelphia: Churchill Livingstone.

U.S. Access Board. (2007). *Accessible play areas: A summary of accessibility guidelines for play areas.* Retrieved from www.access-board.gov/play/guide/guide.pdf

U.S. Department of Health and Human Services. (1980). *Promoting health/preventing disease: Objectives for the nation.* Washington, DC: U.S. Government Printing Office.

U.S. Department of Health and Human Services. (1990). *Healthy People 2000.* Washington, DC: U.S. Government Printing Office.

U.S. Department of Health and Human Services. (2000). *Healthy People 2010: Understanding and improving health* (2nd ed.). Washington, DC: U.S. Government Printing Office.

U.S. Department of Health and Human Services. (2010). *Healthy People 2020* [Brochure]. Retrieved from www.healthypeople.gov/2020/TopicsObjectives2020/pdfs/HP2020_brochure_with_LHI_508.pdf

Wilcock, A. A. (2006). *An occupational perspective of health* (2nd ed.). Thorofare, NJ: Slack.

World Health Organization. (1986). *The Ottawa charter for health promotion.* Retrieved from www.who.int/healthpromotion/conferences/previous/ottawa/en/

Zemke, R., & Clark, F. (1996). *Occupational science: The evolving discipline.* Philadelphia: F. A. Davis.

AUTHORS

S. Maggie Reitz, PhD, OTR/L, FAOTA
Marjorie E. Scaffa, PhD, OTR/L, FAOTA

for

The Commission on Practice
Debbie Amini, EdD, OTR/L, CHT, *Chairperson*

Adopted by the Representative Assembly Coordinating Council (RACC) for the Representative Assembly.

Note. This document replaces the 2007 Statement *Occupational Therapy in the Promotion of Health and the Prevention of Disease and Disability* previously published and copyrighted 2008 by the American Occupational Therapy Association in the *American Journal of Occupational Therapy, 64,* 694–703.

Originally published in the *American Journal of Occupational Therapy, 67*(Suppl.), S47–S59. http://dx.doi.org/10.5014/ajot.2013.67S47

APPENDIX. GLOSSARY OF HEALTH PROMOTION TERMS

Occupational alienation—"Sense of isolation, powerlessness, frustration, loss of control, and estrangement from society or self as a result of engagement in occupation that does not satisfy inner needs" (Wilcock, 2006, p. 343).

Occupational deprivation—"Deprivation of occupational choice and diversity because of circumstances beyond the control of individuals or communities" (Wilcock, 2006, p. 343).

Occupational imbalance—"A lack of balance or disproportion of occupation resulting in decreased well-being" (Wilcock, 2006, p. 343).

Occupational justice—"The promotion of social and economic change to increase individual, community, and political awareness, resources, and equitable opportunities for diverse occupational opportunities that enable people to meet their potential and experience well-being" (Wilcock, 2006, p. 343).

Occupational science—"An interdisciplinary academic discipline in the social and behavioral sciences dedicated to the study of the form, the function, and the meaning of human occupations" (Zemke & Clark, 1996, p. vii).

Social justice—"The promotion of social and economic change to increase individual, community, and political awareness, resources, and opportunity for health and well-being" (Wilcock, 2006, p. 344).

Well-being—A state of flourishing that consists of the following elements: positive emotion, engagement or flow, *meaning* (a sense of belonging to or serving something larger than oneself), positive relationships and accomplishment or achievement (Seligman, 2011).

Subject Index

Note. Page numbers in italic refer to exhibits and figures.

Citation Index

Note. Page numbers in italic refer to exhibits and figures.